Genetics of Asthma and Chronic Obstructive Pulmonary Disease

LUNG BIOLOGY IN HEALTH AND DISEASE

Executive Editor

Claude Lenfant
Former Director, National Heart, Lung, and Blood Institute
National Institutes of Health
Bethesda, Maryland

The opinions expressed in these volumes do not necessarily represent the views of the National Institutes of Health.

Genetics of Asthma and Chronic Obstructive Pulmonary Disease

Edited by

Dirkje S. Postma
University Hospital Groningen
Groningen, The Netherlands

Scott T. Weiss
Harvard Medical School
Brigham and Women's Hospital
Boston, Massachusetts, U.S.A.

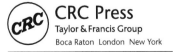

CRC Press
Taylor & Francis Group
Boca Raton London New York

CRC Press is an imprint of the
Taylor & Francis Group, an **informa** business

CRC Press
Taylor & Francis Group
6000 Broken Sound Parkway NW, Suite 300
Boca Raton, FL 33487-2742

First issued in paperback 2019

ISBN-13: 978-0-8493-6966-7 (hbk)
ISBN-13: 978-0-367-39040-2 (pbk)

This book contains information obtained from authentic and highly regarded sources. While all reasonable efforts have been made to publish reliable data and information, neither the author[s] nor the publisher can accept any legal responsibility or liability for any errors or omissions that may be made. The publishers wish to make clear that any views or opinions expressed in this book by individual editors, authors or contributors are personal to them and do not necessarily reflect the views/opinions of the publishers. The information or guidance contained in this book is intended for use by medical, scientific or health-care professionals and is provided strictly as a supplement to the medical or other professional's own judgement, their knowledge of the patient's medical history, relevant manufacturer's instructions and the appropriate best practice guidelines. Because of the rapid advances in medical science, any information or advice on dosages, procedures or diagnoses should be idependently verified. The reader is strongly urged to consult the relevant national drug formulary and the drug companies' and device or material manufacturers' printed instructions, and their websites, before administering or utilizing any of the drugs, devices or materials mentioned in this book. This book does not indicate whether a particular treatment is appropriate or suitable for a particular individual. Ultimately it is the sole responsibility of the medical professional to make his or her own professional judgements, so as to advise and treat patients appropriately. The authors and publishers have also attempted to trace the copyright holders of all material reproduced in this publication and apologize to copyright holders if permission to publish in this form has not been obtained. If any copyright material has not been acknowledged please write and let us know so we may rectify in any future reprint.

Library of Congress Cataloging-in-Publication Data

Genetics of asthma and chronic obstructive pulmonary disease / edited by Dirkje S. Postma, Scott T. Weiss.
    p. ; cm. -- (Lung Biology in health and disease ; 218)
    Includes bibliographical references and index.
    ISBN-13: 978-0-8493-6966-7 (hardcover : alk. paper)
    ISBN-10: 0-8493-6966-5 (hardcover : alk. paper)
    1. Asthma--Genetic aspects. 2. Lung--Diseases, Obstructive. I. Postma, D. S. (Dirkje S.) II. Weiss, Scott T. III. Series.
    [DNLM: 1. Asthma--genetics. 2. Pulmonary Disease, Chronic Obstructive--genetics. W1 LU62 v.218 2006 / WF 553 G3285 2006]

RC591.G46 2006
616.2'38042--dc22   2006048588

Visit the Taylor & Francis Web site at
http://www.taylorandfrancis.com

and the CRC Press Web site at
http://www.crcpress.com

We, the editors, would like to dedicate this book to the late Benjamin Burrows who inspired both of us to pursue the quest for understanding the etiology and natural history of obstructive airway diseases.

Introduction

Surely some—indeed, perhaps, many—people would argue about when precisely the era of the genetics of diseases really began, but the introduction of gene transfer and therapy concepts in the 1980s by French Anderson and colleagues from the National Institutes of the Health, the identification of the cystic fibrosis gene reported in *Science* in 1989 by L. C. Tsui from Toronto and F. S. Collins from the University of Michigan, and then the publication of the human genome in 2001, the "private one" in *Nature* and the "public one" in *Science*, have all been momentous events which have stimulated new and potentially important research. This expectation, but also a word of caution, was quite well articulated by Jean Marx, an editor of *Science*, in her comments in response to the identification of the cystic fibrosis gene: "The discovery ... raises hopes for cystic fibrosis treatments, perhaps even new drugs or even gene therapy to replace the defective gene itself. (However), until a way can be found to deliver a functioning cystic fibrosis gene into lung cells, gene therapy will remain somewhat of a long shot, however" (*Science*. Vol 245, 1989).

Today, so many years later, the goals of better diagnosis and new therapies remain elusive, but the hopes and expectations remain high, even more so than years ago. The reasons for the unrelenting enthusiasm that patients will eventually benefit from the emerging new medicine based on the genome are the commitment of the research community and the productivity of its work, especially with regard to complex diseases such as asthma and chronic obstructive pulmonary disease.

The cardiovascular genetics research area illustrates the potential that we can expect. In the last 15 years or so, we have seen research outcomes which, if applied, would greatly improve the prevention and diagnosis of some cardiovascular diseases. Other research outcomes could help to forecast the course of a disease, and thus direct therapy accordingly. Unfortunately, what has been learned from this research on cardiovascular genes and their polymorphism has not yet found its way into the practice of medicine, or at least on a large scale.

This volume, edited by Dr. Dirkje Postma and Dr. Scott Weiss for the series of monographs Lung Biology in Health and Disease, introduces the reader to what "we know today about the genetics of asthma and chronic obstructive pulmonary disease." The contributions of experts from many countries show how fertile the field is and provide the expectation that if what we know is eventually applied to the practice of medicine, asthma and chronic obstructive pulmonary disease patients will certainly benefit. This volume should be an inspiration to translate this emerging new medicine into practice as quickly and as widely as possible.

As the overall editor of this series of monographs, I am proud to introduce this volume to our readership, and I am grateful to the editors and contributors for opening the door to a new approach to the care of patients.

Claude Lenfant, MD
Gaithersburg, Maryland, U.S.A.

Preface

In the 10 years prior to the sequencing of the human genome (in 2000), much was learned about multifactorial diseases such as asthma and chronic obstructive pulmonary disease. However, as we now begin to apply genetics and genomics to human disease, even more will be gained from this phenomenal step forward, which will improve our insights into the pathophysiology of asthma and chronic obstructive pulmonary disease.

Asthma and chronic obstructive pulmonary disease are diseases that affect the airways and lung parenchyma and are accompanied by respiratory symptoms and reduction in lung function, which is either reversible, as in asthma, or irreversible, as in chronic obstructive pulmonary disease. Asthma—a disease that flourished with the higher standard for living in the 20th century in Western industrialized countries—occurs in about 10% of the population worldwide. Asthma is especially burdensome to an individual patient, given its variability in severity over time and associated morbidity. Finally, childhood asthma may predispose a susceptibility to chronic obstructive pulmonary disease in adult life. We are seeing an astonishing increase in the number of deaths from chronic obstructive pulmonary disease, already surpassing 125,000 worldwide on an annual basis and climbing steadily. Chronic obstructive pulmonary disease affects an individual's life tremendously, given the ongoing and progressive symptoms and associated exacerbations. Both diseases affect hundreds of millions of individuals in the world. Thus, it is of importance to dissect which factors contribute to disease development, progression, and remission. Understanding these factors will eventually contribute to better prevention and management of these diseases and, ultimately, to a cure. Because asthma and chronic obstructive pulmonary disease are multifactorial diseases, i.e., they originate by gene–gene and gene–environment interactions operating in a developmental context, and the genetics of airways disease is proceeding at a rapid pace, it is timely to provide the current state-of-the-art genetic research on airways disease.

This book in the series of Lung Biology in Health and Disease intends to assemble what we know today about the genetics of asthma and chronic obstructive pulmonary disease. It contains chapters on both human and animal studies (including genetic genomics), genome-wide screens, association studies in cases and controls, gene–environment interactions, proteomics, and microarrays. Therefore, we believe this book provides an important and timely update of the broad and rapidly changing field of asthma and chronic obstructive pulmonary disease genetics. In the current book, we hope that the reader finds valuable novel ways to approach the genetics of asthma and chronic obstructive pulmonary disease.

The production of this volume has been helped by the stimulating support from the staff of Informa Healthcare and support from Dr. Claude Lenfant, who as the overall editor of the Lung Biology in Health and Disease series, provided the medium for this communication. We especially thank Mrs. Sandra Beberman who, despite everything that has occurred in her life, was a positive and supportive person behind this book.

Dirkje S. Postma
Scott T. Weiss

Contributors

Irving C. Allen   Department of Genetics, The University of North Carolina at Chapel Hill, Chapel Hill, North Carolina, U.S.A.

Eugene Bleecker   Division of Pulmonary and Critical Care Medicine and Center for Human Genomics, Wake Forest University School of Medicine, Winston-Salem, North Carolina, U.S.A.

H. Marike Boezen   Department of Epidemiology, University Medical Center Groningen, University of Groningen, Groningen, The Netherlands

Juan C. Celedón   Channing Laboratory and Respiratory Disorders Program, Brigham and Women's Hospital, Harvard Medical School, Boston, Massachusetts, U.S.A.

William O. C. Cookson   The National Heart and Lung Institute, Imperial College, London, U.K.

Dawn L. DeMeo   Channing Laboratory and Division of Pulmonary and Critical Care Medicine, Department of Medicine, Brigham and Women's Hospital, Harvard Medical School, Boston, Massachusetts, U.S.A.

Kojo S. J. Elenitoba-Johnson   Department of Pathology, Associated Regional and University Pathologists Institute for Clinical and Experimental Pathology, University of Utah Health Sciences Center, Salt Lake City, Utah, U.S.A.

Stefano Guerra   Arizona Respiratory Center and Mel and Enid Zuckerman College of Public Health, University of Arizona, Tucson, Arizona, U.S.A.

Hakon Hakonarson   Product Development, deCODE Genetics Inc., Reykjavik, Iceland

Eva Halapi   Inflammatory Diseases, deCODE Genetics Inc., Reykjavik, Iceland

Ian P. Hall   Division of Therapeutics and Molecular Medicine, University Hospital of Nottingham, Nottingham, U.K.

Craig P. Hersh   Channing Laboratory and Division of Pulmonary and Critical Care Medicine, Department of Medicine, Brigham and Women's Hospital, Harvard Medical School, Boston, Massachusetts, U.S.A.

Timothy D. Howard   Center for Human Genomics and Department of Pediatrics, Wake Forest University School of Medicine, Winston-Salem, North Carolina, U.S.A.

Machteld N. Hylkema   Department of Pathology and Laboratory Medicine, University Medical Center Groningen, University of Groningen, Groningen, The Netherlands

Takeo Ishii   The James Hogg iCAPTURE Centre for Cardiovascular and Pulmonary Disease, University of British Columbia, Vancouver, British Columbia, Canada

Michael Kabesch   University Children's Hospital, Ludwig Maximilian's University Munich, Munich, Germany

Beverly H. Koller   Department of Genetics, The University of North Carolina at Chapel Hill, Chapel Hill, North Carolina, U.S.A.

Gerard H. Koppelman   Department of Pediatric Pulmonology, Beatrix Children's Hospital, University Medical Center Groningen, University of Groningen, Groningen, The Netherlands

Ingrid A. Laing   Telethon Institute for Child Health Research, Centre for Child Health Research, and School of Paediatrics and Child Health, University of Western Australia, Perth, Western Australia, and Australian Respiratory Council, Sydney, South Wales, Australia

Peter N. Le Souëf   School of Paediatrics and Child Health, University of Western Australia, Perth, Western Australia, Australia

Stephen B. Liggett   Departments of Medicine and Physiology, University of Maryland School of Medicine, Baltimore, Maryland, U.S.A.

Megan S. Lim Department of Pathology, Associated Regional and University Pathologists Institute for Clinical and Experimental Pathology, University of Utah Health Sciences Center, Salt Lake City, Utah, U.S.A.

Thomas J. Mariani Department of Medicine, Brigham and Women's Hospital and Pulmonary Bioinformatics, The Lung Biology Center, Harvard Medical School, Boston, Massachusetts, U.S.A.

Fernando D. Martinez Arizona Respiratory Center and Department of Pediatrics, University of Arizona, Tucson, Arizona, U.S.A.

Miriam F. Moffatt The National Heart and Lung Institute, Imperial College, London, U.K.

Beverly Paigen The Jackson Laboratory, Bar Harbor, Maine, U.S.A.

Benoit Piavaux Laboratory of Allergology and Pulmonary Diseases, and Department of Pathology and Laboratory Medicine, University Medical Center Groningen, University of Groningen, Groningen, The Netherlands

Dirkje S. Postma Department of Pulmonology, University Medical Center Groningen, University of Groningen, Groningen, The Netherlands

Marco F. Ramoni Children's Hospital Informatics Program, Division of Health Sciences and Technology, Harvard Medical School and Massachusetts Institute of Technology, Boston, Massachusetts, U.S.A.

Andrew J. Sandford The James Hogg iCAPTURE Centre for Cardiovascular and Pulmonary Disease, University of British Columbia, Vancouver, British Columbia, Canada

David A. Schwartz National Institute of Environmental Health Sciences, Durham, North Carolina, U.S.A.

Edwin K. Silverman Channing Laboratory and Division of Pulmonary and Critical Care Medicine, Department of Medicine, Brigham and Women's Hospital, Harvard Medical School, Boston, Massachusetts, U.S.A.

Jaspal Singh Duke University Medical Center and National Institute of Environmental Health Sciences, Durham, North Carolina, U.S.A.

Ioannis M. Stylianou The Jackson Laboratory, Bar Harbor, Maine, U.S.A.

Kelan Tantisira Channing Laboratory and Pulmonary Division, Brigham and Women's Hospital, Harvard Medical School, Boston, Massachusetts, U.S.A.

Stephen L. Tilley Division of Pulmonary and Critical Care Medicine, Department of Medicine, The University of North Carolina at Chapel Hill, Chapel Hill, North Carolina, U.S.A.

Cleo C. van Diemen Department of Epidemiology, University Medical Center Groningen, University of Groningen, Groningen, The Netherlands

Antoon J. M. van Oosterout Laboratory of Allergology and Pulmonary Diseases, and Department of Pathology and Laboratory Medicine, University Medical Center Groningen, University of Groningen, Groningen, The Netherlands

Donata Vercelli Arizona Respiratory Center and Department of Cell Biology, University of Arizona, Tucson, Arizona, U.S.A.

Contents

1

Introduction to Genetics

EVA HALAPI

Inflammatory Diseases,
    decODE Genetics Inc.,
Reykjavik, Iceland

HAKON HAKONARSON

Product Development,
    decODE Genetics Inc.,
Reykjavik, Iceland

I. Introduction

In this chapter, we provide an overview of the field of human genetics addressing the key molecular approaches in the study of the role of familial factors and genetic determinants in the causation of complex diseases such as cardiovascular disease, asthma, and diabetes. The genetic complexity of multigenic disorders is outlined underpinning the important need of understanding the linkage disequilibrium (LD) structure of the human genome, ethnic and sex-related differences, and the need for applying approaches that allow for gene–gene and gene–environment interaction studies. While traditional linkage and association studies have been highly successful in uncovering variants that underlie monogenetic disorders and delivered some success in the field of multigenic disorders, the sequencing of the human genome and, more recently, the completion of the International HapMap Project mark the start of a new phase in human genetics. The HapMap project provides an unprecedented resource to investigators by characterizing the patterns of genetic variation and LD structure across four geographical populations, facilitating the design of genome-wide (GW) association

1

studies and unveiling some of the complexity of human genetic diversity. The rapid development in new technology platforms in recent years is now enabling investigators to conduct high-throughput experiments scanning through the whole genome in search for genes and variants that underlie many of the common diseases that affect human beings.

II. Mendelian Traits vs. Complex Diseases

A. Genes and Genetic Diseases

All genetic information about an individual is carried in the linear sequence of nucleotides that line up to form DNA, the structural unit of the genome. In humans, the genome is divided into 24 linear DNA molecules, each contained in a different chromosome. Only four nucleotide bases, adenine (A), cytosine (C), guanine (G), and thymine (T) make up the building blocks of DNA. The discovery in the 1950s that DNA had a helical structure provided one of the major clues to the work of Watson and Crick who won the Nobel price for resolving the structure of double-stranded DNA—one of the most important biological advancements in human genetics in the last century. Strong covalent bonds bind the bases together in the single-stranded DNA, with weaker hydrogen bonds pairing the nucleotide A with T and C with G between the two strands. Each single strand of DNA has two different ends called 5′ and 3′, that are oriented in opposite directions. In a nondividing cell, the DNA in the nucleus of a cell is a double helix. During cell division, double-stranded DNA is replicated by separation of the two strands followed by the formation of a new complementary strand, resulting in two identical copies of the original strand. With the completion of the sequencing of the human genome (1,2), it is estimated that there are at least 20,000 genes (from Greek genos "origin"). The genes carry all the information that is essential for the construction and regulation of proteins (such as enzymes) and other molecules that determine the growth and function of an organism.

Most genes contain alternating regions called exons (regions that are encoded) and introns (noncoding regions between the coded ones). Before a protein is synthesized, a copy of a single strand of DNA is made. The product is called RNA and is similar to DNA, with the exception that T is replaced by U—uracil. This process is called transcription. The RNA that is transcribed is complementary to the whole gene (exons and introns). Mature messenger RNA (mRNA) is then created by posttranscriptional processing, which cuts out the introns and splices the exonic elements to produce mRNA, which encodes for proteins. The synthesis of a protein via mRNA is called translation. Mutations (alterations of the DNA code) within or nearby a gene may cause dysfunctional proteins. Gene mutations can either be inherited from a parent (hereditary or germline mutations), or acquired during a person's lifetime (somatic mutations). Mutations that occur only in an egg or sperm cell or those that occur just after fertilization are referred to as de novo mutations. De novo mutations may explain genetic disorders in which an affected child has a mutation in every cell, but has no previous family history of the disorder. Although there is a high degree of similarity between the genomes of different individuals, no two humans are identical. Sequence variations referred to as polymorphism are responsible for many of the normal differences between people such as eye color, hair color, and blood type. Different types of variations are known to exist in the genome, which consist of single base pair changes, deletion of one or more bases, insertion of one or more bases, or stretches of DNA sequences that are inverted. Simple repeat structure of DNA are interspersed throughout the genome and demonstrate considerable variation between different individuals; these are commonly called micro-satellites. Most frequent are dinucleotide repeats, which account for about 0.5% of the genome sequence and are often highly polymorphic. Most of the variations have no negative effects on a person's health, while others may influence the risk of developing a disease.

The foundation of modern genetics has been greatly influenced by the work of Darwin and Mendel conducted in the late 19th century. In this regard, Charles Darwin's theory of the evolution through natural selection presents one of the cornerstones of modern population studies of genetic disorders, while Mendel's accomplishment in establishing some of the basic laws of inheritance have subsequently unveiled some of the basic principles of heritability known as "Mendel's laws of inheritance."

B. Monogenic Disorders

Genetic diseases where one copy (dominant traits) or two copies (recessive traits) of a variant in a particular gene is sufficient to develop disease are termed "monogenic" or "Mendelian diseases" and typically referred to as Mendelian traits. The Online Mendelian Inheritance in Man (OMIM^{TM}) database is a registry of human genes and genetic disorders (3). The primary focus of OMIN relates to heritable genetic diseases and the registry includes more than 1600 entries for known Mendelian traits that have been resolved (4).

Monogenic diseases are relatively uncommon. However, the frequency of monogenetic disorders often varies with ethnic background and certain Mendelian traits are in higher frequency in certain ethnic groups compared to others. For example, cystic fibrosis has a frequency of about 1 in 2000 births in American descendents of Western European Caucasians, but is much rarer in Americans of African descent.

C. Multigenic Disorders

Multigenic diseases are common and constitute the leading cause of death and disabilities in Western societies. Diseases such as diabetes, heart attack, asthma, anxiety, depression, and cancer are regarded as multigenic and are being referred to as complex genetic diseases because they are believed to arise from the interaction of many genes and the environment, with each gene potentially contributing small effects. Thus, complex diseases are not only dependent on the presence of certain variants in one or more genes. In addition to the genetic makeup in a susceptible individual, exposure to environmental factors is also necessary for the disease to develop. For example, smoking is the major risk factor for developing chronic obstructive pulmonary disease (COPD), a disease that is projected to rise to the third major cause of death in 2020 (5). However, only 15% to 20% of heavy smokers develop COPD, suggesting that genetic factors may also be important. At present, the only proven genetic factor for COPD is the deficiency of the proteinase inhibitor (Pi) alpha-1 antitrypsin (SERPINA1) (6). Premature development of pulmonary emphysema early in the second decade is one of the hallmarks of deficiency of the Pi SERPINA1. The gene has multiple deficient Pi alleles that influence the expression of the protein. The PiZ allele, which differs from the normal variant by a single base mutation of Glu342Lys, is the most common allele responsible for severe SERPINA1 deficiency and obstructive lung disease. Relative to the wild type, the neutrophil elastase activity of the Z protein is markedly reduced. Most individuals (>95%) who present with severe deficiency are homozygotes for the PiZ allele, and their serum SERPINA1 levels are reduced to 10% to 15% of normal values. In contrast, subjects with the PiS (Glu264Val) variant have normal elastase activity despite having only 40% to 60% of normal protein levels. While all PiZZ homozygotes develop pulmonary disease, pulmonary morbidity is more severe and occurs earlier in those who smoke compared to nonsmokers. Recently, the PiSZ genotype was also reported to be a significant risk factor for the development of COPD (7).

III. Familial Risk and Heritability

Many complex diseases cluster in families; however, their pattern of inheritance remains illusive. A higher concordance of disease among monozygotic compared with dizygotic twins or among relatives (e.g., siblings) of cases than among relatives of controls or subjects who are randomly selected from the general population are usually the observations that lead researchers to believe that a disease is familial or may possibly be under genetic influence. If a disease shows equal concordance in both monozygotic and dizygotic twins, it could be caused by either shared genetic or environmental factors or both. This is because both monozygotic and dizygotic twins tend to be brought up in shared environmental conditions. If the concordance rate is higher in the monozygotic than the dizygotic twins, however, then genetic factors are likely to be more important than environmental factors.

Two types of statistical measurements are commonly used to assess the impact of shared genetic factors on specific diseases or disease-related phenotypes. First, the risk ratio (λ), which is defined as the disease prevalence in a first-degree relative of a proband divided by the prevalence in the general population, presents a relatively accurate measure of disease susceptibility. For instance, approximately 20% to 25% of first-degree relatives of asthma patients suffer from asthma compared to the 5% to 7% prevalence in the general population. In this instance, λ for first-degree relatives of asthma patients would be estimated to be about 4. It should be emphasized, however, that the risk ratio is strongly influenced by the disease prevalence in the general population. Thus, the genetic contribution as reported by λ may be underestimated for diseases with higher prevalence. Second, genetic contribution may also be measured by kinship coefficient, a measure of heritability (H). Heritability is defined as the proportion of phenotypic variance in a population that can be attributed to genetic factors (8).

A. Strategies for Gene Discovery: Pros and Cons of Linkage vs. Association Studies

Two main approaches have been used to search for genes contributing to complex traits: (i) linkage analysis and (ii) association analysis. In linkage studies, related probands, either sib pairs or extended families are studied [(9) and references within]. Both linkage and association studies utilize the fact that the genetic variation close to a disease gene is coinherited with the disease. While linkage studies have taught us most of what we know about the genetic causes of diseases, linkage analysis has two major disadvantages:

1. Relatively low statistical power for detecting genes with low to modest risk (RR < 1.5) and poor mapping resolution: Rare alleles with high penetrance and high risk as is typical for monogenetic diseases are more likely to be identified by linkage (10,11). Because the risk conferred by alleles involved in complex diseases is generally modest, linkage studies may not be as suitable for these conditions.
2. The lack of recombination between closely related individuals (where several millions of base pairs of a locus may be shared) can interfere with gene identification even after a chromosomal region has been mapped. Once a region has been identified by linkage, a dense set of markers is typed for association and LD mapping using either family- or population-based case–control studies in search for markers that associate with a given disease or trait (12).

The past two decades were tremendously fruitful in identifying disease-causing genes with over 1600 Mendelian traits being mapped using linkage and positional cloning approaches (12). Despite being described as monogenic, the observed variability in disease severity and age of onset tell us that Mendelian diseases are far from simple. However, scientists have successfully unveiled many of the complex interactions of some Mendelian disease-causing genes and modifier genes in humans, as well as for quantitative traits in plants and other organisms (13–15). Disease-modifying genes can mask or alter the phenotypic effect of another gene (epistasis) by affecting "penetrance" (the proportion of individuals affected by a specific disease of those carrying the same mutation), modifying "expressivity" (the relative capacity of a gene to affect the phenotype), or influencing "pleiotropy" (where a single gene is responsible for producing multiple phenotypic traits). Conversely, mutations at different genetic loci can convey the same disease phenotype, termed "genetic heterogeneity." Although the complexity of the above-mentioned factors are better understood for monogenic diseases (13,14), this is not the case for multigenic disorders, where there has been relative little progress made in identifying disease causative genes (16–19).

IV. Linkage Disequilibrium

A fundamental concept for association analysis relates to LD, the nonrandom association between alleles of markers. Genetic markers that are in proximity on a chromosome are more likely to originate from the same ancestral chromosome, and in extreme cases an allele found at a locus may predict the probability of finding other alleles. Knowing the level of LD at a locus will guide the genotyping effort, thereby avoiding genotyping redundant markers and reducing both time and cost. The further apart markers are located, the greater the chance that they may have different ancestral genealogies because of recombination. The strength of the LD between pairs of markers decreases as a function of the genetic distance between markers. The latter is determined by the recombination fraction and number of generations.

Two important and commonly used measures of LD are the correlation coefficient, r^2, and the disequilibrium coefficient, D prime (D′). Both measure a continuum from 0 (no disequilibrium) to 1 (complete disequilibrium). The D′ gives an estimate of recombination between two sites while the r^2 denotes the statistical correlation between two sites (20–22). Several studies have concluded that the human genome is structured in discrete blocks of limited haplotype diversity that show high level of LD (21,22). These blocks are intersected by possible hotspots for recombination, which disrupt the LD pattern. The extent of LD can span from a few to a few hundred kilobases (kb). While larger LD blocks are rare, they are most commonly seen in founder populations (21,22). A high-resolution mapping of the LD structure in a region is instrumental in the discovery of genes and variations that may underlie linkage and association signals.

V. Genetic Linkage Analysis

Linkage analysis has been widely used to map and positionally clone genes that underlie genetic disorders. The identification of the cystic fibrosis transmembrane conductance regulator in 1989 was the first study in which a Mendelian trait was mapped by linkage analysis alone (23,24). Since then, multiple genes have been mapped by positional cloning following linkage studies, including six potential asthma or atopy genes (*ADAM33*, *PFH11*, *DPP10*, *GPRA*, *HLA-G*, and *CYFIP2*) (25–30). Linkage analysis utilizes the fact that variations that are close to the disease gene are coinherited with the disease. During meiosis, chromosomes line up and exchange parts of their DNA. The further apart two loci are on the same chromosome, the higher is the probability that a recombination may occur. By genotyping markers and studying how they segregate in families, haplotypes (a series of alleles at linked loci on a single chromosome) can be inferred in subjects with a disease or their relatives as exemplified by the representative panel in Figure 1. The distances along chromosomes are expressed in centimorgans (cM). One cM corresponds to a region where a crossover is expected in 1 of 100 meioses. Physical distance refers to the number of base pairs (bp) between two points in the genome. The relation between physical and genetic distance (bp vs. cM) on a chromosome differs between chromosomes and also between males and females (31).

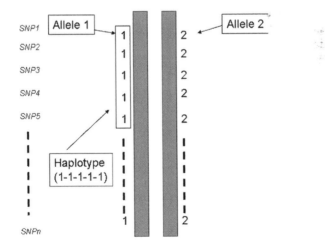

Figure 1 Illustration of alleles, genotypes, and haplotypes. Individual alleles for a given set of polymorphic markers/loci (single nucleotide polymorphism (SNP1 allele 1 or 2; SNP2 allele 1 or 2; etc.) are depicted on each chromosome. Genotype refers to the pair of alleles for a given marker (genotype for SNP1 is 1,2, etc.). A haplotype is an ordered series of alleles for many markers on a single chromosome, here represented by 1–1–1–1 and 2–2–2–2, respectively. *Abbreviation*: SNP, single nucleotide polymorphism.

The markers most commonly used to determine the pattern of genetic variation include single tandem repeats, also called microsatellites, and single nucleotide polymorphisms (SNPs). Microsatellites are simple repeats of DNA. Most microsatellites have multiple alleles (numbers of repeats) and are therefore more informative for linkage analysis than a typical SNP that has only two alleles. SNPs are single-base mutations in which one base is substituted for another. SNPs are highly abundant in the genome. It is estimated that there exists more than 10 million polymorphic sites throughout the genome with frequency greater than 1%. The HapMap project (32) is a multicenter, multination collaborative effort that aims at characterizing patterns of haplotype structure and LD across the human genome from populations with ancestry from Africa, Asia, and Europe. The HapMap effort was built to facilitate the mapping of complex disease genes (33) and is focused on creating a map of evenly spaced SNPs (1 SNP per every 600 bp), each with minor allele frequencies greater than or equal to 5%. Based on the local LD pattern within different ethnic groups, the minimum number of SNPs from each LD block that are needed to capture the genetic variation with acceptable accuracy (i.e., tag SNPs) is currently being used to perform GW association in the search for genes and variants that confer disease susceptibility or variants that potentially influence response to drugs.

Within a given family, individuals who share the disease phenotype will also share alleles at markers near the disease gene. If allele sharing occurs significantly more often than expected by chance, linkage of the particular marker with the disease can be assumed, indicating that the chromosomal region containing the marker also contains a gene that contributes to the disease trait. Results of linkage analysis are reported as logarithm of the odds (LOD) of sharing a chromosomal region. A positive LOD score is indicative of a region linked to the disease. Calculation of LOD score requires specification of the genetic model used, including the mode of inheritance, penetrance, and marker allele frequencies.

In the study of common diseases where the mode of inheritance is unknown, a nonparametric approach is favored. Nonparametric linkage analysis using affected sib pairs or extended multiplex families is focused on identifying regions that are shared by siblings or other relatives who have the disease more often than expected by chance. Founder populations such as Finnish, Amish, Hutterites, Sardinian, Ashkenazi Jews, or the Icelandic population have been successfully used for mapping disease genes (34–37). There are two main advantages of using founder populations for mapping complex traits. First, the gene pool is less complex, which may yield less locus heterogeneity. Second, LD between alleles at linked loci is more likely to exist than in outbred populations. This facilitates gene mapping due to the greater size of shared segments of DNA. An example of use of a founder population is the genealogical linkage and mapping approach of asthma-related traits in the Icelandic population (Fig. 2).

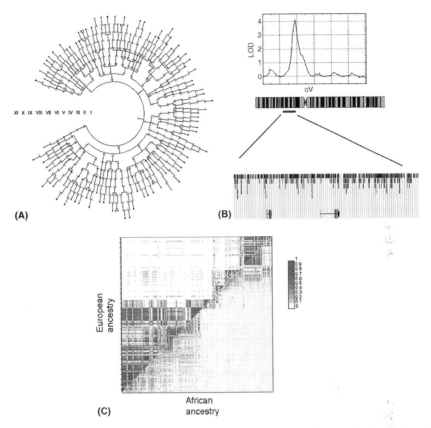

Figure 2 A representative example of the application of linkage in the study of complex disorders. (**A**) Extended families with multiple cases are recruited and markers are typed throughout the genome using a dense set of microsatellites. The diagram shows a large extended pedigree using the genealogy approach in Icelanders. Over 100 asthma patients who trace back to the same forefather born in the 17th Century are shown. (**B**) Haplotypes are inferred and the intervals of sharing are calculated based on nonparametric multipoint analysis and plotted as logarithm of the odds (LOD) scores (*y*-axis) versus cM (*x*-axis). Regions with significant linkage are subsequently mapped with dense set of markers (typically single nucleotide polymorphisms) to establish the local linkage disequilibrium (LD) structure. Markers are selected from the public domain, including the HapMap and dbSNPs and from the de novo sequencing with the aim of discovering novel polymorphisms. Association of single and/or combination of markers is evaluated in cases and controls. Significant haplotypes or single alleles are verified in additional patient cohort(s). (**C**) Pairways evaluation of r^2 in Hapmap dataset: U.S. residents with northern and western European ancestry (*upper left*) and individuals from the Yoruba people of Ibadan, Nigeria (*lower right*). Note the block-like LD structure in Caucasian set while a distinctly more limited LD is evident in the Yorubian population. Strength of r^2 is indicated on right hand side panel with r^2 of 0 (lightest) and r^2 of 1 (darkest). *Source*: From Refs. 35, 38.

Taken together, the success of identifying genes in Mendelian diseases and the relative ease at which the whole genome could be scanned with the introduction of the polymerase chain reaction technology prompted investigators to apply this technology to study complex diseases. This has resulted in numerous linkage reports that in general lack consistency (16). Criteria for the interpretation of the significance of linkage signals have been proposed (39). For a sib pair analysis, an LOD score of 2.2 (or greater) with a p value of 7.4×10^{-4} or less is, in general, regarded as a suggestive signal, while LOD score of 3.6 or greater with corresponding p value of 2.2×10^{-5} or less is considered by most to be of GW significance. However, it is the general consensus that an LOD score of 5.4 or higher and a p value of 3×10^{-7} or lower is the preferred stringency criterion for GW significant linkage (39). Furthermore, confirmation should include a significant linkage from more than one study, and preferably in separate studies conducted by independent investigator groups.

A. Quantitative Trait Loci

A disease can often be categorized as being either present or absent. A heart attack is an example of such phenotype. However, there are several traits such as hypertension and hypercholesterolemia that may contribute significantly to the end phenotype, such as heart attack. A quantitative trait has a measurable phenotypic variation while a quantitative trait locus (QTL) is the allele that affects the variation. In general QTLs are multifactorial and are influenced by several polymorphic genes, and multiple QTLs can influence the same (or different) phenotypic traits. The ability to map a QTL depends on the magnitude of the QTL effect as measured by the proportion of the QT variance explained by the putative QTL (40,41).

B. Admixture Mapping

The identification of genetic variants that are associated with complex diseases by admixture LD mapping approach [matrix-assisted laser desorption (MALD)] is an emerging technology that is gaining popularity (42,43). MALD is a genetic association strategy that uses the outcome of admixture between different ethnic groups such as Caucasians versus African-Americans or Latinos. In many respects, the strategy could be best positioned somewhere between linkage and association analysis. Near a disease gene, patient populations descended from the recent mixing of two or more ethnic groups should have an increased probability of inheriting alleles that are derived from the ethnic group that carries more disease-susceptibility alleles. Recent progress in establishing suitable genetic marker maps, algorithms, and computational power to infer ancestral origin of study subjects has enabled investigations to successfully map disease genes for conditions such as hypertension (44) and multiple sclerosis (45) using this approach. However, more studies are needed before this methodology would be expected to win over users of more standard methods. Admixture mapping is expected to be particularly powerful in uncovering genes for diseases, which differ strikingly in frequency across populations such as lupus, end-stage renal disease, and type 2 diabetes (42).

VI. Genetic Architecture of Complex Diseases

The nature of the genetic variations that underlie complex diseases in humans remains largely unknown. Whether common diseases occur as a result of many rare alleles at numerous loci (46) or the interaction of common risk alleles of a handful of loci (47), or both, remains speculative (48–50). In the event that a few common variants would confer a relatively large fraction of the risk for a given disease trait, existing technologies would have sufficient power and stringency to successfully map such variants. If, on the other hand, common diseases originate from multiple rare mutations, alternative sequence-based methods need to be developed. Based on modeling of human genetic population structure, Reich and Lander (47) deducted that common diseases are most likely the result of common variations in genes, lending support to the common disease/common variant hypothesis (51).

The human population has undergone a dramatic expansion over the past 100,000 years. However, mutation rates are thought to occur at a fairly similar frequency for most genes. A rare allele would be predicted not to have a selective advantage over time and would thus be maintained at a low frequency in the population or may be "overgrown" by newer mutations. In contrast, a disease-risk allele that was common in a founder population some 100,000 years ago would remain at higher frequencies for a longer time period before it would be diluted out by the new alleles generated during population growth. Thus, an allele that was common in the distant past remains common today, and the allelic diversity would be expected to be low. Reich and Lander also estimate that in the future the allelic spectrum for common and rare diseases may become equally diverse. However, at the present time, we are at a stage where rare diseases are more likely to have higher allelic diversity (47). Examples of common disease alleles that confer risk and/or are disease modifying include the APOE E4 allele that is associated with susceptibility to Alzheimer's disease, cardiovascular disease, and the major histocompatibility complex region in autoimmune diseases such as Ankylosis spondylitis, type 1 diabetes, and psoriasis (49,52).

VII. Gene-by-Gene and Gene-by-Environment Interactions

An increased awareness for the importance of gene–gene interaction, or epistasis, in complex genetic diseases is currently emerging (15,53,54). A recent hypothesis proposes that epistasis is a ubiquitous and common component of the genetic architecture of multigenic disorders and that multifaceted interactions are more important than the independent effect of any one susceptibility gene (50). The relative contribution of each gene would not be (statistically) significant but only detected when interaction between loci is investigated. Likewise, there is growing interest in the study of gene–environment interaction in disease etiology. It is the general consensus that nongenetic factors may play a major role in the common late-onset disorders of Western societies, many of which have increased in prevalence over the past few decades (i.e., type 2 diabetes, obesity, hypertension, and coronary artery disease). Indeed, the increasing prevalence of these common disorders is more likely attributed to nongenetic influences triggering the disease in genetically susceptible individuals, because nongenetic factors have undergone a more recent change than common disease alleles in the population (48). A recent example of the importance of incorporating analysis of environmental influences in association studies is the CD14 gene in asthma (55). A polymorphisms in the promoter region of CD14, an endotoxin receptor on monocytes, has been shown to provide protection to asthma and atopy when environmental endotoxin levels are low and confer an increased risk for asthma when endotoxin levels are high (56). Statistical and bioinformatics solutions that incorporate effects of gene-by-gene and gene-by-environment interactions in association studies in complex diseases are emerging and are likely to influence the analytical approach of these disorders in the near future (53,57).

VIII. Genetic Association Studies

Replication of association or linkage is considered to be the gold standard in genetic research. Therefore, it is discouraging that to date, relatively few of the many polymorphisms that are reported to influence the risk to common diseases have been replicated (17–19,58–62). Furthermore, the individual effect of each variant is often small, explaining only a fraction of the overall heritability of the disease. Numerous reports of genes showing association to complex diseases have failed in replication studies, raising considerable concern with respect to design and interpretation of these studies and the data produced (17–19,58–62). Issues that need careful consideration prior to any association testing include calculations of the degree of statistical power needed to detect association, if one exists. This is largely dependent on frequencies of the at-risk alleles, the sample size, and the composition of cases versus controls with respect to any stratification biases (58–60,62). Thus, more rigidity is needed in the study design to minimize potential study bias and reduce the risk of reporting false-positive results due to lack of study power.

Recently, GW association studies, a technology using large number of SNPs in search for variants that contribute to complex diseases (63), have emerged and begun to replace the more traditional microsatellite mapping approach that has dominated the gene discovery process of common diseases for decades. By taking advantage of the knowledge that the genome is organized in discrete LD blocks with limited haplotype diversity within each block, the smallest sets of SNPs necessary for detecting all major haplotypes (haplotype-tagging or tSNPS) can be determined, thus improving genotyping accuracy and reducing genotyping cost. However, the experience with the GW association approach is small and several potential hurdles remain (62,64–66). These include but are not limited to the number and selection of SNPs used (map-based vs. gene-based), population selection, study design, statistical analysis, and study power, Nonetheless, large-scale SNP-based association mapping studies recently conducted have reported discovery of variants that are associated with myocardial infarction (67) and age-related macular degeneration (68). No doubt, the recent success coming from SNP-based GW association will spur gene-hunters of complex diseases to use this approach in their attempt to unveil the genetic causes of these common disorders in the near future.

In conclusion, there has been rapid development in new technology platforms, which has led to increased understanding of the human genome and the discovery of variants that either alone or in combination with other variants in different genes and/or the environment underlie many of the common diseases that affect human beings. While several genes that confer disease susceptibility have been uncovered, the genetic causes of most common diseases remain unresolved. Optimal use of the HapMap dataset in future GW association studies conducted on large cohorts and replicated in different populations present a major challenge for gene-hunters in the coming years.

References

1. Lander ES, Linton LM, Birren B, et al. Initial sequencing and analysis of the human genome. Nature 2001; 409(6822):860–921.
2. Venter JC, Adams MD, Myers EW, et al. The sequence of the human genome. Science 2001; 291(5507):1304–1351.
3. Online Mendelian Inheritance in Man, OMIM^{TM}. McKusick-Nathans Institute for Genetic Medicine, Johns Hopkins University (Baltimore, MD) and National Center for Biotechnology Information, National Library of Medicine (Bethesda, MD).
4. http://www.ncbi.nlm.nih.gov/omim/
5. Murray C, Lopez A. Global health statistics: a compendium of incidence, prevalence, and mortality estimates for over 200 conditions. Global Burden of Disease and Injury Series. Vol. II. Harvard University Press, 1999.
6. DeMeo DL, Silverman EK. (alpha)1-Antitrypsin deficiency 2: Genetic aspects of (alpha)1-antitrypsin deficiency: phenotypes and genetic modifiers of emphysema risk. Thorax 2004; 59(3):259–264.

7. Dahl M, Hersh CP, Ly NP, et al. The protease inhibitor PI*S allele and COPD: a meta-analysis. Eur Respir J 2005; 26(1):67–76.
8. Burton PR, Tobin MD, Hopper JL. Key concepts in genetic epidemiology. Lancet 2005; 366(9489):941–951.
9. Dawn Teare M, Barrett JH. Genetic linkage studies. Lancet 2005; 366(9490):1036–1044.
10. Risch N. Searching for genetic determinants in the new millennium. Nature 2000; 405:847–856.
11. Altshuler D, Daly M, Kruglyak L. Guilt by association. Nat Genet 2000; 26:135–137.
12. Botstein D, Risch N. Discovering genotypes underlying human phenotypes: past successes for Mendelian disease, future approaches for complex disease. Nat Genet 2003; 33(suppl):228–237.
13. Nadeau JH. Modifier genes in mice and humans. Nat Rev Genet 2001; 2(3):165–174.
14. Salvatore F, Scudiero O, Castaldo G. Genotype-phenotype correlation in cystic fibrosis: the role of modifier genes. Am J Med Genet 2002; 111(1):88–95.
15. Carlborg O, Haley CS. Epistasis: Too Often Neglected In Complex Trait Studies? Nat Rev Genet 2004; 5(8):618–625.
16. Altmuller J, Palmer LJ, Fischer G, et al. Genomewide scans of complex human diseases: true linkage is hard to find. Am J Hum Genet 2001; 69(5):936–950.
17. Glazier A, Nadeau J, Aitman T. Finding genes that underlie complex traits. Science 2002; 298(20 December):2345–2349.
18. Ioannidis JPA, Trikalinos TA, Ntzani EE, et al. Genetic associations in large versus small studies: an empirical assessment. Lancet 2003; 361(9357):567–571.
19. Page GP, George V, Go RC, et al. "Are we there yet?": deciding when one has demonstrated specific genetic causation in complex diseases and quantitative traits. Am J Hum Genet 2003; 73(4):711–719.
20. Jorde LB. Linkage disequilibrium and the search for complex disease genes. Genome Res 2000; 10:1344–1435.
21. Ardlie KG, Kruglyak L, Seielstad M. Patterns of linkage disequilibrium in the human genome. Nat Rev Genet 2002; 3(4):299–309.
22. Wall JD, Pritchard JK. Haplotype blocks and linkage disequilibrium in the human genome. Nat Rev Genet 2003; 4(8):587–597.
23. Kerem B, Rommens JM, Buchanan JA, et al. Identification of the cystic fibrosis gene: genetic analysis. Science 1989; 245(4922):1073–1080.
24. Riordan JR, Rommens JM, Kerem B, et al. Identification of the cystic fibrosis gene: cloning and characterization of complementary DNA. Science 1989; 245(4922):1066–1073.
25. Van Eerdewegh P, Little RD, Dupuis J, et al. Association of the ADAM33 gene with asthma and bronchial hyperresponsiveness. Nature 2002; 418(6896):426–430.
26. Zhang Y, Leaves NI, Anderson GG, et al. Positional cloning of a quantitative trait locus on chromosome 13q14 that influences immunoglobulin E levels and asthma. Nat Genet 2003; 34(2):181–186.
27. Allen M, Heinzmann A, Noguchi E, et al. Positional cloning of a novel gene influencing asthma from chromosome 2q14. Nat Genet 2003; 35(3):258–263.

28. Laitinen T, Polvi A, Rydman P, et al. Characterization of a common susceptibility locus for asthma-related traits. Science 2004; 304(5668):300–304.
29. Nicolae D, Cox NJ, Lester LA, et al. Fine mapping and positional candidate studies identify HLA-G as an asthma susceptibility gene on chromosome 6p21. Am J Hum Genet 2005; 76(2):349–357.
30. Noguchi E, Yokouchi Y, Zhang J, et al. Positional identification of an asthma susceptibility gene on human chromosome 5q33. Am J Respir Crit Care Med 2005; 172(2):183–188.
31. Kong A, Barnard J, Gudbjartsson DF, et al. Recombination rate and reproductive success in humans. Nat Genet 2004; 36(11):1203–1206.
32. www.hapmap.org.
33. The International HapMap Project. Nature 2003; 426(6968):789–796.
34. Arcos-Burgos M, Muenke M. Genetics of population isolates. Clin Genet 2002; 61(4):233–247.
35. Hakonarson H, Bjornsdottir US, Halapi E, et al. A major susceptibility gene for asthma maps to chromosome 14q24. Am J Hum Genet 2002; 71(3):483–491.
36. Laitinen T, Daly MJ, Rioux JD, et al. A susceptibility locus for asthma-related traits on chromosome 7 revealed by genome-wide scan in a founder population. Nat Genet 2001; 28(1):87–91.
37. Peltonen L. Positional cloning of disease genes: advantages of genetic isolates. Hum Hered 2000; 50(1):66–75.
38. Gulcher JKA, Stefansson K. The genealogic approach to human genetics of disease. Cancer J 2001; 7:61–68.
39. Lander ER, Kruglyak L. Genetic dissection of complex traits: guidelines for interpreting and reporting linkage results. Nat Genet 1995; 11:241–247.
40. Majumder PP, Ghosh S. Mapping quantitative trait loci in humans: achievements and limitations. J Clin. Invest 2005; 115(6):1419–1424.
41. Members of the Complex Trait C. The nature and identification of quantitative trait loci: a community's view. Nat Rev Genet 2003; 4(11):911–916.
42. Smith MW, O'Brien SJ. Mapping by admixture linkage disequilibrium: advances, limitations and guidelines. Nat Rev Genet 2005; 6(8):623–632.
43. McKeigue PM. Prospects for admixture mapping of complex traits. Am J Hum Genet 2005; 76(1):1–7.
44. Zhu X, Luke A, Cooper RS, et al. Admixture mapping for hypertension loci with genome-scan markers. Nat Genet 2005; 37(2):177–181.
45. Reich D, Patterson N, Jager PLD, et al. A whole-genome admixture scan finds a candidate locus for multiple sclerosis susceptibility. Nat Genet 2005; 37(10):1113–1118.
46. Pritchard JK, Cox NJ. The allelic architecture of human disease genes: common disease-common variant... or not? Hum Mol Genet 2002; 11(20):2417–2423.
47. Reich DE, Lander ES. On the allelic spectrum of human disease. Trends in Genetics 2001; 17(9):502–510.
48. Weiss KM, Terwilliger JD. How many diseases does it take to map a gene with SNPs? Nat Genet 2000; 26(2):151–157.
49. Wright AF, Hastie ND. Complex genetic diseases: controversy over the Croesus code. Genome Biol 2001; 2:(Comment 2007).

50. Moore JH. The ubiquitous nature of epistasis in determining susceptibility to common human diseases. Hum Hered 2003; 56(1–3):73–82.
51. Lander ES. The new genomics: global views of biology. Science 1996; 274(5287):536–539.
52. Lai CQ, Parnell LD, Ordovas JM. The APOA1/C3/A4/A5 gene cluster, lipid metabolism and cardiovascular disease risk. Curr Opin Lipidol 2005; 16(2):153–166.
53. Marchini J, Donnelly P, Cardon LR. Genome-wide strategies for detecting multiple loci that influence complex diseases. Nat Genet 2005; 37(4):413–417.
54. Nagel RL. Epistasis and the genetics of human diseases. C R Biol 2005; 328(7):606–615.
55. Ober C, Thompson EE. Rethinking genetic models of asthma: the role of environmental modifiers. Curr Opin Immunol 2005; 17:1–9.
56. Zambelli-Weiner A, Ehrlich E, Stockton ML, et al. Evaluation of the CD14/-260 polymorphism and house dust endotoxin exposure in the Barbados Asthma Genetics Study. J Allergy Clin Immunol 2005; 115(6):1203–1209.
57. Hahn LW, Ritchie MD, Moore JH. Multifactor dimensionality reduction software for detecting gene-gene and gene-environment interactions. Bioinformatics 2003; 19(3):376–382.
58. Cardon LR, Bell JI. Association study designs for complex diseases. Nat Rev Genet 2001; 2(2):91–99.
59. Cordell HJ, Clayton DG. Genetic association studies. Lancet 2005; 366(9491):1121–1131.
60. Hattersley AT, McCarthy MI. What makes a good genetic association study? Lancet 2005; 366:1315–1323.
61. Lohmueller KE, Pearce CL, Pike M, et al. Meta-analysis of genetic association studies supports a contribution of common variants to susceptibility to common disease. Nat Genet 2003; 33(2):177–182.
62. Palmer LJ, Cardon LR. Shaking the tree: mapping complex disease genes with linkage disequilibrium. Lancet 2005; 366(9492):1223–1234.
63. Risch N, Merikangas F. The future of genetic studies of complex human diseases. Science 1996; 273:1516–1517.
64. Hirschhorn JN, Daly MJ. Genome-wide association studies for common diseases and complex traits. Nat Rev Genet 2005; 6(2):95–108.
65. Wang WY, Barratt BJ, Clayton DG, et al. Genome-wide association studies: theoretical and practical concerns. Nat Rev Genet 2005; 6(2):109–118.
66. Syvanen AC. Toward genome-wide SNP genotyping. Nat Genet 2005; 37(suppl):S5–S10.
67. Ozaki K, Ohnishi Y, Iida A, et al. Functional SNPs in the lymphotoxin-alpha gene that are associated with susceptibility to myocardial infarction. Nat Genet 2002; 32(4):650–654.
68. Klein RJ, Zeiss C, Chew EY, et al. Complement factor H polymorphism in age-related macular degeneration. Science 2005; 308(5720):385–389.

2

Genetic Epidemiology of Reduced Lung Function

CLEO C. VAN DIEMEN and H. MARIKE BOEZEN

Department of Epidemiology,
  University Medical Center Groningen,
  University of Groningen,
Groningen, The Netherlands

I. Introduction

Genetic epidemiology of respiratory disease focuses on identifying genetic determinants of disease development taking environmental factors that preclude, affect, or enhance this development, into account. The respiratory disease chronic obstructive pulmonary disease (COPD) is almost fully attributable to the environmental factor, smoking, with the exception of the genetical predominance of α1-antitrypsine (AAT) deficiency gene, which carriers need no further environmental smoke exposure to develop a phenotypic expression of COPD. However, AAT deficiency is accounting for a minimal number of COPD cases worldwide (< 1%), because the fast majority of COPD does not have ATT deficiency but is attributable to cigarette smoking. The role of smoking as major determinant of COPD has risen above any doubt. However, if "the whole world" would have been smoking, COPD would have been considered to be a genetic disease, because only a minority of smokers develops COPD. Therefore, those smokers who do develop COPD seem to be genetically more susceptible to the deleterious effects of cigarette smoke than smokers who do not develop COPD. This chapter focuses on the genetic determinants of diminished lung function, taking environmental factors that preclude, affect, or enhance this development, into account, with specific emphasis on different study designs that are used in genetic epidemiology.

II. Environmental and Genetic Factors Affecting Lung Function

COPD is the third cause of death worldwide and is expected to increase in prevalence in the forthcoming decades (1,2). Reduced levels of lung function, assessed by lung function measurements, provide the most important and robust phenotypes of COPD and predict progression of the disease and overall mortality (3,4).

The level of lung function is both genetically and environmentally determined. In the past decades, the environmental determinants have been extensively studied, i.e., smoking, air pollution, occupational exposure, childhood respiratory illness, diet, and exposure to respiratory allergens. The genetic determinants have been studied less frequently and consistently, and they are more difficult to study, because COPD is a disease that is merely expressed at later ages. Therefore, the "traditional" types of genetic studies, such as those performed within families, are more difficult to perform, because the parents of individuals with COPD often already have died and the children of subjects with COPD are likely to be too young to manifest airway obstruction already.

Nevertheless, a number of genetic studies on COPD have been performed, usually including small numbers of subjects and various definitions of disease status, which makes it difficult to compare results between such studies. Because of this low interstudy comparability with regard to COPD disease state, it makes sense to choose a robust phenotype-like level of pulmonary function, which can be compared more easily between studies. Moreover, an accelerated decline in FEV_1 is a predictor for mortality from COPD (3,4), and provides additional information compared to taking only the level of FEV_1 into account.

A. Environmental Factors Affecting Lung Function

The rate of decline in lung function is determined by many environmental factors. Cohort studies have shown that adult smokers experience faster decline in FEV_1 than do nonsmokers (5) and that this accelerated decline returns to normal levels of aging-related decline after smoking cessation (6). Additionally, women have a faster decline in FEV_1 in response to cigarette smoke than have men (7). The rate of FEV_1 decline is also related to outdoor and indoor air pollution levels (8,9) and occupational exposure to dust, gasses, and fumes (10–12). A poor level of lung function at a later age is not necessarily caused by excessive lung function decline, but can also be the consequence of a diminished maximal attained level of lung function, which can be due to many causes. Current and cumulative cigarette smoking, the presence of respiratory symptoms, increased numbers of blood eosinophils, and increased airway responsiveness were all found to be significant predictors of reduced level of FEV_1 in a large cohort of the general population (13). Another study demonstrated a 10.7% reduction in FEV_1 among children with a smoking parent compared to children of a nonsmoking parent, thereby emphasizing the importance of environmental tobacco smoke already in childhood (14). To accurately assess decline in lung function or level of lung function at an older age, it is important to keep these environmental factors in mind.

B. Genetic Factors Affecting Lung Function

There are many approaches to determine whether there is a genetic component contributing to a reduced level of lung function, and if such a genetic component can be identified, how big its effect is. In this chapter, we will discuss the different approaches to study genetic epidemiology of reduced level of lung function, together with the major results each method has provided in elucidating the role of genetics in level of lung function.

III. Family and Twin Studies

About 30 years ago, studies already demonstrated that there is a familial resemblance in pulmonary function. Cohen et al. showed in 1977 that first-degree relatives of COPD patients had lower rates of forced expiration than had relatives of patients with nonrespiratory disease or community-derived controls (15). Many studies have addressed the familial component of COPD and found that familial factors account for up to 40% to 50% of variability in cross-sectional lung function levels. For example, Astemborski et al. showed that additive genetic variation accounted for 28% of the variation in residual FEV_1 in 108 adult families and 24% of the variation in residual FEV_1/FVC adjusted for appropriate confounders (16). A number of studies have demonstrated that the risk to develop COPD is two- to threefold greater for smokers who have a first-degree relative with COPD compared to smokers without such a relative (17). Moreover, lower values of $FEF_{25-75\%}$ and $FEF_{25-75\%}/FVC$ in smoking and in nonsmoking first-degree relatives of early-onset COPD patients compared to controls suggest a genetic susceptibility to develop COPD independent of smoking (18). Indeed, this risk may increase according to higher levels of exposure to detrimental environments such as cigarette smoke, because smoking relatives showed lower $FEF_{25-75\%}$ and $FEF_{25-75\%}/FVC$.

Some family studies have addressed the familial correlation in decline of FEV_1 and found no evidence for spousal or parent–offspring correlation for decline in FEV_1 (slope) over the years. However, there was a strong correlation in slope of FEV_1 between siblings, especially in smoking-concordant pairs (19).

Twin studies are an interesting method to study the relative importance of genetic and environmental effects on a trait, because monozygotic (MZ) twins share 100% of their DNA and dizygotic (DZ) twins only 50%. A higher degree of similarities in MZ than in DZ twins suggests a genetic influence, irrespective of environmental influences. MZ twins exposed to opposite environmental influences shed a light on the relative importance of the environment (e.g., cigarette smoking) on a phenotypic trait such as reduced levels of lung function. Several studies have shown that intrapair correlations for spirometric measures between MZ twins are high and highly significant, and smaller between DZ twins (20,21), although one such a study showed no such intrapair difference in pulmonary function between MZ and DZ twins (22). Strong indications for genetic effects on pulmonary function come from a study by Redline et al.(23). They showed that the strength of the correlations in FEV_1 and FVC decreases when relatives share less of their genotype, i.e., correlations of 0.71 for MZ twins (100% shared genotype), 0.16 to 0.29 for relatives with 50% shared genotype, and 0.09 to 0.27 for relatives with 25% shared genotype (23). A study of lung function in 203 twin pairs aged 18 to 34 detected significant genetic variations in females and males (24). There was evidence that the heritability was lower in males (about 0.6) than females (about 0.8). An effect of smoking on lung function was detected but accounted for less than 3% of the variance. The geometry of the airways may also be related to genetic factors, because the difference in V_{max} at 60% of total lung capacity on air and on helium–oxygen is smaller between MZ twins than DZ twins (25).

Two other twin studies have suggested that genetic factors are important in susceptibility to airway disease in reaction to cigarette smoke. Within identical twins who are raised apart, twins concordant for cigarette smoking or nonsmoking have highly similar lung function, whereas twin pairs discordant for smoking status have larger differences in pulmonary function (26,27).

In conclusion, these family and twin studies have demonstrated that there is a familial aggregation of lung function measures, indicating that genetic factors are important for level of lung function. Because twin studies do not require the genotype and phenotype of at least two generations like the other types of family studies, the late onset of the disease is not a problem and twin studies are suitable for studying COPD.

IV. Segregation Analysis and Heritability

Segregation analysis evaluates whether the proportion of affected and unaffected offspring in families is consistent with Mendelian expectations.

It addresses the question whether a disease is caused by a major Mendelian gene or whether different minor gene effects account for the disease.

There are conflicting results for the mode of inheritance of pulmonary function. Rybicki et al. found evidence for a major gene influencing FEV_1 in families ascertained through a proband with COPD, but not in randomly ascertained families (28). The Humboldt family study showed a major genetic mechanism for inheritance of FVC, but environmental factors remained significant in the segregation analyses (29,30). The National Heart, Lung, and Blood Institute (NHLBI) Family Heart study also provided evidence for major genes for FEV_1 and FEV_1/FVC (31). In the 264 members of 26 Utah Genetic Reference pedigrees, major locus inheritance was found for the FEV_1/FVC ratio, although they could not discriminate between a dominant and recessive mode of inheritance. No evidence of major locus inheritance was found for either FEV_1 or FVC (32). Similarly, in the Framingham study (5003 subjects from 1408 families), models with a Mendelian gene for inheritance of FEV_1 were rejected (33). The familial correlation was greater between mothers and offspring than between fathers and offspring in models that assume no major gene. Additionally, sibling correlation exceeded parent–offspring correlation.

The Framingham study is the only study that addresses heritability of longitudinal decline in lung function. The authors describe heritability of longitudinal change in lung function over at least 15 years in two generations of the general population. Heritability factors explained a modest proportion of the population variance, but were higher when analyses were restricted to smoking status (34).

In summary, all studies indicate a significant heritability of pulmonary function, but it is not clear whether a major gene causes this effect or that several minor genes exert the effect, combined with or without environmental factors.

V. Genome-Wide Linkage Analysis

Genome-wide linkage analysis is an approach to identify which chromosomal areas are involved in disease. This method compares the inheritance of disease with inheritance of genetic markers in families with multiple affected members. If the disease is coinherited with the marker, this suggests that a disease susceptibility gene is located close to the marker of that chromosome.

The first studies on linkage analyses for COPD were performed in the Boston severe early-onset COPD population. This population consists of families ascertained through probands with severe early-onset COPD without AAT deficiency. Given the young age of probands, it was possible to include parents to perform these linkage analyses. Multiple chromosomes were identified to be linked to different phenotypes, for example, pre- and postbronchodilator FEV_1 and FVC. These studies will be described in more detail in Chapter 11 of this book.

An overview of the genome-wide linkage analyses that have been performed on lung function measures so far is given in Table 1. The Framingham cohort is based on the general population. In a genome-wide screen on this cohort, FEV_1 was most influenced by the locus on chromosome 6 [Likelihood of disease (LOD) score = 2.4], whereas chromosome 21 contained markers with the strongest linkage to FVC (LOD score = 2.6) (37). In the subsequent fine screen of the linked region, the linkage peak was narrowed to chromosome 6q27 and the LOD score for linkage of FEV_1 increased from 2.4 to 5.0 (38).

A genome-wide scan of pulmonary function measures in the NHLBI Family Heart Study identified regions on chromosomes 4 and 18 with LOD scores above 2.5, and these two chromosomes were further evaluated by incorporating additional marker genotyping. The FEV_1/FVC ratio was linked to chromosome 4 with a LOD score of 3.5. FEV_1 and FVC were suggestively linked to regions on chromosome 18 with multipoint LOD scores of 2.4 for FEV_1 and 1.5 for FVC at 31 cM (D18S843) and a LOD of 2.9 for FVC at 79 cM (D18S858) (39).

In the Utah CPH, suggestive evidence for linkage of FEV_1/FVC was found on chromosome 2 (heterogeneity LOD 2.36, dominant model) and chromosome 5 (heterogeneity LOD 2.23, recessive model). In addition, nonparametric variance component linkage analysis showed linkage of $FEV_1/$ FVC in both of these regions, providing further support to the results (32).

A genome-wide scan for asthma phenotypes was conducted in 295 French Epidemiological study on the Genetics and Environment of asthma, bronchial hyperresponsiveness and atopy (EGEA) families selected through at least one asthmatic subject. Besides linkage of asthmatic phenotypes, they also found linkage for % pred FEV_1 to chromosome 6q14, which appears to be a new region potentially linked to %pred FEV_1 (40). Another genome-wide screen within 200 families ascertained through a proband with asthma was performed by Postma et al. (41), and in addition these authors assessed influences of early-life smoke exposure. Significant evidence for linkage of pre- and postbronchodilator FEV_1/VC was found for chromosome 2q32 (LOD 4.9, increasing to 6.03 with additional fine-mapping markers, and 3.2, respectively), 35 cM proximal from linkage previously observed in families of probands with early-onset COPD. Linkage existed for chromosome 5q for pre- and postbronchodilator VC (LOD 1.8 and 2.6, respectively). Results for pre- and postbronchodilator FEV_1 were less significant (LOD 1.5 and 1.6, chromosomes 11p and 10q, respectively). Results were not affected by passive smoke exposure. Thus, there may be multiple genes on chromosome 2q that are important in determining presence and degree of airflow limitation in families ascertained for obstructive airway disease. Thus far, linkages with lung function on chromosome 2 are on different chromosomal locations in the different studies (Table 1), which makes it difficult to identify a candidate gene is this area.

Table 1 Genome-Wide Linkage Analyses for Lung Function Measures

Study population	Linkage	Chromosome (Cm)	LOD score	References
Boston early-onset COPD (n = 560)	FEV_1	8p23 (2 from pter)	3.30	Palmer, 2003 (35)
	FEV_1	1p21 (136)	2.24	For every linkage, pre-BDR was also linked, but LOD score was lower
	FEV_1,	8q24 (163)	2.01	
	FEV_1, FEV_1/FVC	19q13 (78)	resp. 1.94, 1.67	
	FEV_1, FEV_1/FVC	2q36 (222)	resp. 1.13, 4.42	
	FEV_1/FVC	1p31 (118)	2.52	
	FEV_1/FVC	17q21 (67)	2.44	
	FEV_1/FVC	2q (222)	4.12	Silverman, 2002 (36)
Boston early-onset COPD (n = 585)	FEV_1/FVC	1(120)	1.92	
	FEV_1/FVC	17 (67)	2.03	
	FEV_1	12p (37)	2.43	
	FVC	1 (13)	2.05	
Framingham cohort, 1578 members of 330 families	FEV_1, FVC	4 (76)	resp. 1.6, 1.2	Joost et al., 2002 (37)
	FEV_1, FVC	6 (qterm)	resp. 2.4, 1.1	
	FEV_1, FVC	21 (pterm)	resp. 1.2, 2.6	
Framingham, fine screen	FEV_1	6q27 (184–190)	5.0	Wilk et al., 2003 (38)
NHLBI family heart study (n = 1327, general population)	FEV_1/FVC	4 (28)	3.5	Wilk et al., 2003 (39)
	FEV_1, FVC (31), FVC (79)	18 (31, 79)	resp. 2.4, 1.5, 2.9	

(Continued)

Table 1 Genome-Wide Linkage Analyses for Lung Function Measures (*Continued*)

Study population	Linkage	Chromosome (Cm)	LOD score	References
264 members of 24 Utah CEPH pedigrees	FEV_1/FVC	2 (222)	1.02 (1.55 in dom model)	Malhotra et al., 2003 (32)
	FEV_1/FVC	5 (295)	2.64	
	FEV_1/FVC	5 (297)	1.92	
	FEV_1/FVC	5 (299)	1.06 (1.54 in rec model)	
Boston early-onset COPD (n = 416)	FEV_1/FVC	5 (303)	1.46	DeMeo et al., 2004 (18)
	$FEF_{25-75\%}/FVC$	2 (216)	2.60	
	$FEF_{25-75\%}$	12 (35)	5.03 (smoke only)	
	$FEF_{25-75\%}/FVC$	2 (221)	4.12 (smoke only)	
	$FEF_{25-75\%}/FVC$	12 (35)	3.46 (smoke only)	
	FEV_1/FVC	2 (229)	4.13	
	FEV_1	12 (36)	3.26	
295 French EGEA families, ascertained for asthma (n = 726)	$FEV_1\%$pred	6q14 (89)	2.94	Bouzigon et al., 2004 (40)
200 Dutch families ascertained for asthma (n = 1183)	Pre- and post-FEV_1/FVC	2q32 (195)	resp. 4.9, 3.2	Postma et al., 2005 (41)
	Pre- and post FVC	5q (140)	resp 1.8, 2.6	

Abbreviations: COPD, chronic obstructive pulmonary disease; LOD, Likelihood of Disease; EGEA, Epidemiological study on the Genetics and Environment of Asthma, bronchial hyperresponsiveness and atopy; CEPH, Centre d'Etude du Polymorphisme Humain.

The results from the linkage analyses are clearly inconsistent. Some regions have been replicated, whereas most others have not. This indicates that the genetics of lung function is a multifactorial and complex matter. The logical next step after linkage analyses would be positional cloning of genes in the linked region. Unfortunately, such approaches are lacking in genetics of lung function or COPD. In contrast, in asthma, positional cloning of genes in linked regions has resulted in identification of four candidate genes for asthma, namely *A Disintegrin and Metalloprotease 33* (*ADAM33*), *Dipeptidyle peptidase 10*, *PDH finger protein 11*, and *G protein coupled receptor 154* (42). The only study that examined candidate genes in a region of linkage in COPD (i.e., chromosome 2q) was performed by Celedon et al. (43), in which the *transforming growth factor-β_1* gene was identified as a risk factor for lower FEV_1/FVC. Hopefully, positional cloning will provide more candidate genes for reduced lung function and COPD in the future.

VI. Case–Control Studies

In case–control studies, a large number of candidate genes, chosen for their biological role in pathogenesis in COPD, have been associated with lung function or COPD. However, for every studied gene there is (at least) one study which results contradict the others. Replication is difficult due to population stratification, ethnic differences, and small numbers of cases and controls that are usually included in studies. In Chapter 14, these studies and the candidate genes that have been identified are described in more detail.

VII. Population-Based Longitudinal Studies on Decline in Lung Function

As mentioned earlier, lung function decline is a risk factor for development of COPD, and the progression of asthma. Studies that evaluate genetic influences on lung function decline in combination with environmental factors are important for identifying subjects at risk for these disabling diseases.

The Lung Health Study Group has performed multiple studies on genetics of lung function decline. Participants in the genetics study were selected from a larger cohort, which was designed to describe the natural history of cigarette smoke–associated COPD. They were all smokers with either no decline in FEV_1 ($n = 306$, mean decline $+14.9$ mL/yr) or a fast decline in FEV_1 ($n = 284$, mean decline -153.6 mL/yr) over a follow up period of five years. The reasoning behind selection of such groups was that widely divergent rates of decline in lung function would give robust phenotypes for detection of genes that contribute to COPD severity. In their initial study, they found associations of the α1-antitrypsin gene MZ genotype and microsomal epoxide hydrolase (His113/His139 haplotype), in combination with a family history of COPD, with rapid decline in FEV_1 (44). Subsequent studies with this same population identified associations with rapid decline in FEV$_1$ of haplotypes of *IL-1β* and *IL-1 receptor antagonist* (45), haplotypes of *glutathione S-transferase (GST)-M1, -T1, -P1* (46), single nucleotide polymorphisms (SNPs) in *Matrix metallopnotease 1 (MMP1)* and a haplotype of *MMP1* and *MMP12* (47), a SNP in *IL-4 receptor antagonist* (48), and a SNP in *β2-adrenergic receptor* (49). Because both nondecliners and fast-decliners had continuously smoked during follow up, these studies suggest that SNPs or a combination of risk alleles contribute to the deleterious effects of smoking on FEV$_1$. SNPs or haplotypes in other candidate genes [*tumor necrosis factor-α (TNF-α), vitamin-D–binding protein* (44), *heme oxygenase-1* (46), *MMP9* (47), *IL-13*, and *IL-13 receptor antagonist 1* (48)] were not associated with rapid decline in FEV$_1$. These studies have been described in more detail in Chapter 14.

In a cohort of firefighters (97% males, 75% Caucasian), longitudinal decline in FEV$_1$ was linked to *IL-10* SNPs. A SNP at position 1668 was associated with a more rapid decline in FEV$_1$ (50). In this same population, SNPs in *TNF-α* and *IL-1β* were also associated with a more rapid decline in FEV$_1$, whereas SNPs in *TGF-β1* were not (51).

Hang et al. have shown that gene–environment interactions can influence decline in FEV$_1$ substantially (52). They investigated whether SNPs in microsomal epoxide hydrolase, resulting in a slow and a fast enzyme activity, were associated with rapid decline in FEV$_1$ during 20 years of follow up. They were furthermore able to discriminate between nonexposed subjects and subjects exposed to airborne cotton dust and gram-negative bacteria endotoxin. Endotoxin exposure was associated with faster lung function decline among genotypes with slower enzyme activity but not among other genotypes. This indicates that SNPs can modify the association between occupational exposure and longitudinal lung function decline.

Recently, the effects of *GST* SNPs and daily fruit intake on decline in FEV$_1$ were studied in the Swiss cohort study on air pollution and lung diseases in adults (SAPALDIA) cohort that was followed up for 11 years (53). Both daily fruit intake and SNPs in *GST-M1* and *GST-T1* had an effect on FEV$_1$ decline in men only, not in women. The protective effect of daily fruit intake was restricted to male persistent smokers. These results indicate complex gene–environment interactions with additional gender effects.

After the identification of *ADAM33* as a candidate gene for asthma (54), SNPs in this gene were also associated with excess decline in FEV$_1$ within asthmatics (55). More recently, van Diemen et al. showed that these SNPs were associated with accelerated decline in FEV$_1$ and with development of COPD (56) in the general population.

VIII. Genetically Isolated Populations

Studies in isolated populations can be used in genetic epidemiology to identify candidate regions in a relatively small population because of their decreased genetic heterogeneity, increased linkage disequilibrium, and more homogeneous environmental exposures. Studying isolated populations has the advantage that data collecting for phenotyping (e.g., lung function measurements) and genotyping can usually be performed in a logistically small area, and also at low cost. The Hutterites of South Dakota are an isolated population of European descent from the early 17th to 18th century. Candidate loci for cardiovascular disease had a similar prevalence in this population compared to two samples of outbred populations, indicating that data gathered in a founder population can be extrapolated to the general population (57).

However, it is possible that common variants in the general population are not present in the isolated population. Conversely, it is possible that disease alleles identified in isolated populations may not contribute significantly to susceptibility in outbred populations. This was the case for the identification of the *cysteinyl leukotriene 2* (*CysLT2*) receptor as a candidate gene for asthma in the population of Tristan da Cunha (58). The SNP was frequent in this population (58), but had only a minor effect in outbred populations because of its low frequency (0.01–0.03) (59).

So far, no studies have been performed on COPD in isolated populations, although this might be a potentially efficient approach in identifying candidate regions, which should thereafter be explored further in general population samples.

IX. Conclusion

Several genes have been studied in relation to reduced level of lung function and COPD. Choices about the most appropriate study design, or the population to study, are usually made dependent of the goal of the study, for example, whether one sets out to confirm a previously found association in a different population, or to search for new genes or pathways, that have not been studied before.

We have discussed several study designs used in genetic epidemiology to study determinants of reduced lung function. Overall, every type of design has its restrictions, varying, for example, from high cost to relatively low costs and hypothesis-generating to hypothesis-testing. To our opinion, the most fruitful approach for future research seems to lie in combining the results of different types of study and study designs, and focusing on specific pathways; e.g., identifying candidate regions in isolated or patient populations, sequencing these regions, and testing SNPs in candidate genes in relation to lung function decline in the general population. A logical further step lies in studying functionality of identified SNPs, as well as gene expression in tissue. Moreover, genetic epidemiology studies should warrant attention for the interactions of genes with the major environmental exposure that play a role in the development of disease, being cigarette smoking. Therefore, for future research, excellent longitudinally collected data on phenotype, as well as exposures, are as crucial as improving techniques for genotyping.

References

1. WHO. World Health Report 2002. http://www.who.int/whr/2002, 2004.
2. Murtagh E, Heaney L, Gingles J, et al. The prevalence of obstructive lung disease in a general population sample: the NICECOPD study. Eur J Epidemiol 2005; 20(5):443–453.
3. Ekberg-Aronsson M, Pehrsson K, Nilsson JA, et al. Mortality in GOLD stages of COPD and its dependence on symptoms of chronic bronchitis. Respir Res 2005; 6:98.
4. Sin DD, Man SF. Chronic obstructive pulmonary disease as a risk factor for cardiovascular morbidity and mortality. Proc Am Thorac Soc 2005; 2(1):8–11.
5. Kauffmann F, Drouet D, Lellouch J, et al. Twelve years spirometric changes among Paris area workers. Int J Epidemiol 1979; 8(3):201–212.
6. Camilli AE, Burrows B, Knudson RJ, et al. Longitudinal changes in forced expiratory volume in one second in adults. Effects of smoking and smoking cessation. Am Rev Respir Dis 1987; 135(4):794–799.
7. Xu X, Weiss ST, Rijcken B, et al. Smoking, changes in smoking habits, and rate of decline in FEV1: new insight into gender differences. Eur Respir J 1994; 7(6):1056–1061.
8. Tashkin DP, Detels R, Simmons M, et al. The UCLA population studies of chronic obstructive respiratory disease: XI. Impact of air pollution and smoking on annual change in forced expiratory volume in one second. Am J Respir Crit Care Med 1994; 149(5):1209–1217.
9. Brunekreef B, Fischer P, Remijn B, et al. Indoor air pollution and its effect on pulmonary function of adult non-smoking women: III. Passive smoking and pulmonary function. Int J Epidemiol 1985; 14(2):227–230.
10. Christiani DC, Ye TT, Zhang S, et al. Cotton dust and endotoxin exposure and long-term decline in lung function: results of a longitudinal study. Am J Ind Med 1999; 35(4):321–331.
11. Enarson DA, Vedal S, Chan-Yeung M. Rapid decline in FEV1 in grain handlers. Relation to level of dust exposure. Am Rev Respir Dis 1985; 132(4):814–817.
12. Kauffmann F, Drouet D, Lellouch J, et al. Occupational exposure and 12-year spirometric changes among Paris area workers. Br J Ind Med 1982; 39(3): 221–232.
13. Wang X, Mensinga TT, Schouten JP, et al. Determinants of maximally attained level of pulmonary function. Am J Respir Crit Care Med 2004; 169(8):941–949.
14. Tager IB, Weiss ST, Munoz A, et al. Longitudinal study of the effects of maternal smoking on pulmonary function in children. N Engl J Med 1983; 309(12): 699–703.
15. Cohen BH, Diamond EL, Graves CG, et al. A common familial component in lung cancer and chronic obstructive pulmonary disease. Lancet 1977; 2(8037):523–526.

16. Astemborski JA, Beaty TH, Cohen BH. Variance components analysis of forced expiration in families. Am J Med Genet 1985; 21(4):741–753.

17. Chen Y. Genetics and pulmonary medicine.10: Genetic epidemiology of pulmonary function. Thorax 1999; 54(9):818–824.

18. DeMeo DL, Carey VJ, Chapman HA, et al. Familial aggregation of FEF(25–75) and FEF(25–75)/FVC in families with severe, early onset COPD. Thorax 2004; 59(5):396–400.

19. Kurzius-Spencer M, Sherrill DL, Holberg CJ, et al. Familial correlation in the decline of forced expiratory volume in one second. Am J Respir Crit Care Med 2001; 164(7):1261–1265.

20. Hubert HB, Fabsitz RR, Feinleib M, et al. Genetic and environmental influences on pulmonary function in adult twins. Am Rev Respir Dis 1982; 125(4):409–415.

21. Redline S, Tishler PV, Lewitter FI, et al. Assessment of genetic and nongenetic influences on pulmonary function. A twin study. Am Rev Respir Dis 1987; 135(1):217–222.

22. Ghio AJ, Crapo RO, Elliott CG, et al. Heritability estimates of pulmonary function. Chest 1989; 96(4):743–746.

23. Redline S, Tishler PV, Rosner B, et al. Genotypic and phenotypic similarities in pulmonary function among family members of adult monozygotic and dizygotic twins. Am J Epidemiol 1989; 129(4):827–836.

24. Gibson JB, Martin NG, Oakeshott JG, et al. Lung function in an Australian population: contributions of polygenic factors and the Pi locus to individual differences in lung function in a sample of twins. Ann Hum Biol 1983; 10(6):547–556.

25. Man SF, Zamel N. Genetic influence on normal variability of maximum expiratory flow-volume curves. J Appl Physiol 1976; 41(6):874–877.

26. Hankins D, Drage C, Zamel N, et al. Pulmonary function in identical twins raised apart. Am Rev Respir Dis 1982; 125(1):119–121.

27. Webster PM, Lorimer EG, Man SF, et al. Pulmonary function in identical twins: comparison of nonsmokers and smokers. Am Rev Respir Dis 1979; 119(2): 223–228.

28. Rybicki BA, Beaty TH, Cohen BH. Major genetic mechanisms in pulmonary function. J Clin Epidemiol 1990; 43(7):667–675.

29. Chen Y, Horne SL, Rennie DC, et al. Segregation analysis of two lung function indices in a random sample of young families: the Humboldt Family Study. Genet Epidemiol 1996; 13(1):35–47.

30. Chen Y, Rennie DC, Lockinger LA, et al. Major genetic effect on forced vital capacity: the Humboldt Family Study. Genet Epidemiol 1997; 14(1):63–76.

31. Wilk JB, Djousse L, Arnett DK, et al. Evidence for major genes influencing pulmonary function in the NHLBI family heart study. Genet Epidemiol 2000; 19(1):81–94.

32. Malhotra A, Peiffer AP, Ryujin DT, et al. Further evidence for the role of genes on chromosome 2 and chromosome 5 in the inheritance of pulmonary function. Am J Respir Crit Care Med 2003; 168(5):556–561.

33. Givelber RJ, Couropmitree NN, Gottlieb DJ, et al. Segregation analysis of pulmonary function among families in the Framingham Study. Am J Respir Crit Care Med 1998; 157(5 Pt 1):1445–1451.

34. Gottlieb DJ, Wilk JB, Harmon M, et al. Heritability of longitudinal change in lung function. The Framingham study. Am J Respir Crit Care Med 2001; 164(9):1655–1659.

35. Palmer LJ, Celedon JC, Chapman HA, et al. Genome-wide linkage analysis of bronchodilator responsiveness and post-bronchodilator spirometric phenotypes in chronic obstructive pulmonary diesease, Hum Mol Genet 2003, 12(10): 1199–1210.

36. Silverman EK, Palmer LJ, Mosley JD, et al. Genome wide linkage analaysis of quantitative spirometric phenotypes in severe early-onset chronic obstructive pulmonary disease. Am J Hum Gen 2002, 70(5): 1229–1239.

37. Joost O, Wilk JB, Cupples LA, et al. Genetic loci influencing lung function: a genome-wide scan in the Framingham Study. Am J Respir Crit Care Med 2002; 165(6):795–799.

38. Wilk JB, DeStefano AL, Joost O, et al. Linkage and association with pulmonary function measures on chromosome 6q27 in the Framingham Heart Study. Hum Mol Genet 2003; 12(21):2745–2751.

39. Wilk JB, DeStefano AL, Arnett DK, et al. A genome-wide scan of pulmonary function measures in the National Heart, Lung, and Blood Institute Family Heart Study. Am J Respir Crit Care Med 2003; 167(11):1528–1533.

40. Bouzigon E, Dizier MH, Krahenbuhl C, et al. Clustering patterns of LOD scores for asthma-related phenotypes revealed by a genome-wide screen in 295 French EGEA families. Hum Mol Genet 2004; 13(24):3103–3113.

41. Postma DS, Meyers DA, Jongepier H, Howard TD, Koppelman GH, Bleecker ER. Genomewide screen for pulmonary function in 200 families ascertained for asthma. Am J Respir Crit Care Med 2005; 172(4):446–452.

42. Kere J, Laitinen T. Positionally cloned susceptibility genes in allergy and asthma. Curr Opin Immunol 2004; 16(6):689–694.

43. Celedon JC, Lange C, Raby BA, et al. The transforming growth factor-beta1 (TGFB1) gene is associated with chronic obstructive pulmonary disease (COPD). Hum Mol Genet 2004; 13(15):1649–1656.

44. Sandford AJ, Chagani T, Weir TD, et al. Susceptibility genes for rapid decline of lung function in the lung health study. Am J Respir Crit Care Med 2001; 163(2):469–473.

45. Joos L, McIntyre L, Ruan J, et al. Association of IL-1beta and IL-1 receptor antagonist haplotypes with rate of decline in lung function in smokers. Thorax 2001; 56(11):863–866.

46. He JQ, Ruan J, Connett JE, et al. Antioxidant gene polymorphisms and susceptibility to a rapid decline in lung function in smokers. Am J Respir Crit Care Med 2002; 166(3):323–328.

47. Joos L, He JQ, Shepherdson MB, et al. The role of matrix metalloproteinase polymorphisms in the rate of decline in lung function. Hum Mol Genet 2002; 11(5):569–576.

48. He JQ, Connett JE, Anthonisen NR, et al. Polymorphisms in the IL13, IL13RA1, and IL4RA genes and rate of decline in lung function in smokers. Am J Respir Cell Mol Biol 2003; 28(3):379–385.

49. Joos L, Weir TD, Connett JE, et al. Polymorphisms in the beta2 adrenergic receptor and bronchodilator response, bronchial hyperresponsiveness, and rate of decline in lung function in smokers. Thorax 2003; 58(8):703–707.

50. Burgess JL, Fierro MA, Lantz RC, et al. Longitudinal decline in lung function: evaluation of interleukin-10 genetic polymorphisms in firefighters. J Occup Environ Med 2004; 46(10):1013–1022.

51. Yucesoy B, Johnson VJ, Kashon MK, et al. Cytokine gene polymorphisms and rate of decline in lung function in firefighters. American Thoracic Society 2005:A920.

52. Hang J, Zhou W, Wang X, et al. Microsomal epoxide hydrolase, endotoxin, and lung function decline in cotton textile workers. Am J Resp Crit Care Med 2005; 171(2):165–170.

53. Imboden M, Downs SH, Senn O, et al. GST gene polymorphisms and fruit intake modify lung function decline: a population-based study. American Thoracic Society 2005:A919.

54. Van Eerdewegh P, Little RD, Dupuis J, et al. Association of the ADAM33 gene with asthma and bronchial hyperresponsiveness. Nature 2002; 418:6896–430.

55. Jongepier H, Boezen HM, Dijkstra A, et al. Polymorphisms of the ADAM33 gene are associated with accelerated lung function decline in asthma. Clin Exp Allergy 2004; 34(5):757–760.

56. van Diemen CC, Postma DS, Vonk JM, et al. A disintegrin and metalloprotease 33 polymorphisms and lung function decline in the general population. Am J Respir Crit Care Med 2005; 172(3):329–333.

57. Newman DL, Hoffjan S, Bourgain C, et al. Are common disease susceptibility alleles the same in outbred and founder populations? Eur J Hum Gen 2004; 12(7):584–590.

58. Thompson MD, Storm van's Gravesande K, Galczenski H, et al. A cysteinyl leukotriene 2 receptor variant is associated with atopy in the population of Tristan da Cunha. Pharmacogenetics 2003; 13(10):641–649.

59. Pillai SG, Cousens DJ, Barnes AA, et al. A coding polymorphism in the CYSLT2 receptor with reduced affinity to LTD4 is associated with asthma. Pharmacogenetics 2004; 14(9):627–633.

3

Gene–Environment Interaction in Asthma

GERARD H. KOPPELMAN

Department of Pediatric Pulmonology,
Beatrix Children's Hospital, University
Medical Center Groningen,
University of Groningen,
Groningen, The Netherlands

DIRKJE S. POSTMA

Department of Pulmonology,
University Medical Center Groningen,
University of Groningen,
Groningen, The Netherlands

I. Introduction

Asthma is a genetically complex disease, caused by multiple genes and multiple environmental factors that may interact. Epidemiological studies have provided suggestive evidence for many environmental factors that may contribute to the development of asthma, e.g., indoor and outdoor pollution, allergen exposure, tobacco smoke, and other factors related to the "Western lifestyle" such as contact with microbial products and infections (1,2). The approach to detect, which genetic factors contribute to, asthma is extensively reviewed in this book in Chapters 5, 12, 14, and 15. This chapter focuses on the interaction of variations in the genome and environmental exposures. We will review epidemiological and genetic evidence that addresses gene–environment interaction in asthma (Table 1).

II. Evidence for Gene–Environment Interaction in Asthma

Several lines of evidence from twin and population studies support the presence of gene by environment interaction in asthma development.

33

Table 1 Literature Search for this Manuscript

Papers on original research cited in this chapter were retrieved by Medline searches (final search October 2005) using the keywords *gene, environment, gene-environment, interaction, atopy,* and *asthma.* This literature search focused on studies in human subjects and did not include animal models. Studies on gene and asthma drug interaction (pharmacogenetics) were excluded because these will be discussed separately in Chapter 20. References of the papers retrieved, as well as reviews on this subject, were checked to retrieve additional papers (3–8). Papers were categorized based on design (i.e., family study or case–control study), candidate gene, and environmental exposure. Priority was given to data that was replicated by an independent research group.

Twin studies have been widely used to estimate genetic and environmental contribution to asthma by comparing concordance rates in monozygotic and dizygotic twins. The heritability of asthma ranged between 0.36 and 0.75 in seven different twin studies (9). The nature of environmental factors, whether shared or not shared by cotwins, can be estimated by biometric modeling of twin data. The assumption is that differences in monozygotic twins are caused by individual-specific environmental factors, because the genes and the shared environment are similar. For example, a study by Hanson et al. compared prevalence rates of asthma and atopic characteristics in twins reared apart and together. The concordance rate in monozygotic twins was greater than in dizygotic twins, consistent with genetic effects. Furthermore, the difference in concordance within monozygotic twins compared to dizygotic twins suggested that individual specific, but not shared, environmental factors are important (10). Overall, twin studies provide evidence for the liability for asthma in a model consisting of additive genetic factors interacting with nonshared, individual-specific environmental influences, with no evidence for shared environmental factors (9).

Further evidence for gene by environment interaction in asthma is provided by population studies (3). These studies assessed whether a similar increase in prevalence of asthma occurred in all subjects in the population or preferably in subjects who are genetically susceptible for disease development, as assessed by a family history of the disease (11,12). As an example, this design was chosen by Jaakkola et al. who investigated childhood asthma as an interaction of environmental tobacco smoke (ETS) exposure at birth and parental atopy (asthma or hay fever). Childhood asthma in 2531 Norwegian children was based on questionnaire report of symptoms of bronchial obstruction during the first two years of life or a doctor's diagnosed asthma at age four. Parental atopy alone increased the risk of symptoms of bronchial obstruction [odds ratio (OR) 1.62; 95% confidence interval (CI) 1.10–2.40] and asthma (1.66; 95% CI, 1.08–2.54). In children without parental atopy, there was little effect of exposure to ETS on bronchial obstruction

(1.29; 95% CI, 0.88–1.89) and asthma (0.84; 95% CI, 0.53–1.34). In contrast, in children with parental atopy, exposure to ETS had a substantial effect on both symptoms of bronchial obstruction (2.88; 95% CI, 1.91–4.32) and asthma (2.68; 95% CI, 1.70–4.22). The results are consistent with gene by environment interaction and suggest that genes could confer susceptibility to ETS (13). Recent studies have addressed the chromosomal location and identity of these ETS susceptibility genes and will be discussed further on in this chapter.

III. Concept, Definition, and Methods

A general concept that gene by environment interaction would cause chronic disease was proposed by Gluckman and Hanson (Fig. 1). In this concept, genetic and adult life-style factors act in concert with environmental factors in early life. It introduces the term "developmental plasticity," the ability for an organism to change structure and function in response to environmental stimuli. These responses usually operate during critical developmental time windows and then become irreversible (14). In addition, this model addresses the role of the intrauterine and early life environment on gene expression by epigenetic mechanisms. The term "epigenetics" is used to describe stable alterations in gene expression that arise during development and cell proliferation are heritable in the short term, but do not involve

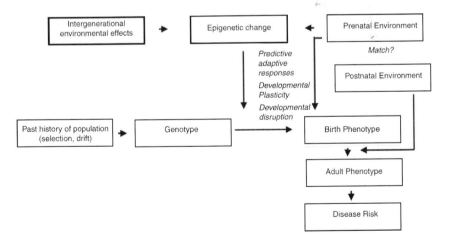

Figure 1 A general model of disease causation by interacting intergenerational, genetic, environmental, and prenatal and postnatal factors. Model of the developmental origins of disease and how intergenerational, genetic and environmental, and prenatal and postnatal factors interact to create a pathway to alter disease risk in adulthood. *Source*: From Ref. 14, excerpted with permission, copyright AAAS.

changes at the DNA level (4). Epigenetic regulation can take place by DNA methylation, or by proteins that associate itself with DNA and influence transcription (i.e., acetylation, methylation, or phosphorylation of histones). Epigenetic regulation can, for instance, be influenced by diet, and has been suggested to be potentially important in gene by environment interaction in asthma as well (4,5).

This concept of the developmental origin of disease may be applicable to asthma. Gene by environment interaction in asthma may include intergenerational and intrauterine environmental effects on epigenetic regulation of gene expression. In addition, environmental factors may act during critical time windows in early childhood when the immunity of children switches from the (intrauterine) Th2 milieu (associated with asthma) to Th1 (4).

Gene–environment interaction can be defined in a statistical or in a biological way. In statistical terms, interaction is present when the effect of genotype on disease risk depends on the level of exposure to an environmental factor (15). Biological interaction refers to the different mechanisms of interactions: epigenetic mechanisms, direct effects on gene transcription or translation, or by an interaction of the environmental factor with the gene product (protein–protein interaction).

Gene–environment interaction can be investigated in four different study designs: a case–control, a case only, a trio, or family design. In a case–control design, cases and controls are stratified for a certain genotype and environmental exposure (Table 2). An OR can be computed for the exposed and the nonexposed subjects. Thus, the ORs as exemplified in Table 2 are ad/bc in the genetically susceptible group and eh/fg in the non-risk group. Interaction can be computed as the OR for the environmental exposure in a multiplicative model; this ratio of these two OR's is calculated as adfg/bceh (15). This design is most useful when risk genotypes and exposures are common (16).

In a case only design, exposed and nonexposed cases are being compared. The null hypothesis of no gene–environment interaction implies that the disease risk is similar in exposed and nonexposed subjects carrying the

Table 2 Case–Control Study Testing for Gene by Environment Interaction

	Risk genotypes		Nonrisk genotypes	
Environmental exposure	Cases	Controls	Cases	Controls
Yes	a	b	e	f
No	c	d	g	h
OR	ad/bc		eh/fg	

Abbreviation: OR, odds ratio.

risk genotype (17). The usefulness of this design remains to be established (15). In a trio or family design, probands of proband-parents-trio or members of a family are stratified by environmental exposures. Risk estimates for disease development are compared in exposed and nonexposed subjects carrying the risk genotype.

IV. Family Studies

Epidemiological studies have consistently shown that ETS exposure in utero and/or in early childhood is associated with development of asthma, bronchial hyperresponsiveness, and reduced lung function later in life (18,19). Two family studies investigated the effect of ETS exposure on linkage results of asthma. These studies assess if certain chromosomal regions cosegregate with asthma in families exposed to ETS, suggesting that these chromosomal regions harbor asthma susceptibility genes that interact with ETS.

In a U.S. collaborative study of 144 families ascertained through two affected sibs, genome-wide linkage results on asthma were compared in children exposed and not exposed to ETS in infancy. Three regions (1p, 5q, and 9q) were identified with modest evidence for linkage of asthma when stratified on the basis of ETS exposure [logarithm of odds (LOD) ≥ 1.18]. The increase in LOD score in those exposed to ETS was significantly different from the LOD score in all asthmatics (simulation, $p < 0.05$). For example, the LOD score for asthma on chromosome 5q increased fourfold from 0.34 in all asthmatics to 1.23 in the ETS-exposed group (20). In this study, significant genome-wide LOD scores (i.e., LOD > 3.3) were not observed.

Strong support for interaction of gene(s) on chromosome 5q and ETS was provided by a genome-wide linkage study of 200 Dutch families ascertained through a proband with asthma. Families were stratified based on the known smoking history of the proband at recruitment, at the time the children were born, which was consistent with ETS exposure in infancy of the children. Smoking habits of both parents were highly correlated. The families with the children exposed to passive smoking accounted for all evidence for linkage of bronchial hyperresponsiveness (BHR) and asthma to 5q. The LOD scores in exposed families were 3.77 and 3.4, respectively, versus 0.7 and 0.21 in nonexposed families (Fig. 2). In contrast, evidence for linkage to 3p was found in both sets of families. The only additional region that showed differences for tobacco smoke–related gene–environment interaction was chromosome 19 (21). A second analysis in these families on measures of pulmonary function did not identify a strong effect of passive smoke exposure in early life on the linkage results (22). Further studies should be directed as to which gene(s), in particular on chromosome 5q, account(s) for this gene by environment interaction and what mechanism of interaction is present.

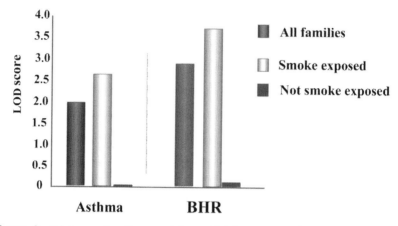

Figure 2 Linkage of asthma and bronchial hyperresponsiveness in 200 Dutch families ascertained through a proband with asthma. Environmental tobacco smoke exposure was assessed by taking the smoking history of the proband: more than or less than or equal to five pack years. All (200) families: 95 smoke-exposed families and 105 not exposed families. *Abbreviations*: BHR, bronchial hyperresponsiveness; LOD, logarithm of odds ratio. *Source*: From Ref. 21.

V. Candidate Gene Studies

Evidence for gene environment interaction in asthma and atopy has been provided by several studies that have used a candidate gene approach and selected environmental factors. Examples are studies of genes interacting with microbial exposure and infections, with cigarette smoke, air pollution, and with allergen exposure. We will discuss these investigations in depth.

A. Innate Immunity Genes Interacting with Microbial Products

Innate immunity genes are situated at the interface between the immune system and microbial products. Many microbes have specific pattern molecules on their surfaces, and these molecules interact with pattern–recognition receptors encoded by innate immunity genes such as CD14 and the Toll-like receptor (TLR) family. CD14 is a high-affinity receptor for lipopolysaccharide (endotoxin), a component of the cell wall of gram-negative bacteria. CD14 does not have a transmembrane domain and thus does not signal itself, but contributes to the affinity of the interaction between microbial products and TLR4 by formation of a receptor complex. TLR2 is part of a receptor complex responsive to a range of microbial products such as gram-positive bacteria, mycobacteria, and yeast. TLR4 more selectively forms the receptor for endotoxin, which is a major component of the bacterial wall of gram-negative bacteria (23). Downstream effects of activation of TLR2 and 4 pathways include the upregulation of accessory molecules and release of cytokines such as IL-10 and IL-12. Innate immunity pathways may control the activation of regulatory T-cells, be involved in the induction of tolerance, and prevent harmful immune pathology (23). These mechanisms are potentially important in directing the adaptive immune response and the development of atopic disease.

CD14

The *CD14* gene has several single nucleotide polymorphisms (SNPs), the most important one being the *CD14/-159* (also called *CD14/-260*) localized in the promoter region. Functional genomic studies showed that monocytic cells with the *CD14/-159* T alleles are transcriptionally more active than cells with the *CD14/-159* C allele. *CD14/-159* affects binding affinity of transcription factors of the Sp family, in particular the transcriptional repressor Sp3 (24). Genetic studies on the association of *CD14/-159* with asthma and atopy have produced conflicting results (25). Studies in US, UK, and Australian children and Dutch adults showed association of the C allele with atopic phenotypes, whereas other studies in the US Hutterite population identified association of the T allele with atopic phenotypes (25–28). Finally, in other populations, the *CD14* gene was not associated with atopy at all (29,30). Vercelli proposed an explanation for these apparent contradictory results by proposing the "endotoxin switch" (31). Different levels of endotoxin exposure would trigger different host responses, resulting in either Th1- or Th2-type responses. The *CD14* genotype may shift this endotoxin response curve (31). The concept of the endotoxin switch is supported by experiments in a rat model of allergen-induced inflammation. In these experiments, the timing and dosage of endotoxin in relation to allergen exposure resulted in either a Th1 or a Th2 inflammatory response in the lung (32).

Several studies have assessed *CD14* gene by environment interaction of proxy variables of microbial exposure (i.e., living on a farm, contact with stable animals, and presence of pets), and endotoxin exposure. Contact with microbial products, such as endotoxin, or infections may modify the immune response in early life and prevent subsequent asthma development (33). This "hygiene hypothesis" is supported by lower prevalence rates of asthma and allergies in children living on farms compared to children from rural populations not living on farms (35). In addition, protective effects on atopic phenotypes have been observed in children with more siblings, early entry at day care, and with dogs in their house (33). The concept of the endotoxin switch proposes that different levels of endotoxin interact with *CD14* genotype in either protecting or augmenting atopy and asthma development. Evidence to support this was provided by studies in central Europe, the United States, and Barbados.

In a sample of 624 children living in rural communities in central Europe, the *CD14* gene was investigated in relation to exposure to farm life (stable animals) and endotoxin exposure in their mattresses. In this study, outcome variables were total and specific immunoglobulin (Ig)E, and no data on asthma was provided. In the complete sample of 624 children, *CD14/-159* genotype was not associated with total and specific IgE. However, different levels of endotoxin significantly modified the association of *CD14/-159* genotype and IgE levels. In the highest tertile of endotoxin exposure, *CD14/-159* T allele was a risk factor for the development of specific IgE (OR 7.00, 95% CI, 1.36–36.02). The *CD14/-159* T allele was also a risk factor for raised total and specific IgE levels in children with regular contact to stable animals (OR 2.56, 95% CI, 1.07–6.15). In contrast, in children with regular contact with pets, the T allele showed a trend toward protection against raised specific IgE levels (OR 0.25, 95% CI, 0.05–1.15). Because these associations remained significant after corrections for endotoxin exposures, other environmental exposures may explain these interactions (35).

Dog ownership could also be a proxy variable of microbial exposures. Several studies have provided evidence for a protective effect of a dog in the house in early childhood on atopy development. Gern et al. studied interaction of dog ownership, *CD14/-159* genotype on atopy development in 285 US children prospectively followed up until the age of one. At the time of birth, 101 of these 285 infants were exposed to dog at home. At age one, atopy development was assessed by measurements of total IgE, specific IgE, self-reported food allergy, and a report of a physician's diagnosis of atopic dermatitis. In addition, supernatants of phytohemagglutinin (PHA) stimulated blood mononuclear cells of peripheral blood were analyzed for interferon-γ (IFN-γ), and interleukin (IL)-5, 10, and 13. The 101 children exposed to dogs were less likely to report a diagnosis of atopic dermatitis and had lower percentages of specific IgE, but not total IgE levels compared to the children not exposed. The dog-exposed children also had higher IL-10 and IL-13 levels in supernatants of PHA stimulated blood mononuclear cells of peripheral blood. When the dog-exposed children were stratified based on *CD14/-159* genotype, it appeared that *CD14/-159* TT homozygotes exposed to dogs had a lower prevalence of atopic dermatitis (one child out of 17) compared to *CD14/-159* TT homozygotes not exposed to dogs (13 out of 30). Low sample sizes and self-reported assessments of the phenotype limit interpretation of this study. Other atopic variables and cytokine responses did not show significant evidence for interaction and a direct assessment of the environmental exposures was not available in this study (36).

In 122 families from the Barbados Asthma Genetics study, asthma (severity) was assessed by questionnaire, and volume flow loops, total IgE, and skin prick tests were performed. In addition, endotoxin levels in dust samples collected from the living room were investigated in 92 households. Interestingly, among the 49 subjects exposed to low endotoxin levels, *CD14/-159* TT genotypes appeared protective for asthma (OR 0.09, 95% CI, 0.03–0.27), whereas the 7 subjects exposed to high endotoxin levels were at increased risk for asthma (OR 11.66, 95% CI, 1.03–31.7). Similar trends were observed for asthma severity scores and total serum IgE levels (37). Although the small number of TT homozygotes limits the generalizability of these results, it provides additional support for dose-dependent gene by environment interaction in asthma development.

Toll-Like Receptor-2 and -4

Both TLR2 and TLR4 form a receptor complex for various microbial products together with CD14. Therefore, several groups have assessed the interaction of genetic variation in TLR genes with the exposure to microbial products leading to atopic responses.

TLR2 and *4* SNPs were investigated in the same populations of farmers' children from central Europe, which were described in the section on *CD14*. The association of *TLR2* and *4* and atopic phenotypes was investigated in 239 farmers' and 387 nonfarmers' children. Atopy was defined by self-reported physician's diagnosis of asthma and allergic rhinitis, and assessed by specific IgE measurements against a panel of aeroallergens. Exposure was assessed by a question inquiring if children lived on farms, and endotoxin levels were measured in dust samples collected from the child's mattress (35). SNPs with allele frequencies over 10% were genotyped in the full sample: three SNPs in *TLR2*, and five SNPs in *TLR4*, adding one rare functional SNP (*TLR4/4434*) that is associated with hyporesponsiveness to endotoxin (38). Allele frequencies of these SNPs did not differ between the farmers' and nonfarmers' children. Farmers' children carrying a T-allele in *TLR2/−16934* were significantly less likely to have a diagnosis of asthma and current asthma symptoms than farmers children with genotype AA (3% vs. 13%, $p = 0.012$, and 3% vs. 16%, $p = 0.004$, respectively). No such association was found in the nonfarming children (Fig. 3). Multivariate logistic regression analysis adjusting for potential confounders confirmed a protective effect in farmers' children (OR for asthma in *TLR2/−16934* 0.17 (95% CI, 0.04–0.77). However, this protective effect was not present when children were stratified based on high and low endotoxin exposure, indicating that endotoxin may not be the environmental factor explaining this gene–environment interaction of the farming environment with *TLR2*. Results for *TLR4* SNPs showed no differences between the prevalence of atopic phenotypes in farmers' and nonfarmers' children. However, when stratified on endotoxin exposure, highly exposed farmers' children with *TLR4/4434* had significantly lower prevalence of specific IgE compared to low-exposed children. There was no significant effect in the nonfarmers' children. It should be noted that the allele frequencies of the *TLR4* SNPs are low in Western populations, which limit power to detect significant interaction. In summary, this study indicates that the environment (either living on farms or any other unmeasured stimulus) modified the association between

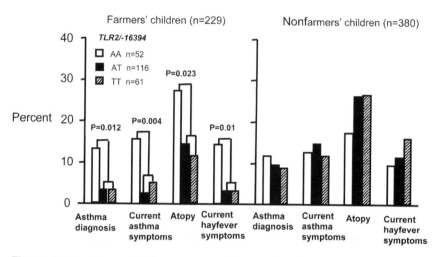

Figure 3 Prevalence of asthma, atopy, and current hay fever symptoms in toll-like receptor-2/−16934 in farmers' and nonfarmers' children. *Source*: From Ref. 39, reprinted with permission from American Academy of Allergy, Asthma, and Immunology.

the *TLR2* gene and asthma whereas endotoxin might interact with *TLR4* gene variants (39).

Two other studies showed evidence for endotoxin–*TLR4* gene interaction. *TLR4* gene has two missense mutations in the region that encodes the extracellular domain of the receptor: D299G and T339I. Healthy volunteers carrying one or two of these missense mutations showed bronchial hyporesponsiveness to endotoxin inhalations (38). These variants were subsequently investigated in a cross-sectional study of the European Respiratory Community Health Survey in Germany. In a total of 334 adult subjects, complete data were available on two *TLR4* gene SNPs (including *TLR4/4434*), endotoxin in house dust, and phenotypes associated with asthma (BHR, lung function measurements) and atopy (total and specific IgE). Allele frequencies of the 2 *TLR4* SNPs were low: 8.3% and 8.6%, respectively, and both risk alleles are in tight linkage disequilibrium in the German population, meaning that these two alleles often occur together in the population and hence it is difficult to separate their effect in an association study. In the total population, *TLR4* gene variants were not associated with asthma or atopy. When stratified on endotoxin exposure in tertiles, carriers of the wild type alleles in *TLR4* exposed to elevated levels endotoxin had increased risk of physician diagnosed asthma [second tertile: 13/97; OR 5.66, 95% CI, 1.23–26.04; third tertile 8/94; OR 4.29 (0.90–20.45)] compared to 2/87 wild type carriers exposed to low endotoxin levels. No clear effect was observed on objective measurements associated with asthma such as BHR and specific and total IgE. In contrast, in carriers exposed to endotoxin (second and third tertile) who carried the mutant allele of one of the two SNPs, lower prevalences of

BHR and elevated total and specific IgE were observed, indicating a protective effect. The low allele frequency inevitably led to small sample sizes; BHR was observed in six out of 24 subjects in the lowest tertile of exposure, compared to one out of 14 in the second and third exposure tertile, respectively (40).

Taken together, these three studies consistently indicate that rare variants in the *TLR4* gene are protective to the development of hyper-responsiveness and asthma in individuals exposed to high levels of endotoxin.

B. Genes Interacting with Infections

The hygiene hypothesis proposed that infections might protect against asthma development. We will now summarize observations on three candidate genes that may be involved in the response to various infections: mannose binding lectin-2 (MBL-2), TIM-1, and NOS3.

MBL-2 is an acute phase reactant produced by the liver and a component of the complement lectin pathway. Various promoter and coding SNPs are associated with loss of function of MBL-2 and are thus related to opsonisation defects. MBL-2 plays a role in the host response to infections with *Chlamydia pneumoniae*; an infection that has been proposed to play a role in asthma development and exacerbation. Association of *MBL-2* gene variants was investigated in 139 children with asthma, and 174 healthy control subjects from Hungary in relation to being infected with *C. pneumoniae* evidenced by serologic measurements. This study did not find a difference in the percentage of asthmatic and nonasthmatic children, who had a positive *S. pneumoniae* serology. However, children infected with *C. pneumoniae* carrying the MBL loss-of-function variants were found to have a higher risk of asthma development than infected children with normal *MBL-2* genotype. This risk was especially high in children with chronic or recurrent infection (positive results for both IgA and IgG; adjusted OR, 5.38; 95% CI, 1.75–14.36; $p = 0.01$) (41). However, in an adult sample of 243 asthma patients and 400 controls, no association of *MBL-2* gene variants and atopic and nonatopic status was detected in the complete sample. No data was available on infectious exposure. Further subgroup analysis provided some evidence of an association of a promoter variant with nonatopic asthma in males and excess lung function decline, although the multiple tests performed in this study limit its interpretation (42).

The *TIM-1* (alias *HAVcr-1*) gene encodes the cell surface receptor used by hepatitis A virus to infect human cells. Previously, it was shown that serologic evidence of hepatitis A infection was inversely associated with atopy in Italian conscripts (43). The *TIM-1* gene was positionally cloned in a mouse model of asthma (44). Activated CD4+ T cells express TIM-1 during the development of Th2 responses that are associated with atopy and asthma development. Therefore, the *TIM-1* – hepatitis A interaction is an attractive pathway for gene by environment interaction. McIntire et al. found a six amino acid insertion (157insMTTTVP) in the *TIM-1* gene. Hepatitis A infection was assessed by serum hepatitis A antibodies, and atopy was defined by IgE levels. In seronegative subjects, the six amino acid insertion was not associated with atopy. However, in seropositive subjects, the six amino acid insertion was associated with a lower prevalence of atopy (OR 0.26, 95% CI, 0.12–0.57). The authors propose that this might represent one mechanism through which infections may protect against atopy development (45). The interaction described in this study has not been replicated, although several recent studies have provided evidence for a role of TIM-1 SNPs in atopy development (46,47).

Daycare exposure in the first six months of life has been associated with decreased asthma and atopy prevalence, presumably because of increased infectious load (33). Gene by environment interaction of daycare exposure in the first six months of life on atopy development was studied in a US cohort of 208 children. 72 SNPs in 45 candidate genes were investigated. Four SNPs at three loci (*NOS3*, *IL-4RA* and *FCERIB*) showed association with multiple phenotypes related to atopy (Th2 cytokine responses) and had at least one interaction with the exposure variable (day care). To interpret the significance of the high number of comparisons, the authors calculated a false discovery rate that indicated that one out of four results could be expected to be false positives. Replication is therefore warranted, as was indicated for the *NOS3* locus (48). The *NOS3_298 Asp* allele was increased in nonasthmatic Hutterites, which is consistent with the protective effect of this allele observed in the daycare environment (49). This study underlines the importance of modeling the interaction between genes and the environment. If that has not been taken into account, no significant associations would have been found (48).

C. Genes Interacting with Tobacco Smoke and Air Pollution

Epidemiological and family studies have indicated that genes predisposed to asthma interact with ETS exposure in early life. At least one of those genes resides on chromosome 5q (20,21). In addition, active smoking may increase asthma severity. Cigarette smoke contains over 4000 different chemical substances (50). Genes that may interact with cigarette smoke are *CD14*, *IL-13*, and *B2AR* on chromosome 5q and Glutathione S transferase (*GST*) genes on chromosome 1 and 22.

The *CD14* gene encodes part of the endotoxin receptor complex. Cigarette smoke contains endotoxin and passive smoking results in exposure levels of endotoxin that are 120 times higher than smoke free air. *CD14* gene–ETS interaction was investigated in 659 Latino families from Puerto Rico and Mexico known to have high ETS exposure (approximately 41% of all children). Three SNPs (*CD14/–810*, *–159*, and *+1437*) were investigated in relation to asthma severity (lung function) and total serum IgE. No associations were found with the presence of asthma. However, two SNPs were significantly associated with low forced expiratory volume in one second (FEV$_1$) in ETS-exposed subjects. One SNP (*CD14/-159*) was also associated with total serum IgE levels in ETS-exposed subjects. This interaction was only significant in the Puerto Rican population. None of these associations were observed in subjects not exposed to ETS. In conclusion, this study shows evidence for a role of *CD14* interacting with ETS resulting in modification of FEV$_1$ and total serum IgE levels in asthmatic children (51). It is however uncertain if the *CD14* gene is responsible for the effects of ETS on the linkage results on 5q, because no significant results were observed for asthma. This could be explained by lower power when using a qualitative instead of a quantitative variable, the absence a healthy control group, and that BHR measurements were not available in these study subjects.

GST genes are implicated in several detoxification pathways, including response to oxidative stress. This gene family consists of four members (designated A, M, P, and T), with each family member having several subtypes (e.g., M1–M5). In white populations, whole gene deletions of *GSTM1* and *GSTT1* are rather prevalent (e.g., genotype frequency in the German population 52% and 17%, respectively). These loss-of-function mutations may result in impaired detoxification of toxic substances such as those present in ETS or air pollution. Association studies of asthma and *GSTP* variants have produced conflicting results, with different *GSTP1* alleles being associated, as well as some negative results (52–55). Therefore, several groups have studied this gene, in relation to ETS exposure and also air pollution.

A first study in 2950 US children assessed effects of *GSTM1* genotype, maternal smoking during pregnancy, and childhood ETS exposure on the presence of asthma and wheezing. The association of maternal smoking in utero on asthma and wheezing occurrence was largely restricted to children with *GSTM1* null genotype. Among *GSTM1* null children, in utero exposure was associated with increased prevalence of asthma with current symptoms (OR 1.7, 95% CI, 1.1–2.8) and persistent asthma (OR 1.6, 95% CI, 1.1–2.4). Among children with *GSTM1* wild type genotype, in utero exposure was not associated with asthma or wheezing (56).

In a second cross-sectional study, 3054 German schoolchildren from two different cities were investigated. Current and past ETS exposure and respiratory symptoms were assessed by questionnaire and children underwent pulmonary function, skin prick, and BHR testing. Interaction of *GSTM1* and *GSTT1* null alleles with ETS was investigated by logistic regression analysis. Prevalence rates of smoke exposure in utero in these cities were 14.2 and 4%, and for current ETS exposure 5.3 versus 2.0%. In utero smoking was significantly associated with lower lung function in children carrying the *GSTT1* null alleles. Moreover, current smoking ($\geq$20 cigarettes per day) was associated with a higher frequency of self-reported asthma and current wheeze in carriers of the GST M1 null genotype compared to the nonsmokers (Table 3) (57).

Table 3 Glutathione S transferase M1 Genotype by Environmental Smoking Interaction (≥20 Cigarettes Per Day) on Self-Reported Asthma and Wheeze in German Schoolchildren

Outcome Numbers	GSTM + ETS − n = 735	GSTM + ETS + n = 33	GSTM − ETS − n = 758	GSTM − ETST + n = 46	OR expected/departure from expected OR
Current asthma					
Percent	3.9%	6.1%	5.1%	8.9%	
OR	1.0	2.94 (0.61–14.05)	1.40 (0.85–2.30)	5.48 (1.62–18.55)[a]	4.10/1.34 ns
Current wheeze					
Percent	6.5%	9.1%	8.9%	1.78%	
OR	1.0%	2.03 (0.55–7.54)	1.50 (1.01–2.22)[a]	4.74 (1.79–12.57)[a]	3.04/1.56 ns

Batto Khoury 2 × 4 table. GSTM + intact gene and −null allele. OR, adjusted odds ratios with 95% confidence interval.
[a]p < 0.05. Column 5 shows the expected OR under a multiplicative effect and the departure from this multiplicative model.
Abbreviations: GST, Glutathione S transferase; ETS, environmental tobacco smoke; ns, statistical interaction not significant.
Source: From Ref. 57, reproduced with permission of the BHJ publishing group.

Table 3 illustrates that even in a large study of over 3000 children, the power to detect statistically significant gene by environment interaction is low. Calculations of the OR ratio for this gene by environment interaction could only be performed in only 3% of the total sample size. Although the combined OR for those exposed to the ETS and carrying the risk genotype is higher than expected based on the individual risks (i.e., risk genotype and environmental exposure only), statistical significant multiplicative interaction was not achieved. The authors calculated that statistical interaction might be significantly proven at sample sizes that were 2.7 to 48 times higher than the original population of their 3054 children (57). Thus, it may be anticipated that future studies on gene–environment interaction should include tens of thousands subjects.

Other studies provided evidence for interaction between cigarette smoke and other genes such as the β2 *adrenoceptor* (58) and *IL-4RA* and *IL-13* (59,60). These interesting observations were done in small study groups and as shown above, they should be followed up in other, preferably larger populations. Consistent replication of these interactions may provide strong evidence how genes interact with ETS and may identify subjects at increased risk for the adverse effects of smoking (6).

Exposure to ambient air pollution has been associated with an increased prevalence of asthma and atopy in various studies. Air pollutants include diesel exhaust particles with particulate matters less than $10\,\mu m$ (PM_{10}) and $2.5\,\mu m$ ($PM_{2.5}$). These diesel exhaust particles are thought to exert their detrimental effects through generation of reactive oxygen species. The *GST* genes are possible protective factors against oxidant stress. Therefore, these genes could play a role in susceptibility or severity of asthma and atopy.

In a cross-sectional study of school children in Taiwan, Lee et al. provided evidence that loss function of the *GSTP1* gene may be associated with increased susceptibility to the effects of air pollution in asthma development. They selected children from three areas in Taiwan, characterized by low, moderate, and high air pollution levels. A nested case–control study was done with a subset of this sample: 61 children with asthma (symptoms and BHR) versus 95 nonasthmatic controls (no symptoms, no BHR, and normal lung function) stratified by area of air pollution. For example, the subset exposed to high air pollution levels consisted of 27 cases and 32 controls. *GSTP1 Ile 105* homozygotes were at significant higher risk of asthma in areas of high air pollution compared to carriers of the *Val 105* alleles (adjusted OR 5.52, 95% CI, 1.64–21.25). This association was not observed in areas of low or moderate air pollution (61).

Further experimental evidence for a role of Glutathione transferase genes in severity of atopic symptoms was provided by a randomized, placebo-controlled study of patients sensitive to ragweed. These patients were challenged in the nose with ragweed allergen in a cross over design with and without diesel exhaust particles. The allergic response to this challenge (IgE, histamine, IL-4, and IFN-γ) was compared in 19 subjects with *GSTM1*, *T1*, and *P1* wild type and null alleles. Subjects with *GSTM1* null and *GSTP 150 Ile* alleles showed increased nasal responses to the ragweed allergen in the presence of diesel exhaust particles compared to carriers of the *GSTM1* wild type or *GSTP1 150 Val* (62). This experiment therefore suggests that *GSTM1* and *GSTP1* genotype modify the effect of diesel exhaust particles on allergic inflammation.

D. Genes Interacting with Allergen Exposure

In a German prospective birth cohort study, SNPs in IL-4, *IL-13*, and *IL-4RA* were investigated for gene–gene and gene–environment interaction on specific IgE development to food and aeroallergens from zero to seven years. Der P1 allergen levels were found to interact with one of these SNPs, a functional promoter SNP in the IL-4 gene, resulting in detectable specific IgE to house dust mite (59).

Human leukocyte antigen (HLA) molecules are membrane-bound glycoproteins that bind processed antigenic peptides and present them to T-cells. Two HLA classes are present: HLA class I is expressed on almost all somatic cells, whereas HLA class II is expressed at B-cells, activated T-cells, and antigen presenting cells such as monocytes, macrophages, and dendritic cells. SNPs in HLA class II genes have been associated with specific IgE responses to several small allergens such as ragweed pollen (63). Other studies have failed to extend this finding to specific IgE responses to common allergens and asthma (63–66). Allergen exposure levels were not taken into account in these studies.

VI. Summary and Future Prospects

Asthma is a complex genetic disease in which multiple genetic and environmental factors are important. The analysis of gene by environment interaction has been recently introduced into genetic studies of asthma. Already by now several studies have provided replicated evidence for these interactions, such as the *CD14* and *TLR4* genes and (proxy variables of) microbial exposure and *GST* and ETS and air pollutants. The majority of these investigations on gene–environment interaction have been derived from cross-sectional studies and small sample sizes. Moreover, multiple testing is a methodological concern in these studies. Nevertheless, these studies illustrate the value of assessing environmental exposure in genetic studies (5).

It is clear that future studies should have large sample sizes (16). For example, a large US prospective study on gene by environment interaction has been proposed that includes over 100,000 subjects (67). Increased power can also be obtained by collaboration between groups and pooling of existing data. Initiatives have been developed to gather all large studies that assess gene and environment (68). For novel studies, the design of choice would be a prospective cohort study that assesses environmental exposures before disease onset (15). This design does not suffer from potential recall bias as in a cross-sectional design, but allows for the observation of incident cases. A drawback from this design is that even larger sample sizes are needed. Now that genetic research has catalogued all prevalent SNPs in humans (69), attention should also be directed at environmental exposures. The studies described in this chapter clearly illustrate that stratification on a uniformly exposed group may enhance the power to detect genetic effects considerably. A recent simulation study suggested that repeated precise measurements of environmental factors result in studies that are as powerful as studies with less precise measurements and 20 times the sample size (70).

A recent workshop of the US national heart, lung and blood institute suggested prioritizing the study of genes and the gene by environment interactions in asthma (71). The application of the detection of gene by environment interaction could be numerous. It could help stratify disease risks and focus interventions to achieve population health benefits, it could identify new environmental factors for disease development or severity, and it could help our understanding of the natural history and severity of the disease (72). This understanding may be increased by further functional studies into the mechanisms of these interactions such as epigenetic effects, and effects of dosing and timing. It may be anticipated that the results of these investigations increase our understanding of the complex etiology of asthma, and open up new possibilities for prevention and treatment.

References

1. Upham JW, Holt PG. Environment and development of atopy. Curr Opin Allergy Clin Immunol 2005; 5(2):167–172.
2. D'Amato G, Liccardi G, D'Amato M, et al. Environmental risk factors and allergic bronchial asthma. Clin Exp Allergy 2005; 35(9):1113–1124.
3. Holgate ST. Genetic and environmental interaction in allergy and asthma. J Allergy Clin Immunol 1999; 104(6):1139–1146.
4. Vercelli D. Genetics, epigenetics, and the environment: switching, buffering, releasing. J Allergy Clin Immunol 2004; 113(3):381–386.
5. Ober C, Thompson EE. Rethinking genetic models of asthma: the role of environmental modifiers. Curr Opin Immunol 2005; 17(6):670–678.
6. Kurz T, Ober C. The role of environmental tobacco smoke in genetic susceptibility to asthma. Curr Opin Allergy Clin Immunol 2004; 4(5):335–339.
7. Ober C. Perspectives on the past decade of asthma genetics. J Allergy Clin Immunol 2005; 116(2):274–278.
8. Kleeberger SR, Peden D. Gene-environment interactions in asthma and other respiratory diseases. Annu Rev Med 2005; 56:383–400.
9. Los H, Postmus PE, Boomsma DI. Asthma genetics and intermediate phenotypes: a review from twin studies. Twin Res 2001; 4(2):81–93.

10. Hanson B, McGue M, Roitman-Johnson B, et al. Atopic disease and immuno-globulin E in twins reared apart and together. Am J Hum Genet 1991; 48(5):873–879.

11. Kjellman NI, Nilsson L. Is allergy prevention realistic and beneficial? Pediatr Allergy Immunol 1999; 10(12 Suppl):11–17.

12. Strachan DP, Cook DG. Health effects of passive smoking 6. Parental smoking and childhood asthma: longitudinal and case-control studies. Thorax 1998; 53(3):204–212.

13. Jaakkola JJ, Nafstad P, Magnus P. Environmental tobacco smoke, parental atopy, and childhood asthma. Environ Health Perspect 2001; 109(6):579–582.

14. Gluckman PD, Hanson MA. Living with the past: evolution, development, and patterns of disease. Science 2004; 305(5691):1733–1736.

15. Clayton D, McKeigue PM. Epidemiological methods for studying genes and environmental factors in complex diseases. Lancet 2001; 358(9290):1356–1360.

16. Hwang SJ, Beaty TH, Liang KY, et al. Minimum sample size estimation to detect gene-environment interaction in case-control designs. Am J Epidemiol 1994; 140(11):1029–1037.

17. Khoury MJ, Flanders WD. Nontraditional epidemiologic approaches in the analysis of gene-environment interaction: case-control studies with no controls. Am J Epidemiol 1996; 144(3):207–213.

18. Cook DG, Strachan DP. Parental smoking, bronchial reactivity and peak flow variability in children. Thorax 1998; 53(4):295–301.

19. Cook DG, Strachan DP, Carey IM. Health effects of passive smoking 9. Parental smoking and spirometric indices in children. Thorax 1998; 53(10): 884–893.

20. Colilla S, Nicolae D, Pluzhnikov A, et al. Evidence for gene-environment inter-actions in a linkage study of asthma and smoking exposure. J Allergy Clin Immunol 2003; 111(4):840–846.

21. Meyers DA, Postma DS, Stine OC, et al. Genome screen for asthma and bron-chial hyperresponsiveness: interactions with passive smoke exposure. J Allergy Clin Immunol 2005; 115(6):1169–1175.

22. Postma DS, Meyers DA, Jongepier H, Howard TD, Koppelman GH, Bleecker ER. Genome wide screen for pulmonary function in 200 families ascertained for asthma. Am J Respir Crit Care Med 2005; 172(4):446–452.

23. Vercelli D. Innate immunity: sensing the environment and regulating the regula-tors. Curr Opin Allergy Clin Immunol 2003; 3(5):343–346.

24. LeVan TD, Bloom JW, Bailey TJ, et al. A common single nucleotide polymorph-ism in the CD14 promoter decreases the affinity of Sp protein binding and enhances transcriptional activity. J Immunol 2001; 167(10):5838–5844.

25. Koppelman GH, Postma DS. The genetics of CD14 in allergic disease. Curr Opin Allergy Clin Immunol 2003; 3(5):347–352.

26. Sackesen C, Karaaslan C, Keskin O, et al. The effect of polymorphisms at the CD14 promoter and the TLR4 gene on asthma phenotypes in Turkish children with asthma. Allergy 2005; 60(12):1485–1492.

27. O'Donnell AR, Toelle BG, Marks GB, et al. Age-specific relationship between CD14 and atopy in a cohort assessed from age 8 to 25 years. Am J Respir Crit Care Med 2004; 169(5):615–622.

28. Ober C, Tsalenko A, Parry R, Cox NJ. A second-generation genomewide screen for asthma-susceptibility alleles in a founder population. Am J Hum Genet 2000; 67(5):1154–1162.

29. Kedda MA, Lose F, Duffy D, et al. The CD14 C-159T polymorphism is not associated with asthma or asthma severity in an Australian adult population. Thorax 2005; 60(3):211–214.

30. Sengler C, Haider A, Sommerfeld C, et al. Evaluation of the CD14 C-159 T polymorphism in the German Multicenter Allergy Study cohort. Clin Exp Allergy 2003; 33(2):166–169.

31. Vercelli D. Learning from discrepancies: CD14 polymorphisms, atopy and the endotoxin switch. Clin Exp Allergy 2003; 33(2):153–155.

32. Tulic MK, Wale JL, Holt PG, et al. Modification of the inflammatory response to allergen challenge after exposure to bacterial lipopolysaccharide. Am J Respir Cell Mol Biol 2000; 22(5):604–612.

33. Strachan DP. Family size, infection and atopy: the first decade of the "hygiene hypothesis." Thorax 2000; 55(Suppl 1):S2–S10.

34. Braun-Fahrlander C, Riedler J, Herz U, et al. Environmental exposure to endotoxin and its relation to asthma in school-age children. N Engl J Med 2002; 347(12):869–877.

35. Eder W, Klimecki W, Yu L, et al. Opposite effects of CD 14/-260 on serum IgE levels in children raised in different environments. J Allergy Clin Immunol 2005; 116(3):601–607.

36. Gern JE, Reardon CL, Hoffjan S, et al. Effects of dog ownership and genotype on immune development and atopy in infancy. J Allergy Clin Immunol 2004; 113(2):307–314.

37. Zambelli-Weiner A, Ehrlich E, Stockton ML, et al. Evaluation of the CD14/-260 polymorphism and house dust endotoxin exposure in the Barbados Asthma Genetics Study. J Allergy Clin Immunol 2005; 115(6):1203–1209.

38. Arbour NC, Lorenz E, Schutte BC, et al. TLR4 mutations are associated with endotoxin hyporesponsiveness in humans. Nat Genet 2000; 25(2):187–191.

39. Eder W, Klimecki W, Yu L, et al. Toll-like receptor 2 as a major gene for asthma in children of European farmers. J Allergy Clin Immunol 2004; 113(3): 482–488.

40. Werner M, Topp R, Wimmer K, et al. TLR4 gene variants modify endotoxin effects on asthma. J Allergy Clin Immunol 2003; 112(2):323–330.

41. Nagy A, Kozma GT, Keszei M, et al. The development of asthma in children infected with *Chlamydia pneumoniae* is dependent on the modifying effect of mannose-binding lectin. J Allergy Clin Immunol 2003; 112(4):729–734.

42. Aittoniemi J, Soranummi H, Rovio AT, et al. Mannose-binding lectin 2 (MBL2) gene polymorphism in asthma and atopy among adults. Clin Exp Immunol 2005; 142(1):120–124.

43. Matricardi PM, Rosmini F, Ferrigno L, et al. Cross sectional retrospective study of prevalence of atopy among Italian military students with antibodies against hepatitis A virus. BMJ 1997; 314(7086):999–1003.

44. McIntire JJ, Umetsu SE, Akbari O, et al. Identification of Tapr an airway hyperreactivity regulatory locus) and the linked Tim gene family. Nat Immunol 2001; 2(12):1109–1116.

45. McIntire JJ, Umetsu SE, Macaubas C, et al. Immunology: hepatitis A virus link to atopic disease. Nature 2003; 425(6958):576.
46. Graves PE, Siroux V, Guerra S, et al. Association of atopy and eczema with polymorphisms in T-cell immunoglobulin domain and mucin domain-IL-2-inducible T-cell kinase gene cluster in chromosome 5 q 33. J Allergy Clin Immunol 2005; 116(3):650–656.
47. Chae SC, Song JH, Lee YC, et al. The association of the exon 4 variations of Tim-1 gene with allergic diseases in a Korean population. Biochem Biophys Res Commun 2003; 312(2):346–350.
48. Hoffjan S, Nicolae D, Ostrovnaya I, et al. Gene-environment interaction effects on the development of immune responses in the 1st year of life. Am J Hum Genet 2005; 76(4):696–704.
49. Bourgain C, Hoffjan S, Nicolae R, et al. Novel case-control test in a founder population identifies P-selectin as an atopy-susceptibility locus. Am J Hum Genet 2003; 73(3):612–626.
50. Lofroth G. Environmental tobacco smoke: overview of chemical composition and genotoxic components. Mutat Res 1989; 222(2):73–80.
51. Choudhry S, Avila PC, Nazario S, et al. CD14 tobacco gene-environment interaction modifies asthma severity and immunoglobulin E levels in Latinos with asthma. Am J Respir Crit Care Med 2005; 172(2):173–182.
52. Nickel R, Haider A, Sengler C, et al. Association study of Glutathione S-transferase P1 (GSTP1) with asthma and bronchial hyper-responsiveness in two German pediatric populations. Pediatr Allergy Immunol 2005; 16(6):539–541.
53. Lee YL, Hsiue TR, Lee YC, et al. The association between glutathione S-transferase P1, M1 polymorphisms and asthma in Taiwanese schoolchildren. Chest 2005; 128(3):1156–1162.
54. Aynacioglu AS, Nacak M, Filiz A, et al. Protective role of glutathione S-transferase P1 (GSTP1) Val105Val genotype in patients with bronchial asthma. Br J Clin Pharmacol 2004; 57(2):213–217.
55. Fryer AA, Bianco A, Hepple M, et al. Polymorphism at the glutathione S-transferase GSTP1 locus. A new marker for bronchial hyperresponsiveness and asthma. Am J Respir Crit Care Med 2000; 161(5):1437–1442.
56. Gilliland FD, Li YF, Dubeau L, et al. Effects of glutathione S-transferase M1, maternal smoking during pregnancy, and environmental tobacco smoke on asthma and wheezing in children. Am J Respir Crit Care Med 2002; 166(4):457–463.
57. Kabesch M, Hoefler C, Carr D, et al. Glutathione S transferase deficiency and passive smoking increase childhood asthma. Thorax 2004; 59(7):569–573.
58. Wang Z, Chen C, Niu T, et al. Association of asthma with beta(2)-adrenergic receptor gene polymorphism and cigarette smoking. Am J Respir Crit Care Med 2001; 163(6):1404–1409.
59. Liu X, Beaty TH, Deindl P, et al. Associations between specific serum IgE response and 6 variants within the genes IL4, IL13, and IL4RA in German children: the German Multicenter Atopy Study. J Allergy Clin Immunol 2004; 113(3):489–495.
60. Liu X, Beaty TH, Deindl P, et al. Associations between total serum IgE levels and the 6 potentially functional variants within the genes IL4, IL13, and IL4RA

in German children: the German Multicenter Atopy Study. J Allergy Clin Immunol 2003; 112(2):382–388.

61. Lee YL, Lin YC, Lee YC, et al. Glutathione S-transferase P1 gene polymorphism and air pollution as interactive risk factors for childhood asthma. Clin Exp Allergy 2004; 34(11):1707–1713.

62. Gilliland FD, Li YF, Saxon A, et al. Effect of glutathione-S-transferase M1 and P1 genotypes on xenobiotic enhancement of allergic responses: randomised, placebo-controlled crossover study. Lancet 2004; 363(9403):119–125.

63. Howell WM, Holgate ST. HLA genetics and allergic disease. Thorax 1995; 50(8):815–818.

64. Aron Y, Swierczewski E, Lockhart A. HLA class II haplotype in atopic asthmatic and non-atopic control subjects. Clin Exp Allergy 1995; 25(Suppl 2):65–67.

65. Holloway JW, Doull I, Begishvili B, et al. Lack of evidence of a significant association between HLA-DR, DQ and DP genotypes and atopy in families with HDM allergy. Clin Exp Allergy 1996; 26(10):1142–1149.

66. Li PK, Lai CK, Poon AS, et al. Lack of association between HLA-DQ and -DR genotypes and asthma in southern Chinese patients. Clin Exp Allergy 1995; 25(4):323–331.

67. Collins FS. The case for a US prospective cohort study of genes and environment. Nature 2004; 429(6990):475–477.

68. Khoury MJ, Dorman JS. The human genome epidemiology network. Am J Epidemiol 1998; 148(1):1–3.

69. Altshuler D, Brooks LD, Chakravarti A, Collins FS, Daly MJ, Donnelly P. A haplotype map of the human genome. Nature 2005; 437(7063):1299–1320.

70. Wong MY, Day NE, Luan JA, et al. The detection of gene-environment interaction for continuous traits: should we deal with measurement error by bigger studies or better measurement? Int J Epidemiol 2003; 32(1):51–57.

71. Busse W, Banks-Schlegel S, Noel P, et al. Future research directions in asthma: an NHLBI working group report. Am J Respir Crit Care Med 2004; 170(6):683–690.

72. Khoury MJ, Davis R, Gwinn M, et al. Do we need genomic research for the prevention of common diseases with environmental causes? Am J Epidemiol 2005; 161(9):799–805.

4

Epistatic Interaction, Age, and Gender Effects

MICHAEL KABESCH

University Children's Hospital, Ludwig Maximilian's University Munich,
Munich, Germany

I. Introduction

Strong evidence exists that genetic predisposition and environmental factors contribute to the development of asthma and other atopic diseases as suggested in Chapter 3 and a number of other sources (1–3). Epidemiology has identified a number of environmental risk factors for asthma and atopy in recent years but still, the presence of asthma in first degree relatives of a child is the single most important risk factor for the development of the disease (3). Thus, it seems that different environments may only influence, trigger, or protect from a disorder, which is predominantly based on an individual's genetic susceptibility. In addition, gender and age effects may modify the interaction between risk factors and genes. Due to these complex interactions, asthma is a truly multifactorial disorder in which the effect of a single genetic factor may be hard to detect and to evaluate. However, models testing environmental as well as genetic influences on the occurrence of a disease over generations have been used in family studies to disentangle genetics from environmental contributions. In asthma, allergic rhinitis, or atopic eczema, these segregation analyses revealed a strong but not exclusive genetic contribution (4–7). Instead of a Mendelian pattern of inheritance, mixed models of genetic and environmental influences gave the best match with the observed distribution of asthma in extended families. When asthma was studied in twins, genetics showed a much stronger impact on disease development than did the environment. Based on these different studies, heritability, the genetic contribution to the development of asthma, was estimated to be between 60% and 80% (8,9).

II. Multiple Genes Involved in Disease Occurrence and Perpetuation

While a major genetic contribution to the development of asthma and atopy cannot be disputed, the nature of these genetic influences has been a matter of debate for a long time. From the inspiration of early and major successes in the genetics of cystic fibrosis (10), it was hoped that similar break-throughs might follow soon in asthma genetics. However, this hope could not be fulfilled and the hypothesis that only a few major genes and gene alterations may contribute to asthma susceptibility seems anachronistic as of today. Rather, the mechanisms underlying asthma are complex. As the phenotypical presentation of the disease is extremely variable, the involvement of multiple sets of genes, such as in many other common diseases of modern man, is most likely.

It is still unclear, however, how many genes contribute to asthma and how strong the specific influence of these genes may be. Theoretically, it could be speculated that it is only a handful of major genes exerting major effects and/or a larger number of genes adding smaller contributions. As shown in Figure 1, an inverse relationship exists: The more genes contribute to a disease the smaller their individual effect on the phenotype may be. So far, no major gene for asthma has been identified and the attributable risk of any single candidate asthma gene so far proposed has been rather small (corresponding to the right side of the scale in Fig. 1). Thus, there may be some strong reason to believe that asthma is a polygenic disease, in which a large number of genetic alterations in many genes contribute to the predisposition for the disease. On the other hand, very similar phenotypical expressions of asthma may be caused by the activation of different patho-mechanisms and there may be little argument that indeed a number of independent immunological or lung-specific pathways may cause the phenotype asthma yet via their specific pathways. However, with increasing knowledge of the complex nature of balance in immunological networks and the lung itself, evidence seems to increase that genetic alterations in asthma genes may not act completely independent from each other. Rather, biological interactions—between genes and the environment as well as between genes—may be crucial for the development of the disease.

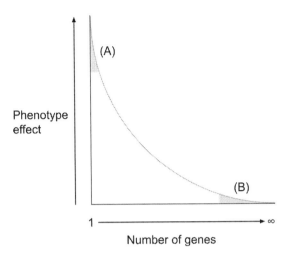

Figure 1 Association between number of genes and phenotype effects. The association between the number of genes associated with a disease and the phenotype effect per gene differs between major gene diseases and polygenic diseases. In the case of major gene diseases, a very limited number of genes affect the phenotype dramatically, while in polygenic diseases a large number of genes exert small effects on the phenotype.

III. A Three-Dimensional Model of Disease Complexity

As if this complexity would not be enough, some other dimensions in disease expression have to be taken into account. As genes may exert their functions differently during the development of the lung and the immune system, changes in susceptibility genes may have different effects at different ages. Windows of opportunity or disadvantage may exist, where the alteration of certain gene combinations may have a profound effect on disease development, for example, when triggered by certain environmental exposures. On the other hand, also effects of gender difference may affect disease development as well as outcome, through direct X-linked genetic influences or through indirect, hormonal differences. Thus, a three-dimensional disease model may be proposed as shown in Figure 2, where genetic susceptibility as the sum of an individual's genetic variability represents one axis, while the environment corresponds to the y-axis, and time dependent vulnerability reflects the third dimension. In this model, disease would occur when the coordinates of the sum of all three parameters fall into a certain area above the threshold layer in the three-dimensional space of the model. An individual may have a strong genetic risk to develop asthma but this risk is modified by the environment in such a way that no clinical symptoms become apparent or their manifestation is drastically diminished.

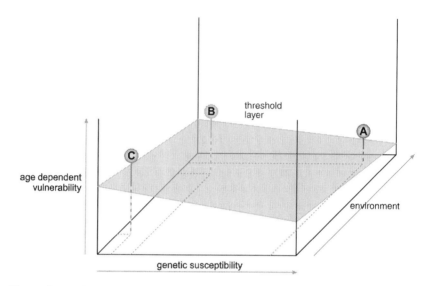

Figure 2 A three-dimensional model of disease complexity. An asthma phenotype may result from an interaction between strong genetic and environmental effects independent of the timing of these effects (**A**). However, genetic predisposition and environmental factors may also cancel each other so that no clinical expression of asthma occurs. As another possibility, asthma may result from strong environmental factors in the absence of a strong genetic predisposition (**B**). On the other hand, weak genetic susceptibility and a relatively mild environmental risk may still add up to produce an asthma phenotype when the expression of these risk factors falls into an extremely vulnerable time, as the first year of life may be (**C**).

Also, the opposite effect of multifactorial interaction may occur, when the environmental component becomes so strong that disease arises almost independently of the genetic background. In addition, even the combination of a minor genetic risk and a minor environmental trigger may lead to disease when these interactions happen at an especially vulnerable time. In this model, gender is not represented in a disease axis, but rather, it may influence the configuration of the threshold layer. While boys may be especially vulnerable for certain gene-by-environment interactions at a young age, this vulnerability may be especially high in girls during puberty. Of course, this model is only an approximation to the complexity of inter-actions leading to asthma and may not be elaborated enough to explain the occurrence of disease in every case.

IV. Complex Challenges and Complex Developments

Taking these levels of comprehensiveness into account, it may seem impos-sible to disentangle the complexity of asthma genetics. However, with increasing knowledge and experience in studying complex traits in different diseases, new study tools have been developed, adapted, and improved over the years. Promising ideas have been proposed, large and informative study populations have been gathered, and an international network for replication studies has evolved. These developments give rise to the hope that the riddle of asthma may be solvable in due time.

Within the last 20 years, asthma genetics has come a long way. Until some years ago, linkage studies relied on a few hundred genetic markers and a limited amount of families available for investigations. Candidate gene studies were limited to assess the correlation between one genetic alteration in a gene and a disease phenotype until recently. In the last years, however, fuelled by the fast advance of the human genome project, projects such as the haplotype mapping project (HAPMAP), have been started to identify haplotype patterns throughout the whole genome. Due to technical improvements in mutation detection and high throughput genotyping, much more sophisticated analyses became not only possible but even more important, they became practicable. Now whole genes of interest and their surroundings are screened for polymorphisms in a high throughput approach in diverse ethnicities, with data instantly available online (11). In many candidate genes for asthma and atopy, multiple polymorphisms have been detected. These polymorphisms, usually single nucleotide polymorphisms (SNPs) equivalent to a single base-change, or deletion and insertion polymorphisms defined by the lack or addition of a single base at a certain position, are identified with a frequency of 1/1000 in most gene regions. This is much more than what was commonly expected only a few years ago, when polymorphic sites were estimated to occur every 10,000 bases. With the development of improved screening techniques, the number of known polymorphisms and the number of candidate genes screened for polymorphisms inflated dramatically. Now the question is not anymore if there is a polymorphism in a specific gene, but how to make sense of the many polymorphisms that are usually detected in a gene. This challenge has been approached by haplotype analyses to assess the combinations of polymorphisms per inherited allele. However, also this technique has limitations and may give best results in combination with single polymorphism analysis. Technical advance in high throughput genotyping methods now allows to genotype large populations for many polymorphisms in a time- and cost-efficient manner. At the same time, large-scale populations of individuals well phenotyped for asthma and atopy have been identified successfully in many countries and are now available for analysis. Thus, more intriguing questions may now be asked emphatically.

V. Does Gene-by-Gene Interaction Really Exist?

As many clues indicate, asthma is a disease of multifactorial nature. The variability in the expression of the disease suggests very clearly that genetic interactions should be expected in such a disease. Gene-by-gene interaction, also called epistasis, is very likely to occur in immunological pathways contributing to the development of asthma. Many studies have shown that the immune system, crucial for the survival, is delicately balanced relaying of numerous feed back loops. Parallel pathways exist to back up important and decisive functions as well as some key regulators of survival and evolution. While an abundance of signals is capable to raise the interest of the immune defence, the progression to an immune response involves numerous steps. Thus, redundancy is coupled with sensitivity and specificity to assure a selective but not overly reactive immune system. Therefore, a genetic alteration in a single gene or step of an immune pathway may not be sufficient to influence or change the direction of an immune reaction decisively. Combinations of genetic alterations may be necessary to reach a certain threshold which only then lead to the manifestation of a specific immune reaction, inflammation, and a clinically relevant manifestation of disease. On the other hand, the genetic alteration of one gene may not only influence one aspect of the immune response but also alter different pathways. In asthma pathogenesis, both effects may be present. Thus, a systematic approach is needed. Genes of signalling pathways and feedback loops relevant to the development of asthma and atopy need to be investigated thoroughly one by one. However, analysis must not stop at the single gene level but the interactions between genes in these pathways need to be analyzed together to evaluate their true impact on the system. A number of alternative effects may theoretically occur when genetic changes in these pathways are analyzed together according to epistasis theory.

- Individual SNPs may only show association with the disease by chance and a combination of these SNPs with other SNPs in the pathway would not influence the outcome.
- The combination of different SNPs would "level out" each other in that combinations of different SNPs in the pathway would not increase above the effect observed with a single SNP. This would be the case if a threshold would exist where SNPs would only be able to influence the system to a certain degree.
- When several SNPs (with individual effects) are combined, an additive effect could occur and the odds ratio would increase accordingly, leading to an additive effect.
- Individual SNPs may actually interact with each other in a biological way. This would lead to a more than additive effect on a logarithmic scale, equivalent to a more than multiplicative effect on a nonlogarithmic scale. In biological terms, this is the most intriguing result possible as this may indicate that putatively functional SNPs are distributed over the pathway and that a combined occurrence leads to interaction between these effects.

Based on these hypotheses, pathway genetics may be crucial in understanding the true nature of genetic influences on the development and natural history of asthma. While the need for these studies has been articulated in many reviews over the last years, very few original studies have actually addressed the issue. Only recently, first steps toward pathway genetics have been taken for some genes and gene families. So far, the pathway, which has been investigated most thoroughly for its role in asthma and atopy, is the interleukin (IL)-4/IL-13 signalling cascade.

VI. Genes of the IL-4/IL-13 Signalling Pathway

Switching from immunoglobulin (Ig) class M to E production in activated B-lymphocytes is a crucial biological event of atopic diseases and asthma, which is strongly influenced by the activation of the IL-4/IL-13 cytokine pathway (see also Chapter 16). Both cytokines, IL-4 and IL-13, signal through a common pathway (12) as shown in Figure 3. On the cell surface, IL-4 or IL-13 may bind to a heterodimeric receptor made up of the IL-4 receptor chain α (IL-4Rα) and either the common γ chain (for binding IL-4 and IL-13) or the IL-13Rα chain (for exclusive IL-13 binding). Activated through the binding of the ligand, intracellular signalling is initiated through the activation of a Janus tyrosine kinase. This in turn allows the phosphorylation of signal transducer and activator of transcription 6 (STAT6), which is previously present in the cytosol in an inactive, unphosphorylated state. Once phosphorylated, STAT6 molecules form homodimers, which,

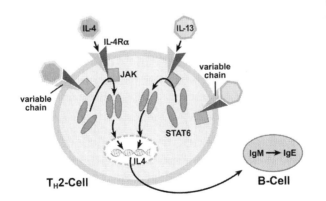

Figure 3 Schematic depiction of the interleukin (IL)-4/IL-13 pathway. Activation of receptors containing IL-4Rα by IL-4 or IL-13 lead to the phosphorylation (by Janus kinases) and transduction of STAT6 into the nucleus inducing target genes and the production of IgE. *Abbreviations*: JAK, Janus tyrosine kinase; IL, interleukin; Ig, immunoglobulin; STAT, signal transducer and activator of transcription.

only now, can penetrate the nucleus. Here, the transcription of target genes is facilitated through the binding of STAT6 molecules to specific transcription factor binding sites in the promoter and regulatory regions of susceptible genes and gene regions. In addition to IgE switching, the IL-4 and IL-13 pathway influences many other immunoregulatory and proinflammatory activities inducing, enhancing, and controlling features of atopic inflammation and asthma as reviewed by Corry and Kheradmand (13).

Genetic variation is present in all major genes of the IL-4/IL-13 signalling pathway (14–19)—IL-4, IL-13, IL-4Rα, IL-13R, and STAT6. Mutation screening has either been performed on the coding and promoter region only (IL-4Rα and IL-13R) or including intronic and surrounding areas (IL-4, IL-13, and STAT6). Association studies have been performed, and for most genes effects of polymorphisms or haplotypes on asthma, IgE regulation or atopy have been studied extensively.

For many of these genes, also functional genetics have been initiated investigating the influence of polymorphisms on gene regulation and the changes in the role of the respective protein (see also Chapter 16 *Interleukin*-13 by Vercelli). For most of the IL-4/IL-13 pathway genes, functional polymorphisms have already been identified.

IL-4 polymorphisms have been associated with elevated IgE levels in asthmatics and nonasthmatics, with asthma and atopy in some (17,20,21) but not all studies published so far (22,23). Preliminary functional studies showed that the T-allele at the proximal promoter site C-589T in the IL-4 gene alters the binding of a transcription factor (20). It was speculated that this SNP may thus lead to an overexpression of the IL-4 gene (which has not yet been shown) and that this may increase the immunological effect of IL-4. However, at least two other SNPs (VE6523 and C-33T) in the IL-4 gene are in close linkage disequilibrium with C-589T and thus show almost the same signals in association studies (17). No functional data exists for these polymorphisms so far and based on association studies alone, the role of these polymorphisms cannot yet be determined.

In the coding region of the IL-4Rα gene, at least 14 polymorphisms have been identified and for some of the more frequent genetic variations, functional data is available. SNP A148G alters an amino acid in the extracellular part of the receptor (I50V), which leads to an increased downstream activation of STAT6, and increased IgE production has been detected in B-cells (24). Polymorphisms T1432C and A1652G lead to amino acid changes Ser478Pro and Gln551Arg in the intracellular domain of the IL-4Rα chain, respectively. The effect of both polymorphisms on the intracellular activation of the signalling cascade has been investigated. As polymorphism A1652G is located very close to a STAT6-recruiting domain in the IL-4Rα, a functional relevance seemed possible. While Kruse et al. showed an effect of the polymorphism on phosphorylation and signalling transduction (25), no such effect was observed in another functional study

(26). Different studies have assessed the effect of these polymorphisms on atopic diseases. But overall the associations between IL-4Rα polymorphisms and asthma as well as serum IgE levels were only minor.

In IL-13, seven frequent polymorphisms exist, of which at least three could be of functional relevance: Polymorphism G2044A alters an amino acid in the protein domain involved with receptor binding (Arg 130Gln) (27). This SNP and two other polymorphisms in the promoter (A-1512C and C-1112T) showed association with asthma and IgE regulation in different populations (19,22). First results from gene expression studies and transcription factor binding analysis on C-1112T strongly support a functional role of this polymorphism in gene expression (28).

For IL-13, two IL-13 receptor chain genes exist: IL-13Rα1 associates with the IL-4Rα chain to form a functional receptor for IL-13, whereas IL-13Rα2 may be a decoy receptor for IL-13 without any downstream activation effects. Both genes have been investigated for polymorphisms and a number of SNPs have been found (16). Association studies have not shown a significant role of the so far identified IL-13 receptor chain SNPs in asthma or atopy.

In contrast, STAT6 is a crucial regulator of the Th2 immune response activating a number of Th2-specific gene promoters. Different studies have consistently shown that the SNP C2892T in the second intron of the STAT6 gene is associated with elevated serum IgE levels (15,29,30). This polymorphism is located in an evolutionary highly conserved region with putative enhancer effects. As the T-allele at position C2892T disrupts an NFκB site, it may very well influence the regulation or expression of the STAT6 gene as indicated by preliminary data from our own laboratory (unpublished data).

Thus, a number of intriguing genetic alterations exist in the IL-4/IL-13 signalling pathway and for some of these genes, functional genetics have progressed considerably. On the protein level, the interaction between the described components of the IL-4/IL-13 signalling cascade is well established. Therefore, it is reasonable to hypothesize from a biological point of view that genetic alterations of the genes coding for the pathway components may influence these interactions. As mentioned before, different consequences may arise from genetically determined alterations of certain pathway genes. These interactions, if present, could lead to additive, multiplicatory, or threshold effects. The question remains, how to assess gene-by-gene interactions in association studies.

VII. How to Assess Gene-by-Gene Interactions?

The term "epistasis" was originally used by William Bateson in 1909 and described a distortion from Mendelian segregation ratios due to one gene masking the effects of others. In other words, it describes "the phenomenon whereby the effects of a given gene on a biological trait are masked or enhanced by one or more other genes" (31). Alternatively, epistasis has been defined as the deviation from additivity in a linear statistical model of genetic interaction. Thus, the terms "epistasis" and also "gene-by-gene interaction" are both used indiscriminately to describe biological as well as statistical interactions. As recently discussed by Moore in his global view of epistasis, this may lead to confusion because these two things are not necessarily the same (31). Statistical significance of interaction may only suggest a biological interaction, and true biological interaction may not always be statistically evident. To measure statistical epistasis, different approaches have been used in population genetics.

In many studies, interactions between genes have been assessed using simple multiple regression models. However, this approach may be restricted to the assessment of a limited number of gene-by-gene interactions and becomes problematic in studying pathways. With every gene added to such a model, the need for extensively large population samples and high-end computing power increases. Alternatively, the effects of certain genotype combinations have been assessed using subgroup analyses in a number of studies in the past. There, carriers of a specific combination of polymorphisms have been compared to either individuals with no genetic alteration in any of the investigated genes (supernormals) or those individuals who did not have all polymorphisms of interest. However, this approach is not assessing interactions but the combined effect of genetic alterations in subgroups. For the evaluation of interaction, specific statistical procedures testing for epistasis have been proposed.

Cordell and Clayton have proposed some methodology to study epistasis in population genetics, assessing the deviation from the expected interaction effects (32–34). This approach is based on a stepwise logistic regression procedure and rather than using full haplotype effects, these procedures use tests with few degrees of freedom to detect relevant determinants. Thus, these tests are powerful tools for studying epistasis in family-based as well as cross-sectional case control settings.

As power decreases with every polymorphism added to an interaction model, a critical step of practical relevance in performing gene-by-gene interaction studies is the selection of polymorphisms for an analysis. Some authors argue that only polymorphisms that show a significant association by themselves should be included in such a gene-by-gene or pathway analysis. While this is a reasonable and pragmatic procedure, some interactions may be missed. The contrary approach—to test all available polymorphisms in a pathway one by one for two-way interactions and then combine all polymorphisms in a pathway that shows significant one by one interaction—may become biased by multiple testing. While the more restrictive approach is advisable in hypothesis-driven research, the later method may be justified in explorative settings.

However, completely new challenges are arising with genome-wide association studies, which will soon also be available for asthma and atopy. In these studies, where more than 100,000 polymorphisms covering the genome are genotyped at a time, the assessment of epistasis may be critical. Here, not only pathways but also networks of pathways consisting of many genes are under investigation. New statistical tools will have to address the issue. In this setting, it may not yet be possible to assign genes to pathways and networks. Thus, exploratory epistatic analysis using random one by one interaction analysis as a screening tool may be needed to assign genes to networks. With the high number of tested polymorphisms in genome wide association studies, anything more than testing two way interactions will exceed today's computing powers. However, the chance that three-way interaction is present without also showing significance in two-way interactions, is extremely rare. According to recently developed theories, this technique may be feasible as a first approach to epistasis in previously unknown networks. However, the exploratory nature of such a method has to be clearly acknowledged and results using this approach have to be verified in a hypothesis-driven approach in a second step.

According to classical guidelines, statistical significance of interactions is reached, only if the observed effect exceeds the expected multiplicative effects. However, this stringent definition of statistical interaction is debated controversially. Additive and multiplicative effects may be different aspects of interaction. Additive interaction may be observed if two terms influence the outcome independently. This may happen when two molecules do not interact physically but subsequently in the pathogenesis of the disease. In contrast, multiplicative effects may be observed if two genes interact directly with each other, e.g., when a polymorphism in a ligand and a receptor gene both reduce the binding capacity of the respective proteins and consecutive signal transduction. In simpler organisms, such as yeast, gene-by-gene interactions have recently been studied extensively in a network of more than 800 genes using a systematic gene-knockout approach (35). These first steps of network genetics in simple organisms, may soon lead to similar approaches in higher organisms, but it may still be a long way until these extensive systems of gene-by-gene interactions may be available for studies in humans.

With all these perspectives in mind, it is important to remember that statistical interaction does not prove biological interaction. On the other hand, biological interaction may be present but not statistically detectable due to overlapping factors in association analyses. Thus, functional studies are not only needed to prove the effects of single polymorphisms on the function of a single gene, but also combinations of pathway alterations have to be tested for their interactive effects in experimental settings. Of which nature such experimental settings need to be, to investigate the subtle changes as observed in most polymorphic genes, is still not clear. However, advance in this direction is crucial to be able to transfer associations into causality. Based on these theoretical considerations, the question is how far have we progressed into epistasis in asthma genetics?

VIII. Evidence for Gene-by-Gene Interactions in the IL-4/IL-13 Pathway

As mentioned previously, epistasis in asthma has to be expected due to the complex nature of the disease. So far, most approaches to study epistasis in asthma have been focused on the IL-4/IL-13 signalling pathway. In 2002, Howard et al. published a combined analysis of two polymorphisms in the IL-4/IL-13 pathway (36). In a longitudinal population of Dutch adults with asthma, one polymorphism in the promoter of IL-13 (C-1112T) and one in the IL-4Rα gene leading to an amino acid change (Pro478Ser) were assessed. Each of these polymorphisms alone showed a statistically significant association with elevated serum IgE. When individuals with polymorphic alleles in both locations were compared to individuals with wildtype alleles, in both locations, the risk for elevated serum IgE levels increased by fivefold. A logistic regression model was used to test for gene-by-gene interaction. Based on the published data, the interaction effect exceeds the expected multiplicative effect of the single gene associations. However, the interaction does not reach statistical significance in terms of deviation from a multiplicative effect, which may be due to the rather small sample size for an interaction analysis. As both tested polymorphisms are known to change the function of their respective genes, a functional interaction may be suspected, but has not been investigated in this report nor has it been shown in any subsequent study so far.

Also the interaction between the polymorphism in the coding region of IL-13 (G2044A) and the promoter polymorphism C-589T in IL-4 has been studied (37). Data from this cohort, containing 368 children at high risk of developing atopy and atopic disorders and 540 parents, suggested that the IL-13 G2044A polymorphism and haplotypes consisting of IL-13 G2044A and IL-4 C-589T were associated with the development of atopy and atopic dermatitis. As children in this analysis were only followed up to the age of 24 months, no information on asthma was available.

In a recent study from Korea, three polymorphisms in the IL-4Rα gene (Arg551Glu, Ile50Val, and Pro478Ser) have been investigated in combination with a promoter polymorphism in the IL-4 gene (C-589T) in a population of 256 asthmatics and 100 healthy controls (38). The risk for asthma increased up to an odds ratio of 1.97 (95%, CI 1.07–3.71) in individuals with the Arg allele at position 551, while the other two SNPs in the IL-4Rα gene did not show any significant effects. The combination of the IL-4Rα Arg allele with the IL-4 589 T-allele further increased the risk for asthma (odds ratio = 3.70, 95% CI = 1.07–12.78). The significance of the gene-by-gene interaction was not assessed in this study, but, rather, a subgroup comparison was performed. Due to missing information on single SNP effects, in this publication, we cannot calculate the size of the interaction. Again, the population size was small for studying gene-by-gene interactions and the results can only be interpreted as suggestive. However, this study extends the initial findings by Howard in the sense that a second combination of genes seems to interact in the IL-4/IL-13 pathway. In a similar British study, two polymorphisms in the IL-4Rα gene (Arg551Glu and Ile50Val) and two in the IL-4 gene (the highly linked SNPs C-589T and C-33T) were analyzed concomitantly. While transmission disequilibrium tests and haplotype analysis showed significant associations with asthma for both genes individually, the authors state that no interaction between the two genes was observed. However, no data and no information on how interaction was tested is provided (39).

Other researchers also failed to replicate interactions between polymorphisms in the IL-4/IL-13 pathway. Liu et al. investigated six polymorphisms in IL-4, IL-13, and IL-4Rα in a longitudinal study of allergy in Germany Multicenter Allergy Study (MAS) where almost 1000 children were followed from birth. In this setting, the effects of genetic variation in the IL-4/IL-13 pathway on specific and total serum IgE levels were analyzed (22,23). While the authors could confirm a role of IL-13 polymorphisms in the regulation of total and specific IgE, SNPs in the IL-4 and the IL-4Rα gene were only associated with the development of specific IgE responses in that study population. While the interaction analysis is not shown, the authors state that no significant interactions between polymorphisms in the three genes were found. A further study of four different components of the IL-4 and IL-13 pathway, namely polymorphisms in IL-4, IL-4Rα, IL-13, and IL-13Rα1 was performed in a British and a Japanese population using a simple factorial analysis of variance (16). While the IL-13 G2044A polymorphism again showed a consistent association with asthma in both populations, no interactions were observed.

Only recently, the genetic analysis of the IL-4/IL-13 signalling pathway has been extended to also include STAT6, a final and crucial transducer of IL-4 as well as IL-13 effects (15,29,30). Due to its function as a bottleneck of IL-4 and IL-13 signals and based on the consistency of association study results in this gene, it seems intriguing to include the STAT6 gene in the analysis of epistasis in the IL-4/IL-13 pathway. Indeed, the addition of STAT6 to gene-by-gene interaction models increased the statistical strength of these interactions significantly in our own data. In a Cordell model including polymorphisms in IL-4 (C-589T), IL-13 (C-1112T), IL-4Rα (I50V), and STAT6 (C2892T), significant gene-by-gene interactions were observed with IgE regulation and asthma exceeding the multiplicative model in a population of more than 1100 children. Affecting approximately 5% of children in a general population sample, the risk for elevated serum

IgE increased by 10.8-fold compared to the maximum individual effect of any tested SNP and by 16.8-fold for asthma (40).

Taken together, these data indicate that genetic alterations in the IL-4/IL-13 pathway may, when seen as an entity, contribute significantly to the overall genetic susceptibility to develop asthma and atopy. In addition, the same alterations in the pathway may or may not be involved in other diseases, such as diabetes (41,42). However, the current interpretation of the results can only be based on statistical association from population genetics, as experimental data on these interactions is not yet published. Also other gene combinations and pathways have been suggested to show epistasis but the data available on these systems is somewhat limited compared to the IL-4/IL-13 signalling cascade. FCER1B 237Gly and NOS2A 346D may interact in determining atopic phenotypes (43). Combinations of CTLA4 and FCER1B polymorphisms may increase total serum IgE levels in patients with asthma (44), and IL-4Rα polymorphisms may interact with IL-1A alterations in conferring the risk of asthma in a population of Finish adults (45). However, replication has to be awaited before the value of these data can be estimated. Now that genetic research has developed the potential to investigate epistasis better, increasing evidence on the role of epistasis in complex diseases is emerging. Studying gene-by-gene and gene-by-environment interactions will be essential to understand the multifactorial nature of asthma genetics in the future.

IX. From Epistasis to Gender and Age

However, complexity in asthma is not restricted to epistasis alone, but also other effects, such as age and gender may modify genetic influences. For instance, polymorphisms in the IL-13Rα1 gene, located on the X chromosome, seem to have different effects in males and females. The polymorphism IL-13Rα1 A1398G was only associated with elevated serum IgE levels in males, hemizygote for the gene, whereas no effect was observed in females (16). While these X-linked gender effects are obvious and expected, they may also have effects on genes not located on the X chromosome due to, for example, hormonal influences. Under their influence, the natural history of asthma may take a different course during puberty in boys and girls. However, these differences during puberty may also be due to the fact that different phenotypes representing different disease entities are summarized under the term asthma. Thus, the pathogenesis (and the genes involved in the pathogenesis) of asthma in young boys may be quite different from asthma in girls during or after puberty. So it has been reported that genetic changes in the b-1 defensin (DEFB1) were only associated with asthma in females (46). For that gene, effects were observed in adults as well as in children, assessed in a family-based cohort. However, DEFB1 alterations had opposite effects on asthma in adult women compared to girls before puberty. While the minor alleles at two polymorphic sites were associated with an increased risk for asthma in the adult population, the same minor alleles were transmitted significantly less frequently to girls with asthma in the family-based cohort. In male subjects, neither such association was observed. So far, no explanation for the distribution of these effects could be given and replication of the results is yet missing.

Similar to these findings, changes in the IL-21 receptor, located on chromosome 16p12, have been reported to influence IgE levels in two cross-sectional population samples of adult females but not males (47). When the same IL-21R polymorphism was studied in German children ($n = 1120$), no such effect was found in girls (unpublished data). Thus, it could be speculated that the role of IL-21R is influenced by gender-specific hormonal triggers, which may only become apparent after puberty. While the asthma phenotype in adulthood may not be the same as during child-hood, the assessment of IgE may be a more stabile phenotype throughout age. Thus, different gender effects at different ages in this study may not be explained by differences in the phenotype. Furthermore, the studied populations were of the same ethnic origin so that population heterogeneity is unlikely to be responsible for the variance in results. How changes in the IL-21R gene could be gender or hormone specific is yet unclear, but it could be speculated that the IL-21 pathway may contribute to the gender-associated differences in females, which, also in other studies, have been linked to hormonal changes (48).

So far, very little is known about asthma in the transition from child-hood to adulthood, as participants in many longitudinal cohorts, which have been started in recent times, have not yet reached adulthood. Thus, compar-isons between genetic effects in children and adults are mostly comparisons between different independent populations or different family members in family studies. Only during the last years, longitudinal data on individuals studied in childhood, puberty, and beyond have become available (49). First results indeed indicate that genetic alterations may have different effects during different stages of life. So it has been reported that a promoter poly-morphism in CD14, involved in the recognition of microbial signals, was associated with early onset asthma, but not with late onset or adult asthma forms within the same group of individuals (50). However, when studied in independent populations of children and adults, no such age-specific effects could be observed (51).

Taken together, we have to admit at this point that we know only very little about the influences of gender and age on asthma and the genetic background of the disease. In addition, phenotype issues may be mixed up with direct and indirect modifications of certain genes by age and gender (52). Genetic alterations in these genes may differ in their effects in females and males and in children and adults. The more we are able to study different aspects of asthma and the better we start to understand the disease, the more complex it becomes. However, as study tools have improved and as the awareness of gender and age effects has increased, it is likely that more genetic studies will address the issues of gender and age interactions.

X. Are We There Yet?

Candidate gene studies have proven to be a powerful tool in asthma genetics in recent years, and the role of alterations in some genes have been newly discovered and proven. However, we are still far from understanding how genetics work in asthma. New approaches, such as genome-wide association studies will increase the knowledge about potentially contributing candidate genes. On the other hand, the need for interconnecting this vastly increasing knowledge and putting it into a common context will further increase. Pathway genetics will play an important role as well as gene environment studies, taking gender and age effects into account. These complex analyses will be crucial to understand the complex mechanisms of genetic regulation in multifactorial diseases, such as asthma. These studies have only recently gained momentum, and new and exciting results can be expected in the near future.

References

1. Bleecker ER, Postma DS, Meyers DA. Genetic susceptibility to asthma in a changing environment. Ciba Found Symp 1997; 206:90–99.
2. Kauffmann F. Post-genome respiratory epidemiology: a multidisciplinary challenge. Eur Respir J 2004; 24(3):471–480.
3. Vercelli D. Genetics, epigenetics, and the environment: switching, buffering, releasing. J Allergy Clin Immunol 2004; 113(3):381–386.
4. Martinez FD, Holberg CJ. Segregation analysis of physician-diagnosed asthma in Hispanic and non-Hispanic white families. Clin Exp Allergy 1995; 25(suppl 2): 68–70.
5. Holberg CJ, Elston RC, Halonen M, et al. Segregation analysis of physician-diagnosed asthma in Hispanic and non-Hispanic white families. A recessive component? Am J Respir Crit Care Med 1996; 154(1):144–150.
6. Townley RG, Bewtra A, Wilson AF, et al. Segregation analysis of bronchial response to methacholine inhalation challenge in families with and without asthma. J Allergy Clin Immunol 1986; 77(1 Pt 1):101–107.
7. Meyers DA, Xu J, Postma DS, Levitt RC, Bleecker ER. Two locus segregation and linkage analysis for total serum IgE levels. Clin Exp Allergy 1995(25 suppl 2): 113–115.
8. Duffy DL, Martin NG, Battistutta D, Hopper JL, Mathews JD. Genetics of asthma and hay fever in Australian twins. Am Rev Respir Dis 1990; 142(6 Pt 1): 1351–1358.

9. Harris JR, Magnus P, Samuelsen SO, Tambs K. No evidence for effects of family environment on asthma. A retrospective study of Norwegian twins. Am J Respir Crit Care Med 1997; 156(1):43–49.

10. Riordan JR, Rommens JM, Kerem B, et al. Identification of the cystic fibrosis gene: cloning and characterization of complementary DNA. Science 1989; 245(4922):1066–1073.

11. www.innateimmunity.net

12. Kelly-Welch AE, Hanson EM, Boothby MR, Keegan AD. Interleukin-4 and interleukin-13 signaling connections maps. Science 2003; 300(5625):1527–1528.

13. Corry DB, Kheradmand F. Induction and regulation of the IgE response. Nature 1999; 402(suppl 6760):B18–B23.

14. Deichmann K, Bardutzky J, Forster J, Heinzmann A, Kuehr J. Common polymorphisms in the coding part of the IL4-receptor gene. Biochem Biophys Res Commun 1997; 231(3):696–697.

15. Duetsch G, Illig T, Loesgen S, et al. STAT6 as an asthma candidate gene: polymorphism-screening, association and haplotype analysis in a Caucasian sib-pair study. Hum Mol Genet 2002; 11(6):613–621.

16. Heinzmann A, Mao XQ, Akaiwa M, et al. Genetic variants of IL-13 signalling and human asthma and atopy. Hum Mol Genet 2000; 9(4):549–559.

17. Kabesch M, Tzotcheva I, Carr D, et al. A complete screening of the IL4 gene: novel polymorphisms and their association with asthma and IgE in childhood. J Allergy Clin Immunol 2003; 112(5):893–898.

18. Rosenwasser LJ. Promoter polymorphism in the candidate genes, IL-4, IL-9, TGF-beta1, for atopy and asthma. Int Arch Allergy Immunol 1999; 118(2–4): 268–270.

19. Graves PE, Kabesch M, Halonen M, et al. A cluster of seven tightly linked polymorphisms in the IL-13 gene is associated with total serum IgE levels in three populations of white children. J Allergy Clin Immunol 2000; 105(3):506–513.

20. Rosenwasser LJ, Borish L. Promoter polymorphisms predisposing to the development of asthma and atopy. Clin Exp Allergy 1998;28(suppl 5):13–15.

21. Basehore MJ, Howard TD, Lange LA, et al. A comprehensive evaluation of IL4 variants in ethnically diverse populations: association of total serum IgE levels and asthma in white subjects. J Allergy Clin Immunol 2004; 114(1):80–87.

22. Liu X, Beaty TH, Deindl P, et al. Associations between total serum IgE levels and the 6 potentially functional variants within the genes IL4, IL13, and IL4RA in German children: the German Multicenter Atopy Study. J Allergy Clin Immunol 2003; 112(2):382–388.

23. Liu X, Beaty TH, Deindl P, et al. Associations between specific serum IgE response and 6 variants within the genes IL4, IL13, and IL4RA in German children: The German Multicenter Atopy Study. J Allergy Clin Immunol 2004; 113(3): 489–495.

24. Mitsuyasu H, Yanagihara Y, Mao XQ, et al. Cutting edge: dominant effect of Ile50Val variant of the human IL-4 receptor alpha-chain in IgE synthesis. J Immunol 1999; 162(3):1227–1231.

25. Kruse S, Braun S, Deichmann KA. Distinct signal transduction processes by IL-4 and IL-13 and influences from the Q551R variant of the human IL-4 receptor alpha chain. Respir Res 2002; 3(1):24.

26. Wang HY, Shelburne CP, Zamorano J, Kelly AE, Ryan JJ, Keegan AD. Cutting edge: effects of an allergy-associated mutation in the human IL-4R alpha (Q576R) on human IL-4-induced signal transduction. J Immunol 1999; 162(8): 4385–4389.

27. Vladich FD, Brazille SM, Stern D, Peck ML, Ghittoni R, Vercelli D. IL-13 R130Q, a common variant associated with allergy and asthma, enhances effector mechanisms essential for human allergic inflammation. J Clin Invest 2005; 115(3):747–754.

28. Vercelli D. Genetics of IL-13 and functional relevance of IL-13 variants. Curr Opin Allergy Clin Immunol 2002; 2(5):389–393.

29. Schedel M, Carr D, Klopp N, et al. A signal transducer and activator of transcription 6 haplotype influences the regulation of serum IgE levels. J Allergy Clin Immunol 2004; 114(5):1100–1105.

30. Weidinger S, Klopp N, Wagenpfeil S, et al. Association of a STAT 6 haplotype with elevated serum IgE levels in a population based cohort of white adults. J Med Genet 2004; 41(9):658–663.

31. Moore JH. A global view of epistasis. Nat Genet 2005; 37(1):13–14.

32. Cordell HJ. Epistasis: what it means, what it doesn't mean, and statistical methods to detect it in humans. Hum Mol Genet 2002; 11(20):2463–2468.

33. Cordell HJ, Clayton DG. A unified stepwise regression procedure for evaluating the relative effects of polymorphisms within a gene using case/control or family data: application to HLA in type 1 diabetes. Am J Hum Genet 2002; 70(1):124–141.

34. Cordell HJ, Todd JA, Hill NJ, et al. Statistical modeling of interlocus interactions in a complex disease: rejection of the multiplicative model of epistasis in type 1 diabetes. Genetics 2001; 158(1):357–367.

35. Segre D, Deluna A, Church GM, Kishony R. Modular epistasis in yeast metabolism. Nat Genet 2005; 37(1):77–83.

36. Howard TD, Koppelman GH, Xu J, et al. Gene-gene interaction in asthma: IL4RA and IL13 in a Dutch population with asthma. Am J Hum Genet 2002; 70(1):230–236.

37. He JQ, Chan-Yeung M, Becker AB, et al. Genetic variants of the IL13 and IL4 genes and atopic diseases in at-risk children. Genes Immun 2003; 4(5):385–389.

38. Lee SG, Kim BS, Kim JH, et al. Gene-gene interaction between interleukin-4 and interleukin-4 receptor alpha in Korean children with asthma. Clin Exp Allergy 2004; 34(8):1202–1208.

39. Beghe B, Barton S, Rorke S, et al. Polymorphisms in the interleukin-4 and interleukin-4 receptor alpha chain genes confer susceptibility to asthma and atopy in a Caucasian population. Clin Exp Allergy 2003; 33(8):1111–1117.

40. Kabesch M, Schedel M, Carr D, et al. Interleukin 4/interleukin 13 pathway genetics strongly influence serum IgE levels and childhood asthma. J Allergy Clin Immunol 2006; 117(2):269–274.

41. Bugawan TL, Mirel DB, Valdes AM, Panelo A, Pozzilli P, Erlich HA. Association and interaction of the IL4R, IL4, and IL13 loci with type 1 diabetes among Filipinos. Am J Hum Genet 2003; 72(6):1505–1514.

42. Maier LM, Chapman J, Howson JM, et al. No evidence of association or interaction between the IL4RA, IL4, and IL13 genes in type 1 diabetes. Am J Hum Genet 2005; 76(3):517–521.

43. Hoffjan S, Ostrovnaja I, Nicolae D, et al. Genetic variation in immunoregulatory pathways and atopic phenotypes in infancy. J Allergy Clin Immunol 2004; 113(3):511–518.
44. Hizawa N, Yamaguchi E, Jinushi E, Konno S, Kawakami Y, Nishimura M. Increased total serum IgE levels in patients with asthma and promoter polymorphisms at CTLA4 and FCER1B. J Allergy Clin Immunol 2001; 108(1):74–79.
45. Adjers K, Pessi T, Karjalainen J, Huhtala H, Hurme M. Epistatic effect of IL1A and IL4RA genes on the risk of atopy. J Allergy Clin Immunol 2004; 113(3): 445–447.
46. Levy H, Raby BA, Lake S, et al. Association of defensin beta-1 gene polymorphisms with asthma. J Allergy Clin Immunol 2005; 115(2):252–258.
47. Hecker M, Bohnert A, Konig IR, Bein G, Hackstein H. Novel genetic variation of human interleukin-21 receptor is associated with elevated IgE levels in females. Genes Immun 2003; 4(3):228–233.
48. Siroux V, Curt F, Oryszczyn MP, Maccario J, Kauffmann F. Role of gender and hormone-related events on IgE, atopy, and eosinophils in the Epidemiological Study on the Genetics and Environment of Asthma, bronchial hyperresponsiveness and atopy. J Allergy Clin Immunol 2004; 114(3):491–498.
49. Nicolai T, Pereszlenyiova-Bliznakova L, Illi S, Reinhardt D, von Mutius E. Longitudinal follow-up of the changing gender ratio in asthma from childhood to adulthood: role of delayed manifestation in girls. Pediatr Allergy Immunol 2003; 14(4):280–283.
50. O'Donnell AR, Toelle BG, Marks GB, et al. Age-specific relationship between CD14 and atopy in a cohort assessed from age 8 to 25 years. Am J Respir Crit Care Med 2004; 169(5):615–622.
51. Kabesch M, Hasemann K, Schickinger V, et al. A promoter polymorphism in the CD14 gene is associated with elevated levels of soluble CD14 but not with IgE or atopic diseases. Allergy 2004; 59(5):520–525.
52. Bottema RW, Reijmerink NE, Koppelman GH, Kerkhof M, Postma DS. Phenotype definition, age, and gender in the genetics of asthma and atopy. Immunol Allergy Clin North Am 2005; 25(4):621–639.

5

Microarray Techniques and Data in Asthma/Chronic Obstructive Pulmonary Disease

THOMAS J. MARIANI

Department of Medicine, Brigham and Women's Hospital and Pulmonary Bioinformatics, The Lung Biology Center, Harvard Medical School, Boston, Massachusetts, U.S.A.

MARCO F. RAMONI

Children's Hospital Informatics Program, Division of Health Sciences and Technology, Harvard Medical School and Massachusetts Institute of Technology, Boston, Massachusetts, U.S.A.

I. Introduction

A. Functional Genomics—The Latest Molecular Technical Revolution

Over the past few years, medical researchers have witnessed the latest in a series of technical innovations, which affects both our approach to and the scope of our work. Such innovations have routinely occurred every 10 to 20 years over the past half-century, beginning with the identification of nucleic acid as the material storing the genetic code, to the advent of molecular cloning, the discovery of the polymerase chain reaction (PCR), and, most recently, the capability of rapidly creating genetically modified animals (in contrast to the slow process of breeding). The latest innovation, which began with the Human Genome Project, has provided us with the tools to observe cells and tissues as a sum of their parts, rather than individual genes or proteins. This is quite a change for a classically reductionistic discipline.

Functional genomics is the practice of assigning biological function to novel genes without previously described functions, as well as assigning additional function(s) to genes with previously known function, utilizing genomics-based information. That such an endeavor is a reality is due to the availability of complete genetic sequence information for dozens of organisms in combination with the ability to rapidly and simultaneously measure the expression of every gene in almost any given cell or tissue. Technologies have been developed, which allow the rapid sequencing of entire genomes (genomics) and parallel measurement of gene expression at the mRNA (transcriptomics) or protein (proteomics) level. These technologies are widely available at a reasonable cost and are, for the most part, highly accurate. The focus of this chapter will be the application of DNA microarray technology to both more fully characterize and accelerate our understanding of the pathogenesis of lung disease, most notably asthma and chronic obstructive pulmonary disease (COPD).

B. A Natural History of Microarray Technology

DNA microarray technology for the purpose of parallel measurement of steady-state mRNA levels rapidly evolved in the 1990s, from standard methods to measure gene expression, through a rational series of technical achievements. The first of these achievements was the capability to generate and organize individual complementary DNA (cDNA) molecules derived from expressed sequences from various biological sources (libraries). This was a simple extension from collections of DNA and cDNA molecules routinely found at the time in every molecular biology laboratory, which was motivated in large part by the effort to sequence complete genomes. The second achievement was the ability to accurately and repeatedly spot these individual cDNAs in a predefined location on a solid support. Initially, this was hardly an achievement, as molecular geneticists had used this concept for decades to identify DNA recombinants through colony hybridization. The true achievement was admittedly the ability to reduce the scale of this solid support by many orders of magnitude; from less than 10 clones per square inch to greater than 100,000 per square inch. Two related issues were the transition of supports (from nitrocellulose to nylon to glass/silica) and the development of optical scanners capable of resolving this number of discrete spots. The third major achievement was the ability to obtain and analyze increasingly smaller amounts of source biological material (RNA). Again, this was a natural progression from other technologies, most notably the use of reverse transcriptase (RT)-PCR to quantify gene expression at the mRNA level. By the beginning of this decade, these methods were so routine that genome-wide expression profiling could be performed using commercially available kits "off the shelf."

In the late 1990s, DNA microarray technology for parallel measurement of 1000 to 10,000 genes was immediately recognized for both its power of resolution and its potential for comprehension of a biological or diseased state. A seminal paper by Iyer et al. (1) applied the technology to define the response of cultured skin fibroblasts to serum stimulation. This biological paradigm had been studied for decades, but the breadth of understanding revealed by this new technology, and the potential for its application garnered a place for this study in the pages of *Science*. Another seminal study by Golub et al. (2) applied the technology to clinical specimens and showed that it was capable of discriminating two distinct disease entities. It was not so much that it was difficult to discriminate between acute lympho-blastic leukemia and chronic myelogenous leukemia using many other objective criteria, but rather that the technology was capable of this discrimination, combined with the appreciation for the potential disease discrimination the technology may also be capable of, that prompted this study to also be published in *Science*.

These and other similar studies introduced us to the power of genome-wide expression profiling. In the short-interceding time, the technology has lived up to much of its potential. Gene expression microarray technology is used by many to pursue diverse goals, to provide biological insight regarding an experimental response, to screen for genetic markers of disease, or to define clinical phenotypes. Microarrays have provided volumes of information regarding numerous biological paradigms including developmental processes and cell/tissue/organism response to stimulation. They have helped identify molecules contributing to the pathogenesis of numerous diseases, either through the analysis of diseased tissue or animal models of disease. Expression profiling has identified distinct classes of histologically identical disease, which have implications for patient morbidity and mortality. DNA microarrays are even under consideration for use by the Food and Drug Administration as a means to determine treatment options for breast cancer. The remainder of this chapter will provide a foundation for understanding DNA microarray technology, the methodology of its application, and the insight it has provided to our current understanding of asthma and COPD pathogenic mechanisms.

II. Basics of Microarray Technology

A. Probes and Targets

At this point, we need to define terminology common for describing microarray-based gene expression analysis. In standard techniques to measure gene expression (e.g., Northern hybridization and quantitative RT-PCR), we are interested in defining expression of a single gene in a complex biological sample. To identify information specific for a single gene in this complex sample, we utilize a specific, traceable "probe." In many instances, the complex sample, or "target" of the probe, is immobilized on a solid support (e.g., Northern blot). For DNA microarray experiments, the "probes" are immobilized, whereas the target is labeled and present in solution. Individual gene-specific information is identified due to a priori knowledge concerning the physical location of the probes upon the solid support.

Labeling of the complex biological sample to produce the labeled "target" follows standard techniques. Typically, this involves reverse transcription of total RNA into cDNA followed by an in vitro transcription (IVT) of this cDNA, in the presence of a "tag" (typically biotin), into labeled RNA. One common variation involves adding a second series of cDNA production and IVT in order to generate a greater abundance of target. This is particularly useful when limiting amounts of biological sample are available. It is currently feasible to perform DNA microarray experiments from as little as a few nanograms of RNA.

B. Microarray Formats

A variety of DNA microarray formats have been and/or are currently available. These formats can be classified in different ways: type of support the DNA is immobilized upon, techniques used to place the DNA on the support, nature of hybridization event, etc. All formats are inherently useful, but each has its own unique benefits/limitations (not all of which will be described), and some are more appropriate for certain applications.

Initial DNA microarray platforms were no more complex than a colony hybridization, consisting of dozens of cDNA clones (probes) placed or spotted onto a nitrocellulose/nylon membrane. This format progressed to include "blots" with 100s of probes. While this early microarray technology did not always function optimally in all hands, a testament to the utility of this platform is that many commercial sources for this type of microarray still exist. The true prospect for genome-wide expression profiling really began with the advent of the technology to rapidly and reproducibly spot thousands of individual cDNA probes onto glass slides. This technology was in large part pioneered by a group of investigators at Stanford University (3–6). Optimizing the reliability and reproducibility of this spotting technique occurred over a number of years. Difficulties included (but certainly were not limited to) reproducibility of spot size and DNA/probe concentration, as well as organization of cDNA clones. While highly challenging to develop this technology, it was at least as difficult to reproduce the method from scratch at additional institutions. Although the reproducibility of replication and hybridization characteristics of large cDNA molecules had advantages, the ability to rapidly synthesize large amounts of cDNAs by PCR led to the near-universal current use of amplification products for probes.

While this technology was being developed at academic institutions, commercial entities also appreciated the potential power of the technology. Numerous companies rapidly developed a variety of microarray platforms that were bought and used by academic and industry scientists. However, one company developed a particular methodology for microarray production, which revolutionized the technology and rapidly promoted its widespread use. Affymetrix developed a proprietary method for in situ synthesis of short (25-mer) oligonucleotides on a silica "chip" at a very high feature (probe) density, which allowed for the simultaneous analysis of more than 100,000 hybridization events (7–9). In addition to advancing the possibility of measuring all transcripts in a given cell/tissue, this probe density initiated a number of unique attributes in the Affymetrix technology. First, Affymetrix uses multiple hybridization events per gene/transcript to be measured. In fact, the incredible probe density allowed the inclusion of "mismatch (MM)" oligonucleotides, differing from the actual probe sequence by a single central nucleotide, to allow for the measurement of background hybridization. Currently, this technology uses 22 hybridization events to define the measurement of gene expression for a single transcript, 11 pairs of correct [perfect match (PM)] and "MM" oligonucleotides. Second, Affymetrix technology promoted single biological sample (target), noncomepetitive hybridization. Most other platforms use a two targets, competitive hybridization strategy to define differential expression between two experimental paradigms. Affymetrix technology developed normalization strategies to compare individual biological samples from different hybridizations. Finally, due to the use of multiple hybridization events for individual measurements, Affymetrix had to develop strategies, algorithms, and software capable of accurately and reproducibly summarizing these data to define gene expression.

One recent technology, which has been developed and widely heralded, is the use of spotted long oligonucleotides (50–70-mer) for custom-made DNA microarrays (10,11). This combines the benefits of high-feature density with rapid, large-scale probe synthesis. One significant limitation of Affymetrix' proprietary photolithographical in situ oligonucleotide synthesis method is the time and effort necessary to develop new microarrays containing new sets of probes. The long oligo format is notable for great flexibility to change features, in part, due to the novel methodology of placing the probes. Feature placement for this microarray format typically relies upon a technology similar to that used by ink-jet printers (12).

An under-appreciated complexity of the transition to oligonucleotide probes was the difficulties associated with determining sequence accuracy and specificity. Individual sequence errors are more forgiving within the context of long cDNA probes, but have significant effects within the context of oligonucleotides. This is of particular relevance for Affymetrix technology, where single-nucleotide MM oligonucleotides are used to define the specificity of hybridization. Novel computational methods to define sequence accuracy and specificity were developed; many of which were reliant upon public sequence databases generated from efforts to sequence the human genome and the genomes of other organisms. As these genome sequence databases are not complete, and their accuracy is continually evolving, oligonucleotide sequence errors exist (13,14). This is additionally

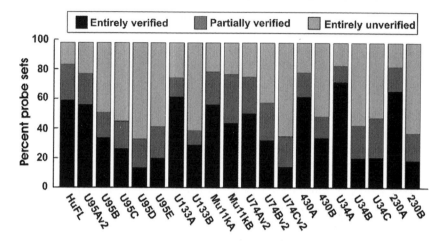

Figure 1 An assessment of microarray probe sequence inaccuracies. An analysis of the commonly used DNA microarrays produced by Affymetrix reveals a substantial number of the probes may not correspond to their anticipated target transcript. Shown is a histogram displaying the percentage of probe sets for which the probe sequences matched the appropriate reference sequence mRNA, for each of the commercially available mammalian microarrays. Probe sets that do not contain at least one probe matching the appropriate reference sequence mRNA (completely unverified) show decreased measurement precision. The most likely explanation of these differences is sequence errors in the databases used to design the probes. *Source*: From Ref. 13.

relevant when relating results from one platform to another, as sequence inaccuracies, can lead to inappropriate measurements (such as the inappropriate measurement of the wrong transcript) (15–17).

III. Microarray Data Processing

Notwithstanding their technical differences, all expression microarray platforms can be regarded as high-resolution arrays measuring the expression level of each gene as a function of the RNA transcript abundance. This abundance is, in turn, measured by the emission intensity of the region where the gene transcript is located in the scanned image of the microarray, and the signal is filtered to remove noise generated by the microarray background and nonspecific hybridization. A comprehensive survey of these statistical techniques can be found in the article by Sebastiani et al. (18).

A. From Images to Data

In both cDNA and oligonucleotide microarrays, hybridization of the target to the probes determines a chemical reaction that is captured into a digital image by a scanning laser device. The next step is to translate the intensity of each hybridization signal into a table with numerical measures. The quality of the image analysis process is crucial for accurate interpretation of the data, and a variety of algorithms and software tools tailored to the different aspects of cDNA and oligonucleotide microarray images have been developed (19).

The analysis of the image of a cDNA microarray consists of three steps (Smyth et al. 2003) (20). The first step, called "gridding," recovers the position of the spot corresponding to a particular probe in the image, taking into account potential translations and rotations of the microarray image. The second step, called "segmentation," identifies which pixels are conveying signal from actual hybridization (foreground) and which are just carrying unspecific signal (background) caused by experimental processing of the microarray or target contamination. This classification can be accomplished using fixed circular areas—like the method implemented in ScanAlyze (89)—or by dynamically identifying the actual diameter of each spot—like the method implemented in GenePix (90). More general methods do not assume a circular form for a spot but try to adaptively identify the geometry of each probe. QuantArray (91) implements the method, developed by Chen et al. (21), which labels groups of eight pixels at a time as background or foreground. The last step (intensity extraction) calculates the intensity of each spot by correcting for background intensity and assessing the quality of the estimation. Most packages calculate the foreground intensity as the mean or the median pixel values, and an estimate of the background intensity is usually subtracted from the foreground intensity. ScanAlyze calculates the corrected intensity as the number of foreground pixels minus the median number of background pixels, whereas QuantArray calculates the corrected intensity as the difference between median foreground pixels and background pixels. Spot computes the background intensity by a nonlinear filter, which creates a background image for the whole microarray, and by sampling this background image at the nominal centers of each spots.

The analysis of oligonucleotide microarray images leverages on the fact that the image produced by the scanning laser device describes the probes as squares of an approximately known number of pixels and that image contains, by design, some recognizable alignment features. Because the approximate physical dimension of each probe in the image is known, once the positions of the alignment features are determined, a basic grid easily identifies the pixels that describe each probe cell through some form of linear interpolation. Notwithstanding these technical devices to simplify gridding and segmentation, a residual risk remains for potential misalignment of the basic gridding procedure. This situation has motivated the development of adaptive pixel selection algorithms (22) and the enhancement of the most recent Affymetrix image analysis software with a new algorithm to account for potential spatial effects in the calculation background intensity (92). Intensity extraction in oligonucleotide microarrays is made more robust and, at the same time, more complex by the choice of sampling the expression of a transcript through a simultaneous sampling of different regions of a transcript. The rationale behind this technology is based on the concept of probe redundancy: a "set" of well-chosen small segments of cDNA not only is sufficient to uniquely identify a specific gene, but also reduces the chances that fragments of the target will randomly hybridize to the probes, thus reducing the chances of cross-hybridization. Therefore, synthetic oligonucleotide microarrays represent each gene not by its cDNA, but by a set of fixed-length independent segments unique to the DNA of the. On the GeneChip® platform, each oligonucleotide (probe) is 25 bases long, and each gene is represented by a number of "probe pairs" ranging from 11 in the new Human Genome U133 set to 16 in the Murine Genome U74v2 set and the Human Genome U95v2. A probe pair consists of a PM probe and a MM probe. Each PM probe is chosen on the basis of uniqueness criteria and proprietary and empirical rules designed to improve the odds that probes will hybridize with high specificity. The MM probe is identical to the corresponding PM probe except for the base in the central position, which is replaced with its complementary base. The inversion of the central base makes the MM probe a further specificity control because, by design, hybridization of the MM probe can be attributed to either cross-hybridization or background signal.

The latest statistical algorithm produced by Affymetrix combines the measurements of each probe into a probe set and returns three measures: a detection call, a detection *p*-value, and a signal value. The detection calls assess the quality of the hybridization, whereas the detection *p*-values represent the confidence in this assessment. The signal is a proxy for the relative expression level of the gene represented by the probe set.

B. Filtering

Several techniques are available to reduce data dimensionality and variability by removing some gene measurements. It is surprising to realize that ad hoc rules are commonly used, and that the choice of the genes to be removed can differ substantially according to the microarray platform and the technique chosen to analyze the data. For expression data measured with a cDNA microarray, it is a common practice to disregard those genes with negative or small expression levels (before or after normalization).

The Affymetrix statistical software assigns a detection call to each probe set to assess the amount and quality of hybridization, and it is suggested to discard all genes that have expression levels labeled as A (absent) or M (marginal) in all samples. This procedure is justified by the empirical evidence that expression levels smaller than 10 are actually measurement errors (Affymetrix, 2002) (23). However, a large proportion of genes would often be discarded by this procedure, and investigators tend to adopt less-stringent criteria to select a subset of the genes to be further analyzed. A common strategy is to retain only those genes that have minimum fold-change that exceeds a particular threshold (typically twofold) in a preset number of experiments (2,24), to limit the analysis to those genes that vary most across experiments by the genes according to their standard deviation.

All these filters depend on arbitrary thresholds used to decide when a value is abnormally large or small, or when the variability of the measurements is too high. The impact of normalization and filtering strategies is unclear, and few systematic studies are available to provide investigators with a description of the properties of these preprocessing techniques and guidance on choosing the one most appropriate for their particular problem. A comprehensive survey of filtering techniques can be found in Ref. 19.

IV. Microarray Data Analysis

The result of a microarray experiment is a numeric representation of the expression of the entire transcriptome of a set of biological samples, to be analyzed using statistical techniques to infer general properties of some biological phenomenon. This section outlines some of the common data processing and analysis techniques currently used to draw experimental conclusions from microarray studies.

A. Comparative Experiments and Differential Expression

Early comparative experiments based on cDNA microarray technology measured differences of gene expression across two conditions in terms of the fold-change: the ratio of the expression levels (4). Particularly, genes that showed a negative or positive fold-change of at least two were deemed to be differentially expressed across the two conditions. The need to choose a threshold to identify significant differentially expressed genes in two conditions through repeated measurements is the motivation of a series of articles focused on statistical fold analysis.

Statistical approaches to ratio-based differential analysis estimate the ratio of the expression levels in two conditions with some statistic, and decide whether deviations of the estimate of such a statistic from one can be attributed to a real difference of the gene expressions in the two conditions or simply to sampling variability. Chen et al. (21) assume that the measurements from the two different conditions are independent and normally distributed, and that they have constant coefficient of variation for all genes in both conditions. Under these assumptions, they derive an approximate distribution of the ratio statistic that can be used to find a $(1-\alpha)\%$ confidence interval for the ratio of the expression in the two conditions.

The main weakness of this approach is that, despite the fact that expression levels should be positive numbers, the expression measurements are assumed to follow normal distributions. This inappropriate distributional assumption is corrected, in Ref. (25), by assuming that the measurements follow Gamma distributions, and a Bayesian method is proposed to estimate the fold-change of each gene to account for the "between-microarrays" variability. Although the second approach is based on sounder distributional assumptions about gene expression measurements, it relies on the unconventional assumption that the experimental error across microarrays also follows a Gamma distribution. Lee et al. (26) used a mixture model to describe the joint distribution of the log ratios of measurements, and the expectation and maximization algorithm to estimate the mixture components to compute the posterior probability that each gene is differentially expressed in the two experimental conditions. When more than one replication is available, this procedure is applied to a summary of the original expression ratios. Several authors have modified this approach by relaxing the parametric assumption on the mixture model, by using a larger number of fixed effects to model dye and spot effects (27) or random effects (28).

To identify the set of genes that are differentially expressed, one needs to test the null hypothesis that no difference of expression exists across the two experimental conditions for each gene, and then select the set of genes for which the null hypothesis is rejected. The standard statistic used to test the null hypothesis is the t-statistic or some modified forms of it (2,29). Large values of the t-statistic would offer evidence in favor of differential expression. The critical problem here is to choose a suitable threshold of the t-statistic to reject the null hypothesis.

The most popular approach to choosing a threshold is distribution-free. The main idea is to compute the value of the t-statistic from the data, in which the sample labels that represent the experimental conditions are randomly reshuffled. By repeating this process several times, it is possible to construct the empirical distribution of the t-statistic under the null hypothesis of no differential expression. From the empirical distribution function, one can select a gene-specific threshold to reject the null hypothesis with a particular significance. This method is implemented in the program GenePattern (92), which conducts the differential analysis based on the signal-to-noise ratio statistic or the standard t-statistics. The program SAM (93) implements a distribution-free differential analysis using a slight-modified version of the t-statistic. Because of the large number of genes, algorithms also have been developed for multiple comparison adjusted p-values. Distribution-free methods tend to be widely used in practice, although few authors have suggested making distribution assumptions on the gene expression data.

B. Molecular Classification

The analysis methods described in the previous section can be regarded as high-throughput screening methods to quickly identify which genes are differentially expressed across two experimental conditions. The procedure of molecular classification takes this approach one step further to perform two new tasks: class prediction and class discovery.

Class Prediction

The experimenter chooses a set of conditions and measures repeatedly the expression level of the same set of genes in each condition (e.g., collects several patient samples sharing the same pathology). Each condition is regarded as a class label, and the goal of the analysis is to detect the genes that are differentially expressed in at least two conditions or that are good predictors of the class. In cancer genomic experiments, for example, the goal may be the development of new diagnostic tools based on the molecular profiles of tumor cells. To do this, the experimenter may collect samples from patients known to be affected by different types of the same tumor class—such as different types of leukemia (2) or breast cancer (30)—and use each patient sample as an instance of the molecular profile of the specific type of tumor. The goal of the analysis would be to determine the molecular profile of each type of tumor to make possible a molecular-based diagnosis of a specific tumor (31).

To accomplish this goal, supervised classification techniques are used to learn a rule from a set of labeled cases (called the *training set*) to classify new unlabeled cases in a "test set." Each condition is regarded as a class label, and each sample is labeled by a class. The goal of the analysis is to identify a molecular profile for each class. The classification can be based on a decision rule that selects a class by minimizing the expected loss. We call this approach model based in contrast to a model-free approach that partitions the space of gene expression data, so that each element of the partition corresponds to one and only one class label. Well-known model-based classification methods are multinomial logistic or probit regression (32) and naive Bayes classifiers (33).

Although model-based approaches provide a quantification of the uncertainty of the predictive model and a principled way to select a subset of the most predictive genes, model-free approaches are currently the most popular. Examples of model-free approaches to classification are methods for discriminant analysis such as Fisher linear discriminant analysis, nearest neighbor classification trees (Hand, 1997) (34) and support vector machines. The selection of genes with predictive properties is often based on heuristic rules, such as filtering out genes with a fold-change that does not exceed a particular threshold (35) or selecting genes that are highly correlated with a dummy pattern of 0s and 1s that mirrors the class partition (2).

Class Discovery

Multiple microarray experiments can also be used to help investigators create new classifications by discovering new classes characterized by a specific molecular profile. There is little doubt that the current taxonomy of cancer lumps together molecularly distinct diseases with distinct clinical phenotypes, with the consequence that patients who receive the same diagnosis can have different clinical courses and treatment responses (36). For example, in the analysis of gene expression data collected from tissues of breast cancer patients, the goal may be the identification of new molecular taxonomies of breast cancers characterized by particular profiles. Again, the advantage of such discovery could be to aid the diagnosis, as well as to tailor treatments to more specific diagnoses. The solution to class prediction problems requires the development of classification rules able to label the molecular profile of a sample, whereas the goal of class discovery studies is to create new classes from the available data. Formally, the distinction between the two tasks is that the former relies on a labeled data set, whereas the latter relies on an unlabeled data set.

Class discovery is typically performed using unsupervised classification techniques, such as clustering or multidimensional scaling, to be used to group either genes with a similar expression profile or samples (e.g., patients) with a similar molecular profile or both. The average-linkage hierarchical clustering, proposed by Eisen et al. (37), is today one of the most popular analytical methods to cluster gene expression data. Relationships among the genes are represented by a tree (dendrogram), the branch lengths of which reflect the degree of similarity between the genes. The similarity measure commonly used is the correlation between pairs of gene expression data, but other measures have been used, such as Euclidean distance or information-theoretic metrics. The resulting tree sorts the genes in the original data array, so that genes or groups of genes with similar expression patterns will be adjacent. The ordered table can be displayed graphically, together with the dendrogram, for the investigators' visual inspection. This method is implemented in the programs Cluster and TreeView (95).

The same approach can be used to cluster samples with a similar molecular profile. Hierarchical clustering applied to the rows and columns of the data array will return a sorted image of the original data. The image of the sorted data is typically used to support the operation of partitioning genes or samples into separated groups with common patterns. This operation is done by visual inspection, by searching for large contiguous patches of color that represent groups of genes that share similar expression patterns or groups of samples that share similar molecular profiles. Identification of these patches allows the extraction of subgroups of genes to be used to recluster the samples and, conversely, the extraction of subgroups of experiments to be used to recluster gene expression patterns. Although the choice of subsets is arbitrary and the final result heavily depends on the genes or samples selected at each step of the procedure, this method has been successfully applied to identify, for example, new molecular classes of non-Hodgkin's lymphoma (36), skin malignant melanoma (38), breast cancer (39), and lung cancer (40).

Notwithstanding these interesting results, this approach is not without problems. The subjective nature of partitioning by visual inspection may lead one to disregard some important information or to include irrelevant information. Permutation tests are sometimes used to validate the partitions found by this procedure (37), and a bootstrap-based validation technique is presented by Kerr and Churchill (41). The gap statistics of Tibshirani et al. (42) can also be used to find the optimal number of groups in the data.

A second problem of this approach is the dilution of distance measures in average-linkage hierarchical clustering. When genes are assigned to the same subtree, the similarity measure between subtrees or between single genes and subtrees is computed by using a subtree profile calculated as the average of the subtree member profiles. As the subtree grows, this average profile becomes a less adequate representation of the subtree members. Relevance networks (43) are a nonhierarchical clustering method, which does not suffer from this dilution problem. For each pair of genes, the method computes a similarity between their expression measures, such as correlation or mutual information on appropriately discretized expression measures, and assigns genes that have a similarity measure above a preset threshold to the same cluster. This method can be regarded as a graphical representation of the matrix of all pair-wise distances between gene expression profiles, because genes assigned to the same cluster are linked by an edge that has a thickness proportional to the similarity between the two elements. Although this method does not rely on visual inspection, the division into clusters is entrusted to an arbitrary threshold.

When some prior knowledge about the number of groups in the data is available, k-means clustering can be used as an alternative to hierarchical clustering to provide an optimal grouping of rows and/or columns of the data array Y into a preset number of clusters. The k-means clustering starts with a random assignment of the rows (columns) of the data matrix into k disjoint groups, and the rows (columns) are iteratively moved among the clusters until a partition with optimal properties is found. Typically, the criterion to find the optimal partition is to minimize the within-cluster variability while maximizing the between-cluster variability. The within-cluster variability is measured by the average distance between cluster members and the cluster profile, whereas the between-cluster variability is a measure of the distance of each cluster member from the other cluster profiles. Tavazoie et al. (44) used k-means clustering to identify groups of genes with similar patterns across different experimental conditions. Similar to k-means clustering are the self-organizing maps. A self-organizing map uses a two-or three-dimensional projection of each cluster profile and provides a straightforward graphical representation of the result. Self-organizing maps have been used to identify classes of genes with similar functions in the yeast cell cycle (35) and have been combined with the nearest neighbor classification method to discriminate between two types of acute leukemia (2).

C. Time Series Analysis

Sometimes, the distinction among different classes is observable only through the dissection of the dynamics of the genomic system. In these cases, the different conditions are represented by time points, and the goal is to identify groups of genes that behave in a similar way. Several applications of genome-wide clustering methods focus on the temporal profiling of gene expression. The intuition behind this analytical approach is that genes that show a similar expression profile over time are acting together, because they belong to the same or, at least similar, functional categories. Temporal profiling offers the possibility of observing the regulatory mechanisms in action and tries to break down the genome into sets of genes that are involved in the same, or at least related, processes. However, the clustering methods described in the previous section rest on the assumption that the set of observations for each gene is exchangeable over time: pair-wise similarity measures, such as correlation or Euclidean distance, are invariant with respect to the order of the observations, and if the temporal order of a pair of series is permuted, these distance measures will not change. While this assumption holds when expression measures are taken from independent biological samples, it may no longer be valid when the observations are a time series.

Although the functional genomic literature is becoming increasingly aware of the specificity of temporal profiles of gene expression data, as well as of their fundamental importance in unraveling the functional relationships between genes, traditional clustering methods are still used to group genes on the basis of their similarity. For example, Holter et al. (45) describe a method for characterizing the time evolution of gene expression levels by using a time translational matrix to predict future expression levels of genes based on their expression levels at some initial time, thus capturing the inherent dependency of observations in time series. This approach relies on the clustering model obtained using a timeless method, such as singular value decomposition (46), and then infers a linear time translational matrix for the characteristic modes of these clusters. The advantage of this approach is that it provides, via the translational matrix, a stochastic characterization of a clustering model that takes into account the dynamic nature of temporal gene expression profiles. However, the clustering model, which this method relies upon, is still obtained by disregarding the dynamic nature of the observations, while we expect that different assumptions on the correlation between temporal observations will affect the way in which gene profiles are clustered together.

When the goal is to cluster gene expression patterns measured at different time points, the observations for each gene are serially correlated, and clustering methods should take into account this dependency. The method of Ramoni et al. (47) is a Bayesian model–based approach to cluster temporal gene expression patterns that accounts for the temporal dependencies using autoregressive models. The method represents gene expression dynamics as autoregressive equations and uses an agglomerative procedure to search for the most probable set of clusters, conditional on the available data. Features of this method are the ability to take into account the dynamic nature of gene expression time series during clustering and a principled way to identify the number of distinct clusters. As the number of possible clustering models grows exponentially with the number of observed time series, a distance-based heuristic search procedure is used to render the search process feasible. In this way, the method retains the important visualization capability of hierarchical clustering, but acquires an independent measure to decide when two series are different enough to belong to different clusters. Furthermore, the reliance of this method on an explicit statistical model of gene expression dynamics makes it possible to use standard statistical techniques to assess the goodness of fit of the resulting model and validate the underlying assumptions. When the autoregressive order is equal to zero, this method subsumes, as a special case, model-based clustering of atemporal (i.e., independent) observations. The method is implemented in the program CAGED (96).

V. Application of Microarrays to Asthma Research

As much as for research of cancer, diabetes, and a few other complex disorders, the development of genomic technology for application to clinical medicine has developed with consideration to potential application for research on asthma. This has been particularly true with respect to human genetics. While the application of DNA microarray technology and genome-wide expression profiling of human asthmatic samples has been curiously limited, significant observations regarding asthma susceptibility and pathogenesis have been made. A considerable proportion of these data have come from studying various animal models of lung inflammation and allergic hypersensitivity. In total, the observations resulting from these studies comprise reasonable expectations for the insight one might anticipate from the application of DNA microarrays to a complex disease state. Here, we will summarize examples of applications of microarray technology to asthma research, which are distinct in their approach and anticipated goals. For comprehensive reviews of the literature, we refer the readers to Tzouvelekis et al. (48), Erle and Yang (49), and Rolph et al. (50).

A common goal of microarray experiments is to comprehensively define changes in gene expression between a diseased state and normal tissue. Such an experimental design is rational for numerous anticipated goals including a desire to identify genes/pathways contributing to disease etiology, to model cell type specificity in the disease response of a complex organ and to identify a molecular signature of a disease or phenotype. In an effort to provide mechanistic insight into the acute response of asthmatics to inhaled allergen, Lilly et al. (51) profiled gene expression in asthmatic airway epithelial cells derived from endobronchial brushings. A major outcome of this study was gene discovery, as a number of those identified as differentially expressed were not previously appreciated as being associated with asthma. This type of study is hypothesis generating and provides candidates for further validation and or mechanistic studies. In a particularly interesting study, Lee et al. (52) investigated the effects of the asthma-associated cytokine IL-13 upon airway epithelial cells, smooth muscle cells, and fibroblasts. Although severely limited by the use of cultured cells treated in vitro, this study represents an excellent example of the capability of genome-wide expression profiling, to define the responsiveness and contribution of specific (airway) cells to disease (asthma) pathogenesis. Interestingly, the set of IL-13 responsive genes identified by Lee et al. in lung epithelial cells in vitro was notably distinct from the allergen-induced genes identified by Lilly et al. in endobronchial brushings. This may reflect the complexity of the disease, differences in the models studied, or a combination of both. Unfortunately, this lack of consistency is seen all too often in microarray studies, and also reflects technical limitations, a large component of which is almost certainly sample size insufficiency (53,54).

Few human diseases involve surgical therapy including the removal of diseased tissue. This fact often makes obtaining sufficient tissue samples for molecular analysis difficult. Therefore, many studies investigating systemic as well as nonsystemic diseases have performed expression profiling of whole or fractionated peripheral blood cells. While it is certainly questionable whether such studies will provide mechanistic insight into the pathways involved in the disease, these studies can define markers for disease type and/or progression. Brutsche et al. (55) profiled gene expression in peripheral blood cells from a total of 40 atopic and nontopic asthmatics as well as healthy controls, using low-density nylon arrays. From the expression data, the authors developed a molecular (gene expression) signature for atopy and asthma, which showed greater predictive power than the gold standard IgE. While it is less than doubtful that this result will have clinical utility, it serves as a powerful proof-of-principle revealing the feasibility of such approaches to define disease state. In a technically similar study, Hansel et al. (56) compared genome-wide expression profiles of CD4+ T-cells from mild and severe asthmatics. Similar to Lee et al., these authors were attempting to identify the contribution of a specific cell type to the pathogenesis of a complex disease involving numerous cell populations. This study, however, showed the potential of using freshly isolated cells, a tremendous advantage over the use of cultured cells exposed to a stimulus in vitro.

Animal models have become a common, if not essential, component to the discovery of disease mechanism(s). Expression profiling of animal models for disease has proven useful to define genes associated with and/or contributing to disease phenotypes. Some of the best examples of this type of application involve the identification of a set of dysregulated genes common to multiple animal models of a particular disease or phenotype. Zimmermann et al. (57) performed genome-wide expression profiling of lung tissue from two distinct animal models of asthma, which show phenotypic overlap. They identified the induction of basic amino acid metabolism pathway genes, arginase I, in particular, in asthma pathogenesis. Arginase I induction was validated in human asthmatic lung tissue. This finding was biologically plausible due to the ability of arginase to generate nitric oxide (NO) and induce collagen synthesis. In fact, earlier work by Meurs et al. (58) had suggested a role for NO synthetase–mediated arginine metabolism in asthma. Subsequent studies by others have confirmed this initial finding (59). This example highlights the power of microarray technology to provide reliable, novel mechanistic insight into genes and pathways contributing to disease pathogenesis.

As mentioned earlier, asthma research has been intimately associated with the development of high-throughput genetics technologies. One example of this is the ability to define loci contributing to (disease) phenotypes in inbred strains of laboratory mice through comprehensive analysis of single nucleotide polymorphism (SNP) markers. Currently, the resolution at which these loci are defined cannot specify among linkage to dozens to thousands of genes. This is completely analogous to the situation with genome-wide linkage scans in humans. In both cases, fine-mapping to identify the causative gene can be extremely laborious and time consuming. Integrative genomics, the combination of genomics technologies, or expression profiling to be specific, can help to expedite the fine-mapping process. Karp et al. (60) provide a classic example of this approach. These authors used quantitative trait locus (QTL) mapping to identify a region of the genome, conferring susceptibility to airways hyperreactivity in a cross between two inbred strains of mice. Concomitant application of expression profiling to the animal model identified a particular gene within the QTL, complement factor 5 (C5), as a candidate asthma-susceptibility gene. Subsequent studies by Hasegawa et al. (61) have revealed a C5 haplotype conferring protection against the development of asthma in children. This study represents an example of the potential power of combining high-throughput genetics and expression profiling to identify susceptibility genes for complex human diseases.

One reason that asthma research has been a focus for genomics-based technology (or vice versa) is the tremendous phenotypic heterogeneity of the disease with respect to clinical symptoms as well as responsiveness to the various therapeutic options. Expression profiling allows for the characterization of not only discrete phenotypes, but also differences in the response to therapy. Asthma pharmacogenetics and pharmacogenomics are areas of significant active research. In a relatively small study, Laprise et al. (62) reported dysregulation of a set of genes in airway epithelial cells

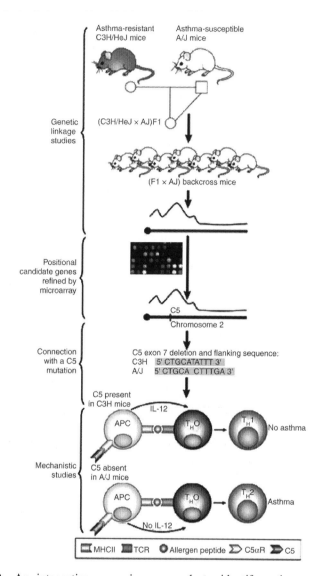

Figure 2 An integrative genomics approach to identify asthma-susceptibility genes. Karp et al. used a combination of QTL and microarray analysis to identify C5 as a gene contributing to airway hyperresponsiveness in an animal model of asthma. Genetic linkage studies were used to define regions of the genome contributing to an asthma-related phenotype in two inbred strains of mice. Microarray analysis of gene expression in these strains, which showed divergent phenotypes, was used to refine positional candidates. This led to the identification of the gene encoding the complement protein C5 in a QTL on chromosome 2, which was shown to have coding sequence differences between the strains. Subsequent in vitro studies suggested mechanistic pathways affected by the distinct alleles that contribute to the phenotypes observed. *Source*: From Refs. 60 and 88.

derived from asthmatic patients when compared to nonasthmatic controls. Importantly, the experimental design of this study sampled the patients before and after steroid therapy. This allowed the authors to show that approximately one-third of those dysregulated genes were affected by therapy. In a similar study using cells in vitro, Hakonarson et al. (63) showed that dexamethasone treatment reverted dysregulation of a majority of genes affected by IL-1β/tumor necrosis factor α treatment of airway smooth muscle cells. Recently, Hakonarson et al. (64) used genome-wide expression profiling of peripheral blood mononuclear cells to investigate severe, steroid-resistant asthma. This study identified a number of genes that may prove to be therapeutic targets for patients with abnormally severe disease and/or those who do not respond to typical asthma therapy.

VI. Application of Microarrays to COPD Research

The application of genomics technologies to research for COPD has lagged behind that for asthma, in part, due to the lack of disease-modifying therapeutic options. However, as COPD prevalence is on the rise, and is predicted to become the third most common cause of death and the fifth most common cause of disability in the world by the year 2020 (65), interest in COPD research and the identification of disease mechanism(s) is growing. The breadth of genome-wide expression profiling in COPD patients is attractive for its potential to identify pathways that may serve as targets for novel therapeutic strategies. Further, a recent increase in the appreciation of phenotypic variability in patients with COPD has provided increased opportunity for microarray technology to distinguish patient populations with respect to risk/susceptibility (both genetic and environmental) and disease heterogeneity. In this section, we will examine notable applications of DNA microarray technology to the response to cigarette smoke exposure and the development of emphysema in human patients and animal models of COPD.

A handful of studies have investigated gene expression in lung tissue samples obtained from COPD patients. Historically, Zhang et al. (66) were the first to describe the application of DNA microarrays to human COPD. This study used low-density cDNA arrays to reveal the induction of EGR1 expression in late-stage emphysema. Golpon et al. (67) used genome-wide expression profiling to investigate changes in *HOX*-gene expression in a small number of emphysema patients. Interestingly, a recent article by Ning et al. (68) confirmed the induction of EGR1 expression in lung tissue from moderate-to-severe COPD patients [global initiative for chronic obstructive lung disease stage 2 (GOLD2)] when compared to normal (GOLD0) lung tissue, using a combination of high-density cDNA arrays and SAGE. This is a rare confirmation, as expression profiling of human COPD patients has typically led to the identification of novel sets of genes, not those identified by previous investigations. It is unclear whether this is a result of sample heterogeneity (sampling from this complex organ results in nonuniform proportion of cell types), phenotypic heterogeneity, or small- and underpowered individual studies.

Two significant studies, which were copublished in 2004, represent examples of the characterization of gene expression in distinct populations of COPD patients. Spira et al. (69) defined changes in gene expression between lung tissue samples obtained from patients with severe emphysema undergoing lung volume reduction surgery to those from patients with mild-to-moderate airflow obstruction. The authors identified a set of genes capable of discriminating patients with severe emphysema, as well as a subgroup of patients with poor outcome. Golpon et al. (70) defined gene expression changes in lung tissue between patients with "usual" emphysema to those with alpha-1-antitrypsin deficiency, and normal controls.

As cigarette smoke exposure is the principal environmental factor contributing to increased risk for COPD, many studies have addressed the effects of cigarette smoke upon gene expression in the lungs of humans and rodents. Hackett et al. (71) performed genome-wide expression profiling of airway epithelial cells isolated by endobronchial brushing from smokers and nonsmokers. This study was noteworthy in the identification of differential expression in antioxidant-related genes in smokers as compared to nonsmokers, as well as significant variability in the expression of these genes between individuals. This suggested to the authors that variability in the response of antioxidant gene expression in response to smoke exposure may play a role in susceptibility to the development of smoke-related lung disease, particularly COPD. A seminal paper by Spira et al. (72) described gene expression from airway epithelial cells, again obtained from endobronchial brushings, in a large cohort of patients including individuals who never smoked, current smokers, and former smokers. These data were used to define the qualitative and quantitative effects of smoke exposure upon human airway epithelial cells in vivo and the temporal effects of smoking cessation. Fuke et al. (73) used laser-capture microdissection to isolate airway epithelial cells from the lungs of smokers with and without airflow obstruction. Microarray analysis of RNA derived from these cells revealed a dysregulation of chemokine receptor 2 in patients with COPD. These approaches are attractive, in that they remove a component of the variability inherent in samples derived from complex tissues composed of multiple cell types, by purifying a particular cell population and investigating only its response in the biological paradigm.

Genome-wide expression profiling from animal models has provided significant mechanistic insight into COPD pathogenesis. Morris et al. (74) applied microarrays in a spontaneous model of emphysema, resulting from deficiency in β6 integrin and subsequent transforming growth factor (TGFβ) insufficiency, to identify changes in gene expression associated with phenotype progression. The most differentially expressed gene in the lungs of emphysematous β6 integrin–deficient mice was identified as matrix metallo-proteinase 12 (MMP-12), a gene shown to be expressed in human emphysema (75–77) and necessary for emphysema in response to chronic cigarette smoke exposure in mice (78). The identification of MMP-12 in this dataset provided novel insight, which was confirmed by showing rescue of the emphysematous phenotype in β6 integrin/MMP-12 compound mutant mice. Rangasamy et al. (79) investigated the effects of both smoke exposure and genetic susceptibility to emphysema, due to deficiency in the transcriptional regulator, Nrf2, upon gene expression in the lung. They identified a cluster of cigarette smoke-induced, Nrf2-dependent genes that were primarily involved in protecting cells from oxidative stress. In an interesting recent report, Woodruff et al. (80) performed expression profiling of alveolar macrophages from smokers and compared gene expression with two animal models of emphysema (IL-13 transgenic and β6 integrin deficient). They identified a single gene, MMP-12, which was dysregulated in all three systems.

Recently, DeMeo et al. (81) used an integrative genomics approach to identify a novel COPD candidate–susceptibility gene. Previous genome-wide linkage studies by the group had identified a number of loci potentially harboring COPD genes (82,83). By investigating existing microarray data sets, the investigators implicated the gene encoding serine protease inhibitor clade E, number 2 (SERPINE2). SERPINE2 was identified as a biologically plausible candidate within one of the loci, due to its pattern of expression in a microarray data set describing lung development (84). Further support for this candidate was provided by the analysis of a data set generated from tis-sue samples obtained from patients with severe emphysema (69). These data revealed significant correlations of SERPINE2 gene expression with quanti-tative lung function measurements representative of COPD phenotypes. Subsequent genetics studies showed significant association between multiple SERPINE2 allelic markers (SNPs) and COPD diagnosis in the family-based population used to define the initial linkage data as well as a case–control population. While disease-specific mutations in the SERPINE2 gene were not reported, this study represents the potential for microarray application in the search for genes conferring susceptibility to complex traits. Both the integration of genetics and genome-wide expression profiling and the use of preexisting microarray data are likely to be common practice for identifying disease-susceptibility/modifying genes.

VII. Challenges and Opportunities for Future Applications

While the application of DNA microarray technology to lung disease research has seen its share of successes as well as failures, clear challenges and real opportunities lay ahead. For the most part, application of the technology has just begun to scratch the tip of the iceberg of potential in the reporting of genes differentially expressed in diseased versus nondisease patients or between conditions of disease models. Tremendous opportunities still exist to define and understand asthma and COPD at a level previously unthinkable. For instance, genome-wide expression profiling retains the potential to define at the molecular level the phenotypic heterogeneity among patients with COPD and the variable responsiveness of asthma patients to the many available therapies.

As the lung is difficult to sample in order to obtain tissue, improvements in some aspects of the technology are necessary to realize its full potential. In this regard, there is reason to remain optimistic. For instance, new techniques are becoming available to allow microarray analysis of smaller biological samples (< 50 ng total RNA). Laser-capture microdissection, though time consuming and laborious in a complex tissue such as the lung, enables the purification of individual cell types that can considerably limit sampling variability. Other technologies are being tested, which would allow the analysis of fixed or otherwise degraded RNA, such as that derived from archival pathology samples. However, many challenges still exist. Many pulmonary cell types, such as alveolar epithelial cells or parenchymal endothelial cells, cannot be purified using current laser capture microdissection (LCM) technology due to limitations in laser resolution. Further, ambitious hopes to molecularly dissect the signature of individual cell types in a microarray data set comprising a complex (multicellular) biological sample have not been realized.

One of the largest potentials to be realized in the future application of microarray technology relates to one of the current biggest concerns, lack of consistency between studies. Although many factors contribute to this problem (such as real population differences between studies), as previously mentioned, this is likely due in large part to two factors: (i) inconsistency in measurement accuracy across studies and (ii) studies of insufficient sample size. Once again, active research in both of these areas promises to significantly limit these problems. A number of studies have helped to identify and catalog accuracies/inaccuracies in the design of specific microarray probes (13,14). Additionally, it has been clearly shown that experimental findings from similar studies are more highly correlated when probe accuracy is considered (15–17).

Other research in bioinformatics has addressed the issue of sample size insufficiency by promoting methods to compile data from multiple sources/studies. This is not a trivial task because variability in microarray technology, data structure, and normalization methods severely limit translatability of gene expression level results (85). Bhattacharya and Mariani (86) recently described a relatively simple, but effective means of translating data across platforms and studies. Using sequence matching of probes

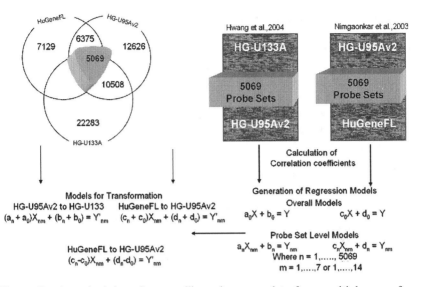

Figure 3 A methodology for compiling microarray data from multiple array formats. An approach was developed to allow the compilation of data from multiple studies performed on more than one array/platform. Probe sequence information is used to confirm measurements on different platforms correspond to the same transcript. A linear regression model, derived from datasets where replicate measurements of the same RNA samples were performed on the relevant arrays, is used to define a transformation procedure. This method was shown to improve correlation in signal intensity measurements and promote sample clustering based upon biological (sample type) rather than technical attributes (array used). *Source*: From Ref. 86.

across generations of Affymetrix platforms, combined with regression modeling of signal intensity measurements made from a set of samples on the multiple platforms, a data integration/transformation method was developed. The methodology was successful in the transformation of signal intensities to allow cluster analysis of data from multiple studies performed on different platforms according to their biological (lung cancer vs. normal lung) rather than technical attributes. Shah et al. (87) have developed a database specific for microarray data sets concerning the effects of cigarette smoke exposure upon lung tissue, termed "smoking-induced epithelial gene expression database." This database is useful for the compilation and thorough analysis of relevant data sets using current, state-of-the-art methods.

Finally, it is worth noting that, in addition to data compilation, the utility of consortia is being realized as a means to design and implement appropriate size genome-wide expression profiling studies of asthma and COPD. This is particularly true in the case of asthma research, where the interest in pharmacogenetics has spurred the development of consortia such as the Severe Asthma Research Network and the Pharmacogenetics

Research Network. Each of these groups of highly collaborative teams provides the opportunity to share patient samples and fund studies of sufficient size. COPD researchers have the opportunity to follow suit with the long-term existence of the National Emphysema Treatment Trial and the inception of the COPD Research Network. That these collaborative networks of researchers are capable of working together to maximize the potential of this technology is a highly anticipated desire which could revolutionize these fields as much as the advent of histological pathology.

References

1. Iyer VR, Eisen MB, Ross DT, et al. The transcriptional program in the response of human fibroblasts to serum. Science 1999; 283(5398):83–87.
2. Golub TR, Slonim DK, Tamayo P, et al. Molecular classification of cancer: class discovery and class prediction by gene expression monitoring. Science 1999; 286(5439):531–537.
3. Shalon D, Smith SJ, Brown PO. A DNA microarray system for analyzing complex DNA samples using two-color fluorescent probe hybridization. Genome Res 1996; 6(7):639–645.
4. Schena M, Shalon D, Davis RW, et al. Quantitative monitoring of gene expression patterns with a complementary DNA microarray. Science 1995; 270(5235): 467–470.
5. Schena M, Shalon D, Heller R, et al. Parallel human genome analysis: microarray-based expression monitoring of 1000 genes. Proc Natl Acad Sci USA 1996; 93(20):10614–10619.
6. Shalon D. Gene expression micro-arrays: a new tool for genomic research. Pathol Biol (Paris) 1998; 46(2):107–109.
7. Chee M, Yang R, Hubbell E, et al. Accessing genetic information with high-density DNA arrays. Science 1996; 274(5287):610–614.
8. Lockhart DJ, Dong H, Byrne MC, et al. Expression monitoring by hybridization to high-density oligonucleotide arrays. Nat Biotechnol 1996; 14(13):1675–1680.
9. Lipshutz RJ, Fodor SP, Gingeras TR, et al. High density synthetic oligonucleotide arrays. Nat Genet 1999; 21(Suppl 1):20–24.
10. Kane MD, Jatkoe TA, Stumpf CR, et al. Assessment of the sensitivity and specificity of oligonucleotide (50mer) microarrays. Nucleic Acids Res 2000; 28(22): 4552–4557.
11. Barczak A, Rodriguez MW, Hanspers K, et al. Spotted long oligonucleotide arrays for human gene expression analysis. Genome Res 2003; 13(7):1775–1785.
12. Hughes TR, Mao M, Jones AR, et al. Expression profiling using microarrays fabricated by an ink-jet oligonucleotide synthesizer. Nat Biotechnol 2001; 19(4): 342–347.
13. Mecham BH, Wetmore DZ, Szallasi Z, et al. Increased measurement accuracy for sequence-verified microarray probes. Physiol Genomics 2004; 18(3):308–315.
14. Gautier L, Moller M, Friis-Hansen L, et al. Alternative mapping of probes to genes for Affymetrix chips. BMC Bioinformatics 2004; 5:111.

15. Barnes M, Freudenberg J, Thompson S, et al. Experimental comparison and cross-validation of the Affymetrix and Illumina gene expression analysis platforms. Nucleic Acids Res 2005; 33(18):5914–5923.

16. Mecham BH, Klus GT, Strovel J, et al. Sequence-matched probes produce increased cross-platform consistency and more reproducible biological results in microarray-based gene expression measurements. Nucleic Acids Res 2004; 32(9):e74.

17. Stec J, Wang J, Coombes K, et al. Comparison of the predictive accuracy of DNA array-based multigene classifiers across cDNA arrays and Affymetrix GeneChips. J Mol Diagn 2005; 7(3):357–367.

18. Sebastiani P, Gussoni E, Kohane IS, et al. Statistical challenges in functional genomics (with discussion). Stat Science 2003; 18(1):33–70.

19. Kohane IS, Kho AT, Butte AS. Microarrays for an Integrative Genomics. Cambridge, MA: MIT Press, 2002.

20. Smyth GK, Speed T. Normalization of cDNA microarray data. Methods. 2003; 31(4):265–273.

21. Chen Y, Dougherty ER, Bittner ML. Ratio-based decisions and the quantitative analysis of cDNA microarray images. Biomedical Optics 1997; 2:364–374.

22. Schadt EE, Li C, Su C, et al. Analyzing high-density oligonucleotide gene expression array data. J Cell Biochem 2000; 80(2):192–202.

23. Affymetrix Inc., Statistical Algorithms Description Document, Santa Clara, CA:Affymetrix Inc. 2002.

24. Sabatti C, Karsten SL, Geschwind DH. Thresholding rules for recovering a sparse signal from microarray experiments. Math Biosci 2002; 176(1):17–34.

25. Newton MA, Kendziorski CM, Richmond CS, et al. On differential variability of expression ratios: improving statistical inference about gene expression changes from microarray data. J Comput Biol 2001; 8(1):37–52.

26. Lee ML, Kuo FC, Whitmore GA, et al. Importance of replication in microarray gene expression studies: statistical methods and evidence from repetitive cDNA hybridizations. Proc Natl Acad Sci USA 2000; 97(18):9834–9839.

27. Kerr MK, Churchill GA. Statistical design and the analysis of gene expression microarray data. Genet Res 2001; 77(2):123–128.

28. Wolfinger RD, Gibson G, Wolfinger ED, et al. Assessing gene significance from cDNA microarray expression data via mixed models. J Comput Biol 2001; 8(6):625–637.

29. Tusher VG, Tibshirani R, Chu G. Significance analysis of microarrays applied to the ionizing radiation response. Proc Natl Acad Sci USA 2001; 98(9): 5116–5121.

30. West M, Blanchette C, Dressman H, et al. Predicting the clinical status of human breast cancer by using gene expression profiles. Proc Natl Acad Sci USA 2001; 98(20):11462–11467.

31. Lakhani SR, Ashworth A. Microarray and histopathological analysis of tumours: the future and the past? Nat Rev Cancer 2001; 1(2):151–157.

32. McCullagh P, Nelder J. Generalized Linear Models. London: Chapman and Hall, 1989.

33. Ramoni MF, Sebastiani P. Bayesian methods. In: Berthold M, Hand DJ, eds. Intelligent Data Analysis: An Introduction. New York: Springer, 2003:128–166.

34. Hand DJ. Construction and assessment of classification rules. In: Chichester. UK: John Wiley and sons, 1997.
35. Tamayo P, Slonim D, Mesirov J, et al. Interpreting patterns of gene expression with self-organizing maps: methods and application to hematopoietic differentiation. Proc Natl Acad Sci USA 1999; 96(6):2907–2912.
36. Alizadeh AA, Eisen MB, Davis RE, et al. Distinct types of diffuse large B-cell lymphoma identified by gene expression profiling. Nature 2000; 403(6769): 503–511.
37. Eisen MB, Spellman PT, Brown PO, et al. Cluster analysis and display of genome-wide expression patterns. Proc Natl Acad Sci USA 1998; 95(25):14,863–14,868.
38. Bittner M, Meltzer P, Chen Y, et al. Molecular classification of cutaneous malignant melanoma by gene expression profiling. Nature 2000; 406(6795):536–540.
39. Sorlie T, Perou CM, Tibshirani R, et al. Gene expression patterns of breast carcinomas distinguish tumor subclasses with clinical implications. Proc Natl Acad Sci USA 2001; 98(19):10,869–10,874.
40. Bhattacharjee A, Richards WG, Staunton J, et al. Classification of human lung carcinomas by mRNA expression profiling reveals distinct adenocarcinoma subclasses. Proc Natl Acad Sci USA 2001; 98(24):13,790–13,795.
41. Kerr MK, Churchill GA. Bootstrapping cluster analysis: assessing the reliability of conclusions from microarray experiments. Proc Natl Acad Sci USA 2001; 98(16):8961–8965.
42. Tibshirani R, Walther G, Hastie T. Estimating the number of clusters in a data set via the gap statistic. J Roy Stat Soc Ser B Stat Methodol 2001; 63:411–423.
43. Butte AJ, Tamayo D, Slonim D, et al. Discovering functional relationships between RNA expression and chemotherapeutic susceptibility using relevance networks. Proc Natl Acad Sci USA 2000; 97:12,182–12,186.
44. Tavazoie S, Hughes JD, Campbell MJ, et al. Systematic determination of genetic network architecture. Nat Genet 1999; 22(3):281–285.
45. Holter NS, Maritan A, Cieplak M, et al. Dynamic modeling of gene expression data. Proc Natl Acad Sci USA 2001; 98(4):1693–1698.
46. Alter O, Brown PO, Botstein D. Singular value decomposition for genome-wide expression data processing and modeling. Proc Natl Acad Sci USA 2000; 97: 10,101–10,106.
47. Ramoni MF, Sebastiani P, Kohane IS. Cluster analysis of gene expression dynamics. Proc Natl Acad Sci USA 2002; 99(14):9121–9126.
48. Tzouvelekis A, Patlakas G, Bouros D. Application of microarray technology in pulmonary diseases. Respir Res 2004; 5(1):26.
49. Erle DJ, Yang YH. Asthma investigators begin to reap the fruits of genomics. Genome Biol 2003; 4(11):232.
50. Rolph MS, Sisavanh M, Liu SM, et al. Clues to asthma pathogenesis from microarray expression studies. Pharmacol Ther 2005.
51. Lilly CM, Tateno H, Oguma T, et al. Effects of allergen challenge on airway epithelial cell gene expression. Am J Respir Crit Care Med 2005; 171(6):579–586.
52. Lee JH, Kaminski N, Dolganov G, et al. Interleukin-13 induces dramatically different transcriptional programs in three human airway cell types. Am J Respir Cell Mol Biol 2001; 25(4):474–485.

53. Wei C, Li J, Bumgarner RE. Sample size for detecting differentially expressed genes in microarray experiments. BMC Genomics 2004; 5(1):87.
54. Yang MC, Yang JJ, Mclndoe RA, et al. Microarray experimental design: power and sample size considerations. Physiol Genomics 2003; 16(1):24–28.
55. Brutsche MH, Joos L, Carlen Brutsche IE, et al. Array-based diagnostic gene-expression score for atopy and asthma. J Allergy Clin Immunol 2002; 109(2): 271–273.
56. Hansel NN, Hilmer SC, Georas SN, et al. Oligonucleotide-microarray analysis of peripheral-blood lymphocytes in severe asthma. J Lab Clin Med 2005; 145(5):263–274.
57. Zimmermann N, King NE, Laporte J, et al. Dissection of experimental asthma with DNA microarray analysis identifies arginase in asthma pathogenesis. J Clin Invest 2003; 111(12):1863–1874.
58. Meurs H, Hamer MA, Pethe S, et al. Modulation of cholinergic airway reactivity and nitric oxide production by endogenous arginase activity. Br J Pharmacol 2000; 130(8):1793–1798.
59. Morris CR, Poljakovic M, Lavrisha L, et al. Decreased arginine bioavailability and increased serum arginase activity in asthma. Am J Respir Crit Care Med 2004; 170(2):148–153.
60. Karp CL, Grupe A, Schadt E, et al. Identification of complement factor 5 as a susceptibility locus for experimental allergic asthma. Nat Immunol 2000; 1(3): 221–226.
61. Hasegawa K, Tamari M, Shao C, et al. Variations in the C3, C3a receptor, and C5 genes affect susceptibility to bronchial asthma. Hum Genet 2004; 115(4): 295–301.
62. Laprise C, Sladek R, Ponton A, et al. Functional classes of bronchial mucosa genes that are differentially expressed in asthma. BMC Genomics 2004; 5(1):21.
63. Hakonarson H, Halapi E, Whelan R, et al. Association between IL-1beta/TNF-alpha-induced glucocorticoid-sensitive changes in multiple gene expression and altered responsiveness in airway smooth muscle. Am J Respir Cell Mol Biol 2001; 25(6):761–771.
64. Hakonarson H, Bjornsdottir US, Halapi E, et al. Profiling of genes expressed in peripheral blood mononuclear cells predicts glucocorticoid sensitivity in asthma patients. Proc Natl Acad Sci USA 2005; 102(41):14,789–14,794.
65. Institute N.H.L.a.B. Data Fact Sheet: Chronic Obstructive Pulmonary Disease. U.S. Department of Health and Human Services NIH, NHLBI, 2002.
66. Zhang W, Yan SD, Zhu A, et al. Expression of Egr-1 in late stage emphysema. Am J Pathol 2000; 157(4):1311–1320.
67. Golpon HA, Geraci MW, Moore MD, et al. HOX genes in human lung: altered expression in primary pulmonary hypertension and emphysema. Am J Pathol 2001; 158(3):955–966.
68. Ning W, Li CJ, Kaminski N, et al. Comprehensive gene expression profiles reveal pathways related to the pathogenesis of chronic obstructive pulmonary disease. Proc Natl Acad Sci USA 2004; 101(41):14,895–14,900.
69. Spira A, Beane J, Pinto-Plata V, et al. Gene expression profiling of human lung tissue from smokers with severe emphysema. Am J Respir Cell Mol Biol 2004; 31(6):601–610.

70. Golpon HA, Coldren CD, Zamora MR, et al. Emphysema lung tissue gene expression profiling. Am J Respir Cell Mol Biol 2004; 31(6):595–600.
71. Hackett NR, Heguy A, Harvey BG, et al. Variability of antioxidant-related gene expression in the airway epithelium of cigarette smokers. Am J Respir Cell Mol Biol 2003; 29(3 Pt 1):331–343.
72. Spira A, Beane J, Shah V, et al. Effects of cigarette smoke on the human airway epithelial cell transcriptome. Proc Natl Acad Sci USA 2004; 101(27):10,143–10,148.
73. Fuke S, Betsuyaku T, Nasuhara Y, et al. Chemokines in bronchiolar epithelium in the development of chronic obstructive pulmonary disease. Am J Respir Cell Mol Biol 2004; 31(4):405–412.
74. Morris DG, Huang X, Kaminski N, et al. Loss of integrin alpha(v)beta6-mediated TGF-beta activation causes Mmp12-dependent emphysema. Nature 2003; 422(6928):169–173.
75. Demedts IK, Morel-Montero A, Lebecque S, et al. Elevated MMP-12 protein levels in induced sputum from COPD patients. Thorax 2005.
76. Molet S, Belleguic C, Lena H, et al. Increase in macrophage elastase (MMP-12) in lungs from patients with chronic obstructive pulmonary disease. Inflamm Res 2005; 54(1):31–36.
77. Grumelli S, Corry DB, Song LZ, et al. An immune basis for lung parenchymal destruction in chronic obstructive pulmonary disease and emphysema. PLoS Med 2004; 1(1):e8.
78. Hautamaki RD, Kobayashi DK, Senior RM, et al. Requirement for macrophage elastase for cigarette smoke-induced emphysema in mice. Science 1997; 277(5334):2002–2004.
79. Rangasamy T, Cho CY, Thimmulappa RK, et al. Genetic ablation of Nrf2 enhances susceptibility to cigarette smoke-induced emphysema in mice. J Clin Invest 2004; 114(9):1248–1259.
80. Woodruff PG, Koth LL, Yang YH, et al. A distinctive alveolar macrophage activation state induced by cigarette smoking. Am J Respir Crit Care Med 2005; 172(11):1383–1392.
81. DeMeo DL, Mariani TJ, Lange C, et al. The SERPINE2 gene is associated with chronic obstructive pulmonary disease. Am J Hum Genet 2006; 78(2):253–264.
82. Silverman EK, Mosley JD, Palmer LJ, et al. Genome-wide linkage analysis of severe, early-onset chronic obstructive pulmonary disease: airflow obstruction and chronic bronchitis phenotypes. Hum Mol Genet 2002; 11(6):623–632.
83. Silverman EK, Palmer LJ, Mosley JD, et al. Genomewide linkage analysis of quantitative spirometric phenotypes in severe early-onset chronic obstructive pulmonary disease. Am J Hum Genet 2002; 70(5):1229–1239.
84. Mariani TJ, Reed JJ, Shapiro SD. Expression profiling of the developing mouse lung: insights into the establishment of the extracellular matrix. Am J Respir Cell Mol Biol 2002; 26(5):541–548.
85. Jarvinen AK, Hautaniemi S, Edgren H, et al. Are data from different gene expression microarray platforms comparable? Genomics 2004; 83(6):1164–1168.
86. Bhattacharya S, Mariani TJ. Transformation of expression intensities across generations of Affymetrix microarrays using sequence matching and regression modeling. Nucleic Acids Res 2005; 33(18):e157.

87. Shah V, Sridhar S, Beane J, et al. SIEGE: Smoking Induced Epithelial Gene Expression Database. Nucleic Acids Res 2005; 33(Database issue):D573–D579.

88. Wills-Karp M, Ewart SL. Time to draw breath: asthma-susceptibility genes are identified. Nat Rev Genet 2004; 5(5):376–387.

89. http://rana.lbl.gov

90. http://www.axon.com

91. http://www.packardbioscience.com

92. http://www.affymetrix.com

93. http://www.broad.mit.edu/cancer/software/genepattern

94. http://www-stat.stanford.edu/~tibs/SAM

95. http://rana.lbl.gov

96. http://www.genomethods.org/caged

6

Mouse Models for Asthma and Mouse Asthma Genetics

BENOIT PIAVAUX and
ANTOON J. M. VAN OOSTEROUT

MACHTELD N. HYLKEMA

Laboratory of Allergology and Pulmonary Diseases, and Department of Pathology and Laboratory Medicine, University Medical Center Groningen, University of Groningen, Groningen, The Netherlands

Department of Pathology and Laboratory Medicine, University Medical Center Groningen, University of Groningen, Groningen, The Netherlands

I. Introduction

Allergic asthma is a heterogeneous disease, which can be characterized by high levels of allergen-specific immunoglobulin (Ig)E in serum, chronic eosinophilic inflammation of the airway tissue and hyperreactivity of the airways (AHR) to bronchospasmogenic stimuli. Genetic susceptibility to asthma appears to be due to multiple genes that interact with each other and the environment. Although genetic linkage and association studies have identified many susceptibility loci for specific asthma traits and identified a number of susceptibility genes, fine-mapping and identification of all the genes involved in asthma-related traits may prove to be extremely difficult not in the least part due to epistatic interactions. Yet, in order to understand the genetic basis of asthma, it is important to identify as many different susceptibility genes as possible and to determine their interactions. Although an animal model of asthma may not exhibit all aspects of human disease, identification of genes involved in certain well-defined characteristics may accelerate further human studies. Given the considerable homology between the human and mouse genome, the mouse may prove to be a useful genetic model organism for complex human diseases. Furthermore, genetic homogeneity and strictly controlled developmental (age) and environmental (infection, food, and climate) conditions are major advantages of a mouse model, as well as the fact that the mouse "toolbox" (gene-targeted mice and genetic and physical map) is very well developed. The possibility to generate congenic lines makes it possible to determine if the phenotypic effect of a locus is caused by one gene or by a combination of multiple closely linked genes at the locus, something that cannot be done in humans.

An illustration of the relevance of comparative genetics is the quantitative trait loci (QTL), which determine plasma lipid concentrations, risk factors for atherosclerosis, in mice and humans. Most of the human QTLs-controlling plasma lipids have concordant QTLs in mice, suggesting that many genes identified in mice may also regulate the same traits in humans (1). Furthermore, if a gene controlling an experimental asthma trait in mice is not genetically linked to asthma in humans, understanding the biological function of this gene and the pathway leading to the asthma trait in mice may still be relevant for asthma in humans. In this chapter, we will discuss some of the mouse models for experimental asthma and the genetic tools available to study asthma genetics in the mouse. Furthermore, genetic studies of asthma-related traits in the mouse will be discussed.

II. Mouse Models for Asthma

A. Allergens

Various allergens including ovalbumin (OVA), house dust mite (HDM), and *Aspergillus fumigatus* are being used in the mouse in an attempt to provide insights into the complex immunological and pathophysiological mechanisms of human IgE-mediated allergic diseases.

Ovalbumin

In the majority of current models for allergic airway inflammation, OVA is used as a model allergen, though it is a food, instead of an aeroallergen. In most protocols, mice are sensitized by an intraperitoneal (i.p.) injection of OVA, often together with a Th2-skewing adjuvant such as aluminium hydroxide (2). Sensitization in itself induces the production of OVA-specific IgE-resembling allergic sensitization in atopic individuals.

Sensitized animals can subsequently be exposed to allergen, administered to the target organ, the lung, via inhalation, intranasal, or intratracheal routes. The mouse is not the most suitable model to measure immediate bronchoconstrictive responses upon allergen provocation, although a small bronchoconstrictive reaction can be measured, which is associated with mast-cell degranulation (3,4). Furthermore, the late-phase bronchoconstriction is absent or mild compared to the response in patients with allergic asthma (4,5).

Without prior systemic sensitization, repeated exposure to aerosolized OVA results in inhalation tolerance and no or very low serum levels of OVA-specific IgE (6,7). Following repeated airway allergen challenge, OVA-sensitized mice gradually develop AHR and recruit eosinophils, T-cells, and some neutrophils into the airways, which can be monitored by histologic examination of airway tissue, bronchoalveolar lavage (BAL), or single-cell suspension after enzymatic digestion of lung tissue (5). Th2 cytokines such as interleukin (IL)-4, IL-5, and IL-13 can be measured in BAL fluid (8,9) or upon antigenic restimulation of thoracic lymph node cells (10).

AHR is most often determined in response to the acetylcholine analogue, methacholine, but other nonspecific bronchospasmogenic agents such as serotonin have also been used (11). Different methods to measure airway constriction and AHR in the mouse have been described as reviewed by Drazen et al. (12). Whole-body barometric plethysmography, which determines the empirical variable "enhance pause," has become extremely popular during the last decade because of its ease of use; however, criticism regarding this technique has been accumulating (13). At present, this technique is no longer recommended, unless as a preliminary technique for screening purposes. Fortunately, other techniques are available, such as the airway pressure time index (APTI), forced oscillations, and the classic approach of measuring dynamic lung compliance and resistance (12).

Importantly, most of the OVA mouse models described in the literature show differences with respect to levels of airway inflammation and AHR. This is probably due to the fact that mouse models differ with respect to the genetic background of the mice, the route, dose and frequency of exposure to the allergen, and the type of adjuvant being used. In particular, the route of OVA administration has an important impact on the quality of the immune response. Development of allergic airway disease can also be induced by the administration of antigen-pulsed dendritic cells into the airways following limited inhaled allergen exposure (14). However, virtually all of the protocols, which avoid systemic sensitization with adjuvant, elicit less-prominent airway inflammation when compared to sensitization with adjuvant. Importantly, the percentage of eosinophils in BAL of patients with allergic asthma ($\sim$ 5–20%) is more close to the percentages observed in models without adjuvant (20%) than those with alum as adjuvant (50–80%) (2,15). One has to be aware that there are no perfect mouse models that fully reflect all aspects of human asthma.

House Dust Mite

HDM are the most common sources of aeroallergens, which, in genetic susceptible individuals, can cause symptoms ranging from atopic dermatitis to bronchial asthma. In Europe, *Dermatophagoides pteronyssinus* (*Der p*) is the most frequently encountered HDM, and their fecal particles contain several groups of molecules acting as allergen. The most important is *Der p* 1, a cysteine protease derived from the mite's intestinal tract (16,17). A number of studies have demonstrated that *Der p* 1 is capable of cleaving human proteins with potentially immunomodulatory effects including α1-proteinase inhibitor (18), CD23 (the human low-affinity IgE receptor) (19), CD25 (the α subunit of the IL-2 receptor) (20), and tight junctions of bronchial epithelium, leading to increased bronchial epithelial permeability (21). In contrast to the OVA model, in which robust allergic sensitization relies on the introduction of OVA in the peritoneum in conjunction with an adjuvant, for HDM it has been shown that intranasal exposure generated acute (22) as well as chronic (23) airway inflammation and AHR to methacholine, with the characteristic hallmarks of a Th2-type immune-inflammatory response. Interestingly, a recent study showed that HDM facilitates OVA-specific allergic sensitization and airway inflammation (24). In order to study the impact of concurrent allergen exposure on the development of allergic responses, mice were exposed to HDM concurrently with OVA for five weeks. Subsequently, mice were allowed to rest for eight weeks, at which time they were then reexposed to aerosolized OVA alone. This in vivo OVA recall elicited a robust airway inflammatory response in the lung but also systemically (OVA-specific IgE). Collectively, these data demonstrate that HDM is able to subvert OVA's intrinsic innocuous nature and to privilege a Th2 inflammatory response over the default tolerogenic bias.

HDM is also used in a protocol in which mice are sensitized with an i.p. injection of HDM/aluminium hydroxide and exposed to HDM via trachea instillation (25,26).

Aspergillus fumigatus

Among the allergic fungi, *A. fumigatus*, a saprophytic mold, distributed widely in the environment, is a frequently recognized etiologic agent in a number of allergic conditions. Inhalation of *A. fumigatus* antigens complicates a number of pulmonary diseases ranging from infective (invasive aspergillosis), allergic bronchopulmonary aspergillosis, and allergic exacerbation of asthma. Allergic responses to *A. fumigatus* involve a number of immunologic abnormalities including elevated IgE, enhanced Th2 cytokines such as IL-4, IL-5, and IL-13 (27), eosinophilic and T-cell inflammation, AHR to methacholine, and profound airway remodeling (28). Currently over 20 recombinant allergens from *A. fumigatus* have been cloned and expressed. However, in spite of the recombinant antigens available in pure form, soluble, crude *A. fumigatus* antigen extract is still most commonly used for the induction of allergic airway disease by intranasal instillation in animals (29). Crude extracts are highly antigenic and contain biologically active substances such as ribotoxin and proteases (30). In the models for *A. fumigatus*–induced allergic airway inflammation, potent sensitization to the extract occurs in the absence of exogenous adjuvants. Enzymes such as proteases may serve as adjuvants, perhaps, by inducing epithelial damage and allowing normally excluded antigens to bypass the mucosal barrier (30).

B. Gender

A striking common feature of many autoimmune and inflammatory diseases is that females are more susceptible to specific immunological disorders than males (31). In general, females have better B-cell–mediated immunity than age-matched male counterparts. They have higher Ig levels and stronger antibody responses to various foreign antigens (32,33). For asthma, it also has been described that, after puberty, asthma occurs more frequently among women who also have a higher risk of more severe asthma (34,35). We have used an OVA mouse model of allergic airway inflammation to characterize gender differences in mice, with respect to the local immune response in the lung (36). We found that female mice are evidently more susceptible to allergic airway inflammation than males. They have higher numbers of eosinophils and (activated) T-cells and B-cells in lung tissue. In addition, they have higher levels of IL-4, IL-5, and IL-13 in lung homogenates. Serum levels of total and OVA-specific IgE were also higher in females than in males. Our study is in accordance with Hayashi who also found a clear difference with respect to eosinophilia (37) and studies from Seymour et al. and Corteling et al. who both found elevated IgE levels in female mice sensitized and challenged with OVA as compared to males sensitized and challenged with OVA (38,39). Preliminary data from our group indicate that gender differences in mice with respect to allergic airway inflammation also exist in a HDM mouse model of asthma (Hylkema et al. manuscript in preparation).

C. Models for Chronic Airway Inflammation and Hyperreactivity

Typical features of asthma are recurrent episodes of airway inflammation and airway obstruction, and some patients experience a gradual decline in lung function and fixed obstruction. These fixed alterations have been attributed to structural changes in the airways, which are apparent on histologic sections and have been termed "airway remodeling." To create a chronic model with features of airway remodeling, different approaches have been tried, mainly by sustaining airway challenges over weeks to months following the initial acute response. However, there have been relatively few descriptions of satisfactory mouse models of chronic antigenic challenge associated with airway inflammation and remodeling resembling human asthma. Experimental protocols have involved repeated exposure by OVA inhalation (40,41) and repeated bolus delivery of antigen intratracheally using OVA (42) or *A. fumigatus* (29) or intranasally using OVA (43) or HDM (23). In these chronic mouse models, marked inflammatory processes, mucus hypersecretion, epithelial cell hyperplasia, and thickening of the basement membrane are found in the bronchi in response to repeated airway challenges with the allergen. However, in most chronic models, structural changes in the proximal airways have been described, and structural changes in small airways were usually absent. Recently, a protocol was developed by the group of Renz that demonstrated chronic allergic inflammation of both proximal and distal airways (44). Airway inflammation was associated with subepithelial fibrosis, goblet cell hyperplasia, and increased mass of α-smooth muscle actin-positive cells in small airways. Furthermore, the inflammatory and structural changes in this model were associated with stable airflow limitation and increased AHR. Interestingly, compared with acute allergic inflammation, the chronic inflammation was dominated by lymphocytes and not by eosinophils.

Assessment of chronic changes in the airways and lung tissue cannot be quantitated without very careful tissue preparation and morphometry. Given discrepancies in methodological approaches, problems of tolerance induction and issues related to differences among certain strains and allergens, more thorough studies of "chronic" models, are needed to critically judge their applicability and usefulness.

III. Mouse Asthma Genetics

A. Mouse Toolbox for Gene-Hunting

For geneticists, inbred mouse strains are powerful tools to identify new disease-related genes. Each mouse is "completely" homozygous and genetically identical to all other mice of the same strain, and the environment can be controlled throughout the experiments. Additionally, mice can be crossed at discretion of the investigator, and they have a very short generation time, three weeks gestation and eight weeks to sexual maturity.

In human genetics, linkage, association, and DNA microarray studies are the only tools available. These tools were also extensively used in mice. However, in mice, other approaches are possible. For example, recombinant inbred (RI) and recombinant congenic (RC) strains, which are derived from two inbred strains, have shown to be a powerful tool in the identification of QTLs in all kind of multigenic diseases and traits (45,46). Another interesting technique is transgenesis with artificial chromosomes, by which effects of human loci can be investigated in mice (47).

As there is almost no genetic or phenotypic variation within one strain, all genetic and phenotypic variation has to be introduced by outcrossing two inbred mouse strains. The selection of these two mouse strains is critical. There are many mouse strains, but only few are regularly used for genetics. These are well-characterized strains, from which single nucleotide polymorphisms (SNP) and microsatellite markers polymorphisms are known. The best option is to phenotype these strains first. If no phenotypic difference in the trait of interest is found in these well-known strains, other strains can be screened. Choosing strains with extreme phenotypic differences can make phenotyping easier and linkage or association analysis more powerful.

Induced mutagenesis was widely used in the genetics of microorganisms and *Caenorhabditis elegans* and can also be used in mice. As part of the Program for Genetic Applications (PGA) project of the NHLBI (48), the Jackson Laboratory is screening *N*-ethyl-*N*-nitrosourea (ENU)-induced mutants for naïve AHR and other heart, lung, and blood disease-related phenotypes (49). Direct comparison of both mutant and wild-type strains is difficult because there is not enough genetic variability between both strains for classical mapping methods (linkage, association, RC, and RI strains). Without introducing genetic variability by outcrossing with another inbred strain only microarray comparisons and sequencing can be used to identify the mutation. By outcrossing both mutant and wild-type strains with the same strain, the mutation can be mapped using conventional techniques. As the only difference between both mapping experiments is the presence of a mutation in one of the parental strains, the differences in results can only be due to this mutation and experimental variability. The mutant strain can of course also be used as any other inbred strain in conventional mapping experiments. Despite these mapping difficulties, a big advantage of ENU-induced mutagenesis is that it can lead to new interesting mutations which are not present in any inbred strains. The biggest advantage, however, is that mutant strains are a very powerful tool to study the biological implications of the mutation, once it is mapped and identified.

Linkage and Association Analysis

Linkage and association studies have massively been performed in human and mouse to identify genes involved in multigenic traits. In mice, these studies are largely facilitated by the short generation time with large nest sizes and the homozygous genotypes. However, less resolution is obtained due to twice as low recombination frequencies in mice compared to human.

The power of the analysis can be increased by selecting strains with extreme phenotypic differences or by the selection of the extreme phenotypes for analysis.

DNA Microarray Experiments

DNA microarray experiments have become a powerful tool to explore the transcriptome. As RNA levels are measured, functional mutations, which do not lead to altered RNA expression levels, cannot be detected.

Microarrays have also been used in combined approaches. The expression QTL (eQTL) strategy is a good example, which is described below (50).

Recombinant Congenic and Recombinant Inbred Strains

Both RI and RC strains are obtained by outcrossing two inbred strains (46). In RI strains, offspring is intercrossed (heterozygote × heterozygote) a few times, and part of the offspring is then inbred in order to obtain a series of strains that contain a random 50% of the donor genome. For RC strains, two backcrosses (heterozygote offspring × homozygote parental) are done with one of the parental strains (the background strain) in order to reduce the fraction of genome inherited from the donor strain to 12.5% (Fig. 1). Generally an RC series of strains is composed of approximately 20 strains.

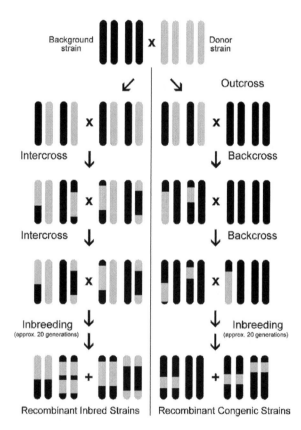

Figure 1 Breeding scheme for recombinant inbred strains and recombinant congenic strains. Only two chromosome pairs showed.

Mapping loci with RC strains is easy and straightforward. The strains from which the genotype is known, and thus also the genomic fragments inherited from the donor strain, are all phenotyped.

The loci of interest are the chromosomal fragments inherited from the donor strain in the strains with the donor's phenotype. Fine-mapping can be done by the analysis of the overlapping regions and by backcrossing with the background strain to obtain more recombination in the region of interest.

RI strains can be used for mapping in the same way as RC strains, but it will require more backcrossing because 50% of the genome is donor inherited compared to 12.5% in RC strains. RI strains are also a very good starting point for association analysis because many intercrosses were already done before inbreeding.

For this, RI strains can be outcrossed, but, generally, it is preferred to backcross them, especially when recessive traits are studied. Backcrossing with the parental strain carrying the recessive allele will raise the fraction of genome of this strain and by this the probability to have an affected recessive phenotype.

The Complex Trait Consortium (CTC), a group of research labs working on genetics of multigenic traits, is planning to make a very large panel of RI strains (~ 1000 strains), derived from eight common inbred strains. Seen the large number of strains, these could be used directly for association-type studies without the need for additional crosses between the RI strains. As each mouse within a strain is genetically identical, mice would have to be genotyped only once. Phenotyping also becomes easier and more robust because more than one mouse with the same genotype can be tested. For this same reason, gene–environment interaction would be also easier to study (51).

Artificial Chromosomes

With artificial chromosomes, human loci or parts of it are added to the mouse genome on a separate small chromosome. A major disadvantage of this technique is that no gene replacement occurs, the mouse loci are still present and unaltered. The fact that human-encoded proteins are expressed in a foreign host (mouse) is the second big disadvantage but also the power of this technique. This second disadvantage could be circumvented by using a syntenic mouse locus.

Interesting "proof of concept" experiments were done by Symula et al. (47) who used Yeast artificial chromosomes (YACs) to explore the effect of a human locus in mice. For this, a panel of YAC transgenic mice containing 1 Mb of the human locus (5q31) was made. Multiple transgenic lines that showed a lowered IgE response in an OVA model of asthma had a 180 kb shared region of human chromosome, encoding five genes including genes for human IL-4 and IL-13, both cytokines involved in B-cell isotype switching. The presence of this 180 kb fragment of the locus appeared to downregulate mouse IL-4 and IL-13. This downregulation can explain the lowered amount of IgE as was already demonstrated in mice using gene inactivation (52,53) or by using transgenesis (54,55). The mechanisms by which both IL-4 and IL-13 are downregulated were not investigated.

Combined Approaches

All methods described above, except microarrays, can identify QTLs with a maximal resolution of approximately 1 cM.

Linkage and association studies are generally faster to map a locus as there is no inbreeding required (typically 20 generations). These techniques are also more able to detect interacting genes, as more different genotypes are analyzed, compared to RC strains. Fine-mapping, however, works best by backcrossing RC strains because it requires fewer mice. Interesting recombinants can be made homozygous in only two generations, which allows fast and efficient testing even when recessive traits are studied.

Combined approaches are therefore most used. In their discovery of the *Tim* gene family McIntire at al. screened RC strains (BALB/c × DBA/2). Then they used one congenic strain that had BALB/c as background and a chromosomal fragment syntenic to human asthma locus 5q23–q35 from DBA/2 for fine-mapping using linkage analysis (56). In another successful gene-hunting study, Karp et al. used linkage analysis in C3H/HeJ × A/J cross as a first step. Then they used microarrays to compare mice from a (C3H/HeJ × A/J)× A/J backcross to A/J. Complement factor 5 was significantly downregulated in A/J mice, the susceptible strain. Sequencing allowed the identification of relevant polymorphisms (57). Both these studies are discussed in more detail below.

eQTL analysis is a new combined approach in which DNA microarray experiments and QTL-mapping are combined. In eQTL analysis, expression levels of genes are used as quantitative traits in a QTL-mapping experiment. First two parental mouse strains with difference in the trait of interest are selected, and a microarray experiment is done to compare the expression levels between both strains. From this experiment, the genes for the eQTL-mapping are chosen. The two strains are then intercrossed a few times. The offspring of the last intercross is then used in a QTL-(trait of interest) and an eQTL (differentially expressed genes)-mapping experiment. QTL and eQTL maps can then be compared. Of particular interest are the regions of the chromosome in which both QTL and eQTL maps show a peak in logarithm of odds ratio (LOD)-score, especially, if the gene of the eQTL maps to that region too. The pool of genes selected this way is enriched for genes with expression levels related to the trait (QTL-peak = eQTL-peak) and that are encoded within the region of the QTL-peak. This eQTL mapping technique is mathematically very complex and still under development. There are still a few statistical issues related to multiple testing to be addressed. However, it has already produced some nice results, especially, in genetics of obesity (58) and hematopoietic stem cell function (59). It has not been used in mouse models of allergic asthma yet.

B. Mouse Asthma Genetics

Allergic asthma, in both human and mouse models, is characterized by AHR, eosinophilic inflammation of the lungs, and elevated allergen-specific serum IgE levels. These three important traits in asthma do not always correlate and can even be mapped to different regions of the genome of both human and mice.

A simple but nice illustration of this is the experiments by Ewart et al. (60). They measured airway responsiveness, OVA-specific serum IgE levels, and eosinophil content of the BAL fluid after OVA sensitization and challenge in five inbred strains of mice. A/J and AKR/J both show equally high airway reactivity. In A/J, both eosinophil and IgE levels were also high compared to the other strains, but in AKR/J only low levels of IgE and eosinophils were detected. C57BL/6J and C3H/J are both unresponsive, except for a mild eosinphilia in C3H/J. BALB/cJ showed intermediate phenotype for all three traits.

Loci and Genes Involved in AHR

AHR in both naïve and sensitized animals has been used as quantitative traits for mapping. An overview of AHR loci is given in Table 1. Interestingly the chromosome 6 locus for naïve AHR found in a A/J×C3H/HeJ is not found in the same cross when mice were sensitized with OVA, while in this same cross the suggestive locus on chromosome 7, with synteny to human 19q13, is found in both naïve and OVA sensitized mice (63). A good candidate gene for this locus is kallikrein, because bronchial tissue kallikrein is highly correlated to the appearance of histamine and kinin after allergen exposure (67), and the BAL levels are highly associated with immediate-type hypersensitivity events. Additionally, kallikrein inhibitors were shown to significantly reduce eosinophilia (68).

Nicolaides et al. identified IL-9 as a candidate AHR-susceptibility gene in naïve mice, using a series of RI strains derived from C57BL/6 and DBA/2. The RI strains were used in a QTL-analysis in order to identify a locus on chromosome 13. Only two candidate genes were selected in the region of linkage: CamL and IL-9. The selection was based upon proximity to the marker and the presence of the human homologue in syntenic region 5q31–q33, a region with high LOD-score for AHR and IgE levels in human (69). The selected RI strains as well as the parental strain C57BL/6 showed significantly lower IL-9 production by splenocytes compared to DBA/2. The IL-9 ORF and the 5′ and 3′ flanking regions were sequenced in both parental strains, but no polymorphisms in coding neither in regulatory

Table 1 Airway Hyperreactivity Loci Identified in Mice

Position [chromosome (cM)]	Name	Cross	Naïve/sensitized	Human synteny[b]	References
2 (10.0)	Abhr1	A/J × C3H/HeJ	OVA-sensitized	10p11–13, 2q12–q14, 9q22–q34	60, 61
2 (30.0)	Abhr2/C5	A/J × C3H/HeJ	OVA-sensitized	9q33–q34, 2q14–q24	60
2 (74.0)	Bhr1	A/J × C57BL6J	Naïve		62
6 (50.5)	Bhr5	A/J × C3H/HeJ	Naïve		63, 61, 64
7 (1.5)[a]	Abhr3	A/J × C3H/HeJ	OVA-sensitized	19q13	60
7 (16.0)[a]	Bhr4	A/J × C3H/HeJ	Naïve		63
9 (18)		BP2 × BALB/c	OVA-sensitized	11q23	65
10 (44)	Asthm1	BP2 × BALB/c	OVA-sensitized	12q22–q24	65
11 (7)		BP2 × BALB/c	OVA-sensitized	5q31	65
11 (23.0)	Tapr/Tim1	BALB/c × DBA/2	KLH-sensitized	5q33.2	56
11 (52)	Asthm2	BP2 × BALB/c	OVA-sensitized	17q12–q22	65
13 (38.0)	Bhr6	A/J × C3H/HeJ	Naïve		63
15 (47.1)	Bhr2	A/J × C57BL6J	Naïve		62
17 (10)		BP2 × BALB/c	OVA-sensitized	6p21	65
17 (7.6–55.7)	Sea-1	BALB/c × C57BL/6 RC	OVA-sensitized	6p21	66
17 (14.0)	Bhr3	A/J × C57BL6J	Naïve		62

[a]Only suggestive linkage.
[b]Corresponding to human QTLs.
Abbreviations: KLH, keyhole limpet hemocyanin; OVA, ovalbumin.

sequences can explain such a drastic loss of IL-9 expression. As no significant polymorphisms are found only a, as yet, undiscovered cis-acting mechanisms could explain the loss of IL-9 expression on the C57BL/6 allele (70).

The group of van Oosterhout used RC strains to map asthma susceptibility loci in an OVA mouse model of asthma. In a first "proof of concept" study CcS/Dem strains, which are RC strains with BALB/c as background and STS as donor, were used (71). From this study, it appears that the different phenotypes related to asthma, i.e., AHR, airway inflammation, and elevated IgE levels, can be separately mapped in the mouse, using RC strains, as no correlations between these asthma-related phenotypes could be found in every strain (72). CcS/Dem-5, which was previously reported to be resistant to *Leishmania major* infection (73), appeared to be almost completely resistant to experimental asthma (72). In a second study, the c.lmr RC strains (BALB/c as background and C57BL/6 as donor) were used (74). The c.lmr.1 strain appears to be resistant to all three major experimental asthma phenotypes (66). Interestingly, the congenic fragment inherited from C57BL/6 (D17Mit57–D17Mit129) maps to the same chromosomal region as the QTL identified by the group of Vargaftig in a BP2 × BALB/c cross (65). Also CcS/Dem-5 inherited a chromosomal fragment (D17Mit19–D17Mit10) from STS, which can be mapped to the same chromosomal region. Currently the group of van Oosterhout is using c.lmr.1 subcongenics (obtained by backcrossing c.lmr.1 with the background strain BALB/c) to narrow down this chromosome 17 locus.

Ackerman et al. used a backcrossing approach to identify two interacting loci involved in naïve AHR. First A/J (susceptible strain) and C57BL/6 (resistant strain) were outcrossed. The most susceptible offspring was then selected for backcrossing with the resistant strain (C57BL/6). Using this backcrossing strategy, the susceptible alleles for the trait of interest are selected, while the resistance alleles are lost during breeding. As traits encoded by other genes are not used for the selection of offspring to cross, the alleles of these genes are still randomly distributed. The trait can now be mapped in the offspring of the last backcross by genotyping and searching for conserved chromosomal regions (61).

Using this strategy, Ackerman et al. identified two interacting loci, one on chromosome 2 and one on chromosome 6. They confirmed these results with chromosome substitution strains with C57BL/6 as background and A/J as donor strain. Interestingly the chromosome 2 locus corresponds to Bhr1, and the locus on chromosome 6 corresponds to Bhr5, which were both identified in a C3H/HeJ × A/J cross (Table 1).

Adam33, a gene that was previously identified as a susceptibility gene for AHR in humans (75) could have been a good candidate gene for the chromosome 2 locus. However, no polymorphisms between both strains can be found in the sequence of Adam33 and its flanking regions suggesting that, at least in the mouse, another closely linked gene is contributing to AHR (61).

Loci and Genes Involved in Airway Inflammation: A Few Success Stories

Only few groups use mouse models to study the genetics of asthma, and most of the work is done on AHR. Despite this, one gene family, *Tim*, and one other gene, C5, related to airway inflammation and AHR were identified using combined approaches as already mentioned above.

The Tim-Gene Family Identified

The first step in the identification of the *Tim*-gene family was the screening for AHR and Th2 cytokines in the BAL fluid in a BALB/c (sensitive, background) × DBA/2 (resistant, donor) RC series of inbred strains, which were sensitized and challenged with OVA. Only one strain was unresponsive (HBA). Interestingly, the DBA/2-inherited fragment is syntenic to human 5q23–35 (56).

The linkage analysis for fine-mapping was done by backcrossing this unresponsive congenic strain with the susceptible BALB/c background strain. Mice were then genotyped, and only mice with interesting recombinations in the DBA/2-inherited locus were phenotyped (IL-4 expression after keyhole limpet hemocyanin immunization). To obtain a resolution able to distinguish the locus from other genes nearby, as, for example, IL-4 and IL-12p40, more than 2000 mice were genotyped. Screening for AHR was done the same way. Both QTLs mapped to the same region on chromosome 11 (56).

Once this mapping was performed, the search for a candidate gene could start. First the human sequence was aligned to identify the genes present in both human and mouse loci, but none of the known genes identified this way showed coding polymorphisms. *Tim-1* the homologue of rat *Kim1* and human *HAVcr-1* was another possible candidate gene. Coding sequences for *Tim-1* from both BALB/c and DBA/2 were compared, and major polymorphisms identified. DBA/2 has a 15-bp deletion and a three amino acid polymorphism. *Tim-3*, identified by expression sequence tags (EST) alignment, does also map to the same locus, but shows no polymorphisms between both strains. From these EST databases, it also appeared that *Tim-1* was mainly expressed by T-cells (56).

Transgenic mice with a T-cell receptor specific to OVA were generated in both BALB/c and DBA background. DBA CD4[+] T-cells showed significantly less IL-4 and IL-13 production in an in vitro assay (76).

In a recent paper, the same group reports the role of *Tim-1* in the regulation of Th-cell differentiation and Th2-cell proliferation. When *Tim-1* is cross-linked on CD4[+] T-cells using a Tim-1, monoclonal antibody IL-4 and IFN-γ expression is significantly upregulated. *Tim-1* expression is maintained only on Th2-cells, where cross-linking results in increased Th2 cytokine production. Cross-linking of *Tim-1* by antibody in vivo was able to prevent the induction of tolerance, leading to more severe AHR and airway inflammation compared to untreated mice (76).

Complement Factor 5

Also the group of Wills-Karp used a combined approach in the identification of complement factor 5 (C5) as asthma susceptibility gene. First they performed a QTL analysis for AHR in a A/J (susceptible strain) × C3H/HeJ (resistant strain) cross and found two loci on chromosome 2, Ahr1 and Ahr2 (Table 1) (60).

In the second step microarrays were used to compare gene expression in the lungs of both resistant [C3H/HeJ and (C3H/HeJ × A/J)× C3H/HeJ backcross low responders] and susceptible [A/J and (C3H/HeJ × A/J) × C3H/HeJ backcross high responders] mice. From the 21 differentially expressed genes, only one, C5, could be mapped to one of both loci identified in the first step (Ahr2) (57).

A significant correlation ($p < 0.005$) between AHR and C5 mRNA expression levels is observed in the (C3H/HeJ × A/J) × C3H/HeJ backcross, confirming the role of C5 in the development of AHR in this OVA model of asthma. Additionally, the lowered expression levels of C5 significantly correlated with the presence of a 2-bp deletion in the 5′exon of the C5 gene in low and high responders from the backcross and the parental strains but also some other inbred strains (57).

The group of Wang further studied the role of C5 on the development of airway inflammation and AHR and its effects on the early and late allergic responses using anti-C5 antibodies and C5-deficient mice. Their results show that C5 is involved, but not critical in the development of airway inflammation, as airway inflammation is inhibited partially when anti-C5 antibodies are administered. In contrast to these observations, there is no difference in airway inflammation in mice carrying the C3H/HeJ resistant allele compared to mice with the A/J allele, suggesting C5 is not involved in asthmatic airway inflammation. AHR however, is largely inhibited by C5 depletion by anti-C5 antibody or in C5 deficient mice. In these C5-deficient mice, AHR could be restored by intravenous injection of recombinant C5. The late and early allergic responses are both lower when mice are treated with anti-C5 antibody, indicating a role for C5 in these processes too (77).

IV. Concluding Remarks

Several genome-wide screens for asthma-related traits, in particular, AHR, have been carried out in mice. These studies have generated many susceptibility loci, some of which are concordant with loci that have been linked with the same trait in humans (78,79). Despite the advantages of mice over humans to find susceptibility gene(s) in a locus, so far only two susceptibility genes, *C5* and *Tim-1*, have been identified. Many of the initial linkage studies in mice appear to be discontinued or are not yet completed. One of the reasons may be that genetics takes time and this is a disadvantage in open competition for research grants that are often focused on short-term results. Nevertheless, there is still a strong need for mouse asthma genetics, in particular, for finding genes in QTLs that have human homologous counterparts, because this is more cost-effective. Once a mouse gene is identified, it can be directly tested in humans. Furthermore, mice can be used to dissect the genetics of different steps in the disease process such as allergic sensitization, progression to allergic disease and asthma, and severity and persistence of the disease.

One of the alleged advantages of mouse asthma genetics is to find interacting genes that are difficult to identify in human genetic studies. For instance, using a set of congenic strains, it was possible to demonstrate that a locus on mouse chromosome 3, which is linked to the development of autoimmune diabetes in the nonobese diabetic mouse, consisted of three different loci, *Idd3*, *Idd10*, and *Idd17*, and that *Idd10* interacted with both *Idd3* and *Idd17* (80). Again, the benefits of mouse genetics have not been exploited extensively in asthma research. At present, only one study has described, interacting loci involved in AHR (61). Future research on mouse asthma genetics should therefore focus on gene–gene interactions and on gene–environment interactions. In contrast to human asthma genetics studies, the environment can be well controlled in mouse studies. However, selecting the relevant environment to carry out these types of mouse asthma genetics studies is rather challenging because the potential environmental variation is tremendous. Therefore, mouse asthma genetic studies involving gene–environment interaction should carefully take into account what is already known regarding the role of the environment in the pathogenesis of asthma-like exposure to endotoxin or cigarette smoke. Furthermore, the environment to which humans are exposed is continuously changing, and, consequently, new genes will be implicated in the development of asthma in these new (micro) environments.

Acknowledgment

B. Piavaux was supported by a research grant from the Dutch Asthma Foundation (3.2.03.55).

References

1. Wang X, Paigen B. Genome-wide search for new genes controlling plasma lipid concentrations in mice and humans. Curr Opin Lipidol 2005; 16(2):127–137.
2. Deurloo DT, van Esch BC, Hofstra CL, et al. CTLA4-IgG reverses asthma manifestations in a mild but not in a more "severe" ongoing murine model. Am J Respir Cell Mol Biol 2001; 25(6):751–760.
3. Hessel EM, Van Oosterhout AJ, Hofstra CL, et al. Bronchoconstriction and airway hyperresponsiveness after ovalbumin inhalation in sensitized mice. Eur J Pharmacol 1995; 293(4):401–412.
4. Cieslewicz G, Tomkinson A, Adler A, et al. The late, but not early, asthmatic response is dependent on IL-5 and correlates with eosinophil infiltration. J Clin Invest 1999; 104(3):301–308.
5. de Bie JJ, Kneepkens M, Kraneveld AD, et al. Absence of late airway response despite increased airway responsiveness and eosinophilia in a murine model of asthma. Exp Lung Res 2000; 26(7):491–507.
6. Holt PG, Batty JE, Turner KJ. Inhibition of specific IgE responses in mice by pre-exposure to inhaled antigen. Immunology 1981; 42(3):409–417.
7. Swirski FK, Gajewska BU, Alvarez D, et al. Inhalation of a harmless antigen (ovalbumin) elicits immune activation but divergent immunoglobulin and cytokine activities in mice. Clin Exp Allergy 2002; 32(3):411–421.
8. Li J, Saito H, Crawford L, et al. Haemopoietic mechanisms in murine allergic upper and lower airway inflammation. Immunology 2005; 114(3):386–396.
9. Herz U, Braun A, Ruckert R, Renz H. Various immunological phenotypes are associated with increased airway responsiveness. Clin Exp Allergy 1998; 28(5):625–634.
10. Hofstra CL, Van AI, Nijkamkp FP, Van Oosterhout AJ. Antigen-stimulated lung CD4+ cells produce IL-5, while lymph node CD4+ cells produce Th2 cytokines concomitant with airway eosinophilia and hyperresponsiveness. Inflamm Res 1999; 48(11):602–612.
11. de Bie JJ, Hessel EM, Van AI, et al. Effect of dexamethasone and endogenous corticosterone on airway hyperresponsiveness and eosinophilia in the mouse. Br J Pharmacol 1996; 119(7):1484–1490.
12. Drazen JM, Finn PW, De Sanctis GT. Mouse models of airway responsiveness: physiological basis of observed outcomes and analysis of selected examples using these outcome indicators. Annu Rev Physiol 1999; 61:593–625.
13. Bates J, Irvin C, Brusasco V, et al. The use and misuse of Penh in animal models of lung disease. Am J Respir Cell Mol Biol 2004; 31(3):373–374.
14. Lambrecht BN, De VM, Coyle AJ, et al. Myeloid dendritic cells induce Th2 responses to inhaled antigen, leading to eosinophilic airway inflammation. J Clin Invest 2000; 106(4):551–559.
15. De Monchy JG, Kauffman HF, Venge P, et al. Bronchoalveolar eosinophilia during allergen-induced late asthmatic reactions. Am Rev Respir Dis 1985; 131(3):373–376.
16. Roche N, Chinet TC, Huchon GJ. Allergic and nonallergic interactions between house dust mite allergens and airway mucosa. Eur Respir J 1997; 10(3):719–726.

17. Tovey ER, Chapman MD, Platts-Mills TA. Mite faeces are a major source of house dust allergens. Nature 1981; 289(5798):592–593.

18. Kalsheker NA, Deam S, Chambers L, et al. The house dust mite allergen Der p1 catalytically inactivates alpha 1-antitrypsin by specific reactive centre loop cleavage: a mechanism that promotes airway inflammation and asthma. Biochem Biophys Res Commun 1996; 221(1):59–61.

19. Hewitt CR, Brown AP, Hart BJ, Pritchard DI. A major house dust mite allergen disrupts the immunoglobulin E network by selectively cleaving CD23: innate protection by antiproteases. J Exp Med 1995; 182(5):1537–1544.

20. Schulz O, Sewell HF, Shakib F. Proteolytic cleavage of CD25, the alpha subunit of the human T cell interleukin 2 receptor, by Der p 1, a major mite allergen with cysteine protease activity. J Exp Med 1998; 187(2):271–275.

21. Wan H, Winton HL, Soeller C, et al. Der p 1 facilitates transepithelial allergen delivery by disruption of tight junctions. J Clin Invest 1999; 104(1):123–133.

22. Cates EC, Fattouh R, Wattie J, et al. Intranasal exposure of mice to house dust mite elicits allergic airway inflammation via a GM-CSF-mediated mechanism. J Immunol 2004;173(10):6384–6392.

23. Johnson JR, Wiley RE, Fattouh R, et al. Continuous exposure to house dust mite elicits chronic airway inflammation and structural remodeling. Am J Respir Crit Care Med 2004; 169(3):378–385.

24. Fattouh R, Pouladi MA, Alvarez D, et al. House dust mite facilitates ovalbumin-specific allergic sensitization and airway inflammation. Am J Respir Crit Care Med 2005; 172(3):314–321.

25. Zuleger CL, Gao X, Burger MS, et al. Peptide induces CD4(+) CD25+ and IL-10+ T cells and protection in airway allergy models. Vaccine 2005; 23(24): 3181–3186.

26. Cheng KC, Lee KM, Krug MS, et al. House dust mite-induced sensitivity in mice. J Allergy Clin Immunol 1998; 101(1 Pt 1):51–59.

27. Skov M, Poulsen LK, Koch C. Increased antigen-specific Th-2 response in allergic bronchopulmonary aspergillosis (ABPA) in patients with cystic fibrosis. Pediatr Pulmonol 1999; 27(2):74–79.

28. Greenberger PA, Patterson R. Allergic bronchopulmonary aspergillosis. Model of bronchopulmonary disease with defined serologic, radiologic, pathologic and clinical findings from asthma to fatal destructive lung disease. Chest 1987; 91(6 Suppl):165S–171S.

29. Hogaboam CM, Blease K, Mehrad B, et al. Chronic airway hyperreactivity, goblet cell hyperplasia, and peribronchial fibrosis during allergic airway disease induced by *Aspergillus fumigatus*. Am J Pathol 2000; 156(2):723–732.

30. Tomee JF, Wierenga AT, Hiemstra PS, Kauffman HK. Proteases from *Aspergillus fumigatus* induce release of proinflammatory cytokines and cell detachment in airway epithelial cell lines. J Infect Dis 1997; 176(1):300–303.

31. Ansar AS, Penhale WJ, Talal N. Sex hormones, immune responses, and autoimmune diseases. Mechanisms of sex hormone action. Am J Pathol 1985; 121(3):531–551.

32. Whitacre CC, Reingold SC, O'Looney PA. A gender gap in autoimmunity. Science 1999; 283(5406):1277–1278.

33. Da Silva JA. Sex hormones and glucocorticoids: interactions with the immune system. Ann N Y Acad Sci 1999; 876:102–117.

34. Watson L, Boezen HM, Postma DS. Differences between males and females in the natural history of asthma and COPD. In: European Respiratory Monograph. UK: Sheffield, 2003:50–73.
35. The ENFUMOSA cross-sectional European multicentre study of the clinical phenotype of chronic severe asthma. European network for understanding mechanisms of severe asthma. Eur Respir J 2003; 22(3):470–477.
36. Melgert BN, Postma DS, Kuipers I, et al. Female mice are more susceptible to the development of allergic airway inflammation than male mice. Clin Exp Allergy 2005; 35:1496–1503.
37. Hayashi T, Adachi Y, Hasegawa K, Morimoto M. Less sensitivity for late airway inflammation in males than females in BALB/c mice. Scand J Immunol 2003; 57(6):562–567.
38. Seymour BW, Friebertshauser KE, Peake JL, et al. Gender differences in the allergic response of mice neonatally exposed to environmental tobacco smoke. Dev Immunol 2002; 9(1):47–54.
39. Corteling R, Trifilieff A. Gender comparison in a murine model of allergen-driven airway inflammation and the response to budesonide treatment. BMC Pharmacol 2004; 4:4.
40. Neuhaus-Steinmetz U, Glaab T, Daser A, et al. Sequential development of airway hyperresponsiveness and acute airway obstruction in a mouse model of allergic inflammation. Int Arch Allergy Immunol 2000; 121(1):57–67.
41. Sakai K, Yokoyama A, Kohno N, et al. Prolonged antigen exposure ameliorates airway inflammation but not remodeling in a mouse model of bronchial asthma. Int Arch Allergy Immunol 2001; 126(2):126–134.
42. Blyth DI, Pedrick MS, Savage TJ, et al. Lung inflammation and epithelial changes in a murine model of atopic asthma. Am J Respir Cell Mol Biol 1996; 14(5):425–438.
43. Henderson WR Jr., Tang LO, Chu SJ, et al. A role for cysteinyl leukotrienes in airway remodeling in a mouse asthma model. Am J Respir Crit Care Med 2002; 165(1):108–116.
44. Wegmann M, Fehrenbach H, Fehrenbach A, et al. Involvement of distal airways in a chronic model of experimental asthma. Clin Exp Allergy 2005; 35(10): 1263–1274.
45. Groot PC, Moen CJ, Dietrich W, et al. The recombinant congenic strains for analysis of multigenic traits: genetic composition. FASEB J 1992; 6(10): 2826–2835.
46. Demant P. Cancer susceptibility in the mouse: genetics, biology and implications for human cancer. Nat Rev Genet 2003; 4(9):721–734.
47. Symula DJ, Frazer KA, Ueda Y, et al. Functional screening of an asthma QTL in YAC transgenic mice. Nat Genet 1999; 23(2):241–244.
48. http://www.nhlbi.nih.gov/resources/pga/index.htm
49. http://pga.jax.org/
50. Broman KW. Mapping expression in randomized rodent genomes. Nat Genet 2005; 37(3):209–210.
51. Churchill GA, Airey DC, Allayee H, et al. The Collaborative Cross, a community resource for the genetic analysis of complex traits. Nat Genet 2004; 36(11):1133–1137.

52. McKenzie GJ, Emson CL, Bell SE, et al. Impaired development of Th2 cells in IL-13-deficient mice. Immunity 1998; 9(3):423–432.
53. Kopf M, Le GG, Bachmann M, et al. Disruption of the murine IL-4 gene blocks Th2 cytokine responses. Nature 1993; 362(6417):245–248.
54. Tepper RI, Levinson DA, Stanger BZ, et al. IL-4 induces allergic-like inflammatory disease and alters T cell development in transgenic mice. Cell 1990; 62(3):457–467.
55. Emson CL, Bell SE, Jones A, et al. Interleukin (IL)-4-independent induction of immunoglobulin (Ig)E, and perturbation of T cell development in transgenic mice expressing IL-13. J Exp Med 1998; 188(2):399–404.
56. McIntire JJ, Umetsu SE, Akbari O, et al. Identification of Tapr (an airway hyperreactivity regulatory locus) and the linked Tim gene family. Nat Immunol 2001; 2(12):1109–1116.
57. Karp CL, Grupe A, Schadt E, et al. Identification of complement factor 5 as a susceptibility locus for experimental allergic asthma. Nat Immunol 2000; 1(3):221–226.
58. Schadt EE, Lamb J, Yang X, et al. An integrative genomics approach to infer causal associations between gene expression and disease. Nat Genet 2005; 37(7):710–717.
59. Bystrykh L, Weersing E, Dontje B, et al. Uncovering regulatory pathways that affect hematopoietic stem cell function using 'genetical genomics'. Nat Genet 2005; 37(3):225–232.
60. Ewart SL, Kuperman D, Schadt E, et al. Quantitative trait loci controlling allergen-induced airway hyperresponsiveness in inbred mice. Am J Respir Cell Mol Biol 2000; 23(4):537–545.
61. Ackerman KG, Huang H, Grasemann H, et al. Interacting genetic loci cause airway hyperresponsiveness. Physiol Genomics 2005; 21(1):105–111.
62. De Sanctis GT, Merchant M, Beier DR, et al. Quantitative locus analysis of airway hyperresponsiveness in A/J and C57BL/6J mice. Nat Genet 1995; 11(2):150–154.
63. De Sanctis GT, Singer JB, Jiao A, et al. Quantitative trait locus mapping of airway responsiveness to chromosomes 6 and 7 in inbred mice. Am J Physiol 1999; 277(6 Pt 1):L1118–L1123.
64. Ewart SL, Mitzner W, DiSilvestre DA, et al. Airway hyperresponsiveness to acetylcholine: segregation analysis and evidence for linkage to murine chromosome 6. Am J Respir Cell Mol Biol 1996; 14(5):487–495.
65. Zhang Y, Lefort J, Kearsey V, et al. A genome-wide screen for asthma-associated quantitative trait loci in a mouse model of allergic asthma. Hum Mol Genet 1999; 8(4):601–605.
66. Jeurink PV, Van Esch ECAM, Groot PC, et al. A Novel Susceptibility to Experimental Asthma (Sea-1) Locus on Mouse Chromosome 17. Am J Respir Crit Care Med 2004; 169:A579.
67. Christiansen SC, Proud D, Sarnoff RB, et al. Elevation of tissue kallikrein and kinin in the airways of asthmatic subjects after endobronchial allergen challenge. Am Rev Respir Dis 1992; 145(4 Pt 1):900–905.
68. Evans DM, Jones DM, Pitt GR, et al. Synthetic inhibitors of human tissue kallikrein. Immunopharmacology 1996; 32(1–3):117–118.

69. Postma DS, Bleecker ER, Amelung PJ, et al. Genetic susceptibility to asthma-bronchial hyperresponsiveness coinherited with a major gene for atopy. N Engl J Med 1995; 333(14):894–900.
70. Nicolaides NC, Holroyd KJ, Ewart SL, et al. Interleukin 9: a candidate gene for asthma. Proc Natl Acad Sci U S A 1997; 94(24):13175–13180.
71. Stassen AP, Groot PC, Eppig JT, Demant P. Genetic composition of the recombinant congenic strains. Mamm Genome 1996; 7(1):55–58.
72. Jeurink PV, Groot PC, Hofman G, et al. Recombinant congenic mouse strains as a genetic model for antigen-induced airway manifestations of asthma. Am J Respir Crit Care Med 2004; 169:A579.
73. Lipoldova M, Svobodova M, Krulova M, et al. Susceptibility to Leishmania major infection in mice: multiple loci and heterogeneity of immunopathological phenotypes. Genes Immun 2000; 1(3):200–206.
74. Roberts LJ, Baldwin TM, Speed TP, et al. Chromosomes X, 9, and the H2 locus interact epistatically to control Leishmania major infection. Eur J Immunol 1999; 29(9):3047–3050.
75. Howard TD, Postma DS, Jongepier H, et al. Association of a disintegrin and metalloprotease 33 (ADAM33) gene with asthma in ethnically diverse populations. J Allergy Clin Immunol 2003; 112(4):717–722.
76. Umetsu SE, Lee WL, McIntire JJ, et al. TIM-1 induces T cell activation and inhibits the development of peripheral tolerance. Nat Immunol 2005; 6(5):447–454.
77. Peng T, Hao L, Madri JA, et al. Role of C5 in the development of airway inflammation, airway hyperresponsiveness, and ongoing airway response. J Clin Invest 2005; 115(6):1590–1600.
78. Wills-Karp M, Ewart SL. Time to draw breath: asthma-susceptibility genes are identified. Nat Rev Genet 2004; 5(5):376–387.
79. http://cooke.gsf.de/asthmagen
80. Podolin PL, Denny P, Lord CJ, et al. Congenic mapping of the insulin-dependent diabetes (Idd) gene, Idd10, localizes two genes mediating the Idd10 effect and eliminates the candidate Fcgr1. J Immunol 1997; 159(4):1835–1843.

7

Generation of Genetically Manipulated Mouse Lines for the Study of Asthma

STEPHEN L. TILLEY

Division of Pulmonary and Critical Care
  Medicine, Department of Medicine,
  The University of North Carolina at
  Chapel Hill,
Chapel Hill, North Carolina, U.S.A.

**IRVING C. ALLEN and BEVERLY
H. KOLLER**

Department of Genetics, The University of
  North Carolina at Chapel Hill,
Chapel Hill, North Carolina, U.S.A.

I. Introduction

Over the past 20 years, our ability to manipulate gene expression in the mouse has increased tremendously. It is not only possible to increase expression of a particular gene in the lung, but also to regulate when and where this increase in expression occurs. These methods have been used extensively to determine whether or not a specific gene product can, when expressed at high levels, induce pathologies similar to those observed in the asthmatic lung. Conversely, methods have been developed which allow removal of gene expression to test the function of the gene in disease development and pathogenesis in the context of models of antigen-induced allergic lung disease. These methods have more recently been refined to allow expression to be either enhanced or removed in a temporal and tissue-specific manner. In this chapter, we present common approaches for phenotyping mice in models of asthma, then discuss standard as well as state-of-the-art methods used to manipulate gene expression in mice. Throughout each section, we provide relevant examples of how this approach has been useful for studying asthma pathogenesis.

II. Allergic Lung Disease in Mice

Unlike other diseases such as diabetes or lupus, no laboratory mouse spontaneously develops asthma. Allergic lung disease as a surrogate model of asthma can be induced in mice by sensitization and challenge with simple protein antigens [e.g., ovalbumin (OVA)], complex microorganisms (e.g. Aspergillus), or chemical compounds [e.g., Toluene diisocyanate (TDI)]. Environmentally relevant protein antigens derived from cockroaches and house dust mite have also been employed (1–3). Short-term exposure models utilizing these antigens, in particular OVA, have been evaluated extensively and reproduce many features observed in human asthma, including increases in antigen-specific immunoglobulin (Ig)E, increases in Th2 cytokines interleukin (IL)-4, IL-5, and IL-13, eosinophilic lung inflammation, goblet cell metaplasia, and airway hyperresponsiveness (AHR) (4). However, it is important to recognize that these short-term exposure models also show many important differences from human asthma, including acute peribronchiolar and perivascular inflammation in the lung parenchyma (rather than acute-on-chronic inflammation within the airway wall), lack of activation, degranulation, or intraepithelial accumulation of eosinophils, significantly less plasma exudation in murine versus human airways, and lack of structural changes in the airway other than goblet cell metaplasia (5). To address these concerns, several chronic inhalation challenge models have been developed, consisting of systemic sensitization followed by two to three airway challenges each week for 8 to 12 weeks (6,7). These chronic models recapitulate more features of human asthma than the acute models including (i) the complete absence of parenchymal inflammation, (ii) intraepithelial eosinophils, (iii) chronic Th2 inflammation in the lamina propria, and (iv) airway remodeling including epithelial hypertrophy, smooth muscle hypertrophy, subepithelial fibrosis, and goblet cell hyperplasia/metaplasia.

III. Phenotyping Methods and Principles

Physiological, histopathological, and biological phenotyping of genetically altered mice is now commonly used to determine the contribution of candidate genes to asthma pathogenesis. Despite the incomplete recapitulation of the precise histopathology of human asthma in these models, they have contributed substantially to the paradigm that a large number of bioactive mediators produced by a number of immune and parenchymal cells act together to orchestrate allergic inflammation in the lung. Development of allergic lung disease, produced by either an acute or chronic model, is compared between normal "wild type" mice and mice with the genetically engineered changes in gene expression; most commonly, mice carry a null allele of the gene. Three characteristic phenotypes are routinely examined:

1. Airway hyperresponsiveness
2. Inflammatory response
3. Structural changes in the lung

Prior to discussion of the assessment of these phenotypes, it is important to recognize the significant impact of strain, sex, and environment on the development of these phenotypic changes. Thus, careful selection of control animals is crucial to adequate interpretation of experimental results.

A. Airway Hyperresponsiveness

Reversible airflow obstruction and AHR are two cardinal features of human asthma, the latter of which has been shown to develop in many mouse strains following the induction of allergic pulmonary inflammation. Assessment and quantification of AHR can be performed by both noninvasive and invasive means, each with their own distinct advantages and limitations. While many homemade and commercially available machines have been used to quantify AHR in mice, a comprehensive description of these methods is beyond the scope of this chapter. Rather, we will provide an overview of three methods that have been commonly used in the evaluation of AHR in genetically altered mice.

Whole-Body Plethysmography

Many investigators have attempted to evaluate AHR in conscious, unrestrained mice utilizing barometric whole-body plethysmography (WBP), after Hamelmann et al.'s report suggesting that the measurement of responsiveness to inhaled methacholine by WBP was a valid indicator of AHR after allergic sensitization in mice (8). In this system, mice are placed in a plethysmographic chamber capable of measuring inspiratory and expiratory pressures and time spent in each phase of the respiratory cycle. A unitless parameter termed "Penh" is derived from these measured variables utilizing the following equation:

$$\text{Penh} = \text{PEP}/\text{PIP} \times (T\text{e} - T\text{r})/T\text{r}$$

where PEP is peak expiratory pressure, PIP is peak inspiratory pressure, $T\text{e}$ is exhalation time, and $T\text{r}$ is relaxation time (8). Mice evaluated after OVA sensitization and challenge typically show an elevated baseline Penh and an exaggerated response to methacholine (AHR) compared to sham-treated controls. Analysis of the determinants of Penh reveals that both prolongation of the expiratory time and decrease in $T\text{r}$ relative to $T\text{e}$ plus increased

PEP/PIP are the primary contributors to changes in Penh both at baseline and in response to cholinergic and other contractile stimuli (e.g., adenosine and thromboxane). Advantages of this methodology include ease of measurement, capacity to measure serial changes over time, and evaluation of mice during normal physiological conditions where reflex neurological pathways remain intact. Disadvantages of WBP include the lack of specificity of the Penh parameter, as it can be influenced by other perturbations in mechanical properties of the lung other than changes in airway resistance, and the inability to distinguish contributions of upper (nose) vs. lower airways to the observed response (9). While some investigators have challenged the usefulness and meaning of the Penh parameter because of its empirical correlations with resistance (rather than representing a true measurement of lung mechanics) (10), when used and interpreted appropriately, it can provide useful information about the genetically modified mouse. For example, the constrictor response of several agents known to elicit bronchoconstriction in humans is not detectable by traditional mechanical measurements of airway physiology, but detectable in conscious mice by WBP. One example of this is adenosine-induced bronchoconstriction. While no or little response to adenosine is observed in anesthetized, mechanically ventilated naive and sensitized mice, respectively, a more robust response is observed by WBP. Mast cell degranulation in the lower airway concomitant with rises in Penh following aerosolized adenosine challenge suggests that lower airway constriction may be contributing to the response (11). This effect of adenosine, dependent on an intact neuronal–mast cell loop and large numbers of mast cells in the upper airway, is not observed in anesthetized, mechanically ventilated mice in which neural pathways are blunted and the upper airway bypassed.

Airway Pressure Time Index

While WBP, under certain circumstances, may reflect changes in lower airway tone, the true mechanical properties of the lung can only be assessed in intubated or tracheostomized animals. The airway pressure time index (APTI) has been frequently used to assess responses to bronchoconstrictor stimuli in anesthetized tracheostomized mice. During mechanical ventilation with a fixed frequency and tidal volume, airway pressure can be recorded via a pressure transducer attached to the ventilator circuit near the airway opening. Changes in airway pressure over time during a methacholine challenge can be graphed and the area under the curve defined as the APTI (12). Because peak airway pressure increases proportionally with the degree of bronchoconstriction, it has been assumed that APTI reflects changes in airway resistance during such a challenge. One advantage of this technique is that it only requires measures of respiratory pressures, not volumes or flows. Its disadvantage is that the pressure measured reflects both airway and tissue resistance; thus APTI is really a measure of total respiratory system impedance, which is influenced by airway, parenchyma, and chest wall. In allergic mice, airway pressures are greater during each second of exposure to methacholine relative to sham-treated controls, resulting in a greater APTI at each dose, displacing the dose–response curve up and to the left. As with WBP, it has been widely assumed but not established that these measurements reflect resistance of the airways.

Dynamic Resistance and Compliance

Classical respiratory system mechanics uses the equation of motion to describe the single compartment model of the lung. By measuring flow, volume, and pressure; resistance (R_L), elastance (E_{dyn}), and compliance ($C_{dyn} = 1/E_{dyn}$) can be calculated. Despite their small size, Martin et al., in 1988, first demonstrated that pulmonary resistance and compliance could be measured in the mouse by this method (13). Over the subsequent decade, this methodology became very popular and was perhaps considered the gold standard for measures of airway mechanics in mice.

Oscillatory Mechanics

A fourth method for assessing AHR in mice is the forced oscillation technique, developed by Hantos et al. in larger animals (14) but successfully adapted to the mouse by Schuessler and Bates (15). Using this technique, a series of mutually primed frequencies from 0.1 to 20 Hz is applied to the airway by a computer-controlled small animal ventilator, and changes in pressure recorded at the airway opening. By measuring respiratory system impedance at multiple frequencies, this data can be fit to a more complex model of the lung, termed the "constant-phase model," which makes a clear distinction between central and peripheral physiology. This capacity to differentiate physiological changes occurring in various parts of the respiratory tree is due to the fact that certain resonant frequencies are reflected by the large airways while other frequencies are only reflected by the most distal small airways and lung parenchyma. Using the constant phase model of the lung, three important variables are derived: airway resistance (*R*aw), tissue resistance (*G*), and tissue elastance (*H*). Due to central airway constriction and peripheral airway closure, *R*aw, *G*, and *H* all increase during graded methacholine challenge. AHR is represented by a shift up and to the left in the dose–response curves. As technology continues to advance our capacity to conduct more precise physiological measurements in these small animals, new techniques will undoubtedly emerge, which will further enable pathophysiological correlations important to our understanding of AHR, a phenotype of significant functional importance to individuals with asthma.

IV. Inflammatory Response

The inflammatory response to allergic sensitization and challenge can be characterized in many ways but is most commonly evaluated by analysis of cells, cytokines, and specific immunoglobulin production.

A. Immune Cells

Whole-lung lavage, commonly termed "bronchoalveolar lavage (BAL)," through a tracheal cannula is performed to obtain cells for quantitative (total cells) and qualitative (cellular differentials) analysis. The numbers of eosinophils, neutrophils, lymphocytes, and macrophages are compared between wild type and genetically modified animals. Inflammatory cells within the whole lung are generally evaluated by hematoxylin and eosin (H&E) staining of fixed, paraffin-embedded sections. Degree, nature, and distribution of inflammation can be evaluated qualitatively and quantitatively by various scoring systems or with digital imaging programs. An alternative method employed by some investigators is to analyze total lung cells by fluorescence-activated cell sorter. By this method, immune cells from the entire lung are isolated and labeled with antibodies specific for a given cell population. Histological analysis of the mouse lung following acute challenge protocols has revealed similarities, but also important differences from the human asthmatic lung, as detailed above.

B. Inflammatory Mediators

Cytokines

Lavage fluid supernatant is used by some investigators for analysis of cytokines, and is generally representative of the cytokine environment within the lung itself. Whole-lung homogenates, however, will provide better representation of the cytokine milieu within the entire lung as cytokines detectable in lung lavage supernatant may only reflect production by cells within the alveoli and airway lumen. Cytokine mRNA is frequently analyzed from whole lung or lung lobes, as this provides a quantitative assessment of cytokine expression levels in the lung.

Immunoglobulins

One hallmark of allergic disorders including allergic asthma is elevations in IgE. The switch to IgE production by B-cells is dependent on IL-4 and associated with the transition from a Th1- to Th2-dominated response. Thus, it is not surprising that most investigators have included in their analysis an evaluation of IgE levels. Some have specifically measured the levels of IgE to the sensitizing antigen while others measure total IgE. When both have been measured, it is clear that in pathogen-free animals the vast majority of the IgE is directed against the sensitizing antigen. Less frequently, the levels of other antibodies have been evaluated. Antigen-specific IgE and IgG1 are elevated following virtually all immunization protocols, with levels significantly higher in the serum than in the lung lavage fluid. IgE is believed to contribute to asthma pathogenesis by serving as a principle activator of mast cells, through its binding to the FcεRI receptor (16). Cross-linking of the receptor through antigen–antibody interaction results in mast cell activation and degranulation—releasing a number of proinflammatory and bronchoactive mediators including histamine, LTC_4, PGD_2, and IL-4. Thus, it came as some surprise when it was shown using mast cell–deficient mice that IgE-mast cell activation was not required for the development of AHR, Th2 response, or eosinophilic lung inflammation in mice systemically sensitized and airway challenged with antigen (17). Consistent with this observation, it has also been demonstrated that neither IgE nor B-cells are required for the development of allergic airway disease in mice when alum-boosting sensitization protocols are employed (18,19). However, with less robust immunizations with antigen alone, mast cell–dependent phenotypes were uncovered using mast cell- and FcεRI-deficient animals (20). These studies suggest that mast cells are necessary for amplification and full manifestation of the allergic response with less potent allergen sensitization models, but unnecessary for the full expression of allergic lung disease when more potent protocols are employed. The variable efficacy of anti-IgE therapy in allergic asthmatics suggests the possibility of a human correlate to these observations in mouse.

C. Airway Remodeling

It is now well recognized that asthma is a disease characterized by chronic inflammation of the airways resulting in variable degrees of airway remodeling over time. The term "airway remodeling" refers to the development of specific structural changes to the airway wall in patients with asthma. These structural changes are now believed to be involved in the pathogenesis of AHR and the progressive loss of lung function that occurs in some asthmatics, as a result of decreasing caliber of the airway lumen. The pathological changes constituting airway remodeling include (i) epithelial shedding, (ii) subepithelial fibrosis, (iii) hypertrophy of airway smooth muscle (ASM), and (iv) mucous gland and goblet cell hyperplasia. While only the latter structural change is typically observed in acute allergen models, chronic allergen exposure models demonstrate most of the pathological changes characteristic of airway remodeling in man (21). Both histopathological and biochemical methods are available for quantifying these remodeling changes in the murine airway. Morphometric analysis of Mason-trichrome–stained sections can be used to measure thickness of the airway wall including the subepithelia and smooth muscle layers, and total lung collagen levels can be determined by analysis of hydroxyproline content. Finally, the expression of alpha smooth muscle actin can also be used to gauge the degree of smooth muscle hypertrophy elicited by chronic allergen exposure (7). These chronic exposure models, tools for quantitating the remodeled airway, and mice under- or overexpressing candidate genes are being used collectively to determine the factors involved in this important aspect of asthma pathogenesis.

V. Manipulating the Mouse Genome

The two strategies, the over expression of genes in the lung and assessment of the impact of gene loss on the development of allergic lung disease in the mouse, have been extensively used to investigate the biological mediators and pathways important to asthma pathogenesis. In Table 1, we list and summarize some of the findings obtained on over expression of candidate asthma genes in mice. In Tables 2–5, we list mouse lines, each carrying a null mutation in a particular gene, which have been examined in allergic asthma models. Two points are worth noting. First, while the list contains some experiments in which no impact of loss of expression is noted, the list is clearly biased toward experiments in which loss of gene expression altered at least one phenotype. Unfortunately, it is likely that an equal number of mouse lines have been tested in which loss of gene expression resulted in no change in the development of allergic airway disease, and because of the difficulty in publishing negative results, this information is largely unavailable to the research community. While, in general, there is good agreement in results when similar mice were generated and studied by different research groups, a few exceptions are noted.

A. Overexpression of Genes and the Development of Phenotypes with Some Aspects of Asthma

It is now over 26 years since the first transgenic mouse was generated. Generally, a transgenic mouse is one in which the expression of the gene is "added" to the normal repertoire of genes expressed. The biological roles of IL-4 and IL-5 in vivo were first elucidated using transgenic mice overexpressing these cytokines in lymphocytes. In Figure 1A, we show a schematic for a typical transgene used in these types of studies. In 1990, Tepper et al. used an immunoglobulin promoter/enhancer to drive IL-4 transgene expression in lymphocytes (22,23). Mice constitutively expressing increased amounts of IL-4 developed a marked increase in serum IgE and IgG1 levels as well as allergic inflammation in the eyes. In the same year, Dent et al. reported their findings with transgenic mice overexpressing IL-5 (24). The expression of IL-5 was driven by its own promoter.

(*Text continues on page 142.*)

Table 1 Transgenic/Gene Transfer Mouse Models

Gene	Mouse strain	Promoter	Inflammation model	AHR	Eosinophilia	Airway remodeling	References
hIL-1β	Mixed	Rat CC10	Naïve	NA	↔	↑	Lappalainen, 2005
hIRAP	FVB/N	SP-C	IL-1 alpha	NA	↔	NA	Wilmott, 1998
IL-4	CBA	Rat CC10	Naïve	NA	↑	↑	Rankin, 1996
IL-9/IL-4Rα⁻/⁻	BALB/c	Rat CC10	Naïve	NA	NA	↓	Whittaker, 2002
IL-5	BALB/c	Metallothionein	OVA	NA	↑	NA	Tanaka, 2004
IL-5	C57BL/6	Rat CC10	Naïve	↑	↑	↑	Lee, 1997
IL-5	BALB/c	IL-5/DCR	IL-13	NA	↑	↔	Pope, 2001
IL-5	C3H/HeN	Metallothionein	OVA	↑	↑	NA	Kobayashi, 2003
IL-6	BALB/c	Rat CC10	Naïve	NA	↓	NA	Wang, 2000
IL-6	C57BL/6	Rat CC10	Naïve	NA	↓	NA	Wang, 2000
IL-9	FVB/NJ	PIM-1	AF	↑	↑	NA	McLane, 1998
IL-9	B10.D2	Rat CC10	Naïve	↑	↑	↑	Temann, 1998
IL-9	Mixed	Rat CC10	Naïve	NA	↑	↑	Temann, 2002
IL-10	C57BL/6	Rat CC10	Naïve	NA	↑	↑	Lee, 2002
IL-11	Mixed	Rat CC10	Naïve	↑	↑	NA	Tang, 1996
IL-12	BALB/c	adenovirus	Naïve	NA	↓	↑	Stampfli, 1999
IL-12	BALB/c	adenovirus	OVA	NA	↓	↑	Stampfli, 1999
IL-13	Mixed	Rat CC10	Naïve	↑	↓	↑	Zhou, 1999
IL-15	C57BL/6	H2K	OVA	NA	↓	NA	Ishimitsu, 2001

(Continued)

Table 1 Transgenic/Gene Transfer Mouse Models (*Continued*)

Gene	Mouse strain	Promoter	Inflammation model	AHR	Eosinophilia	Airway remodeling	References
GM-CSF	BALB/c	adenovirus	OVA	NA	↑	↑	Stampfli, 1998
CXCL 10	129/SV	Keratin 5	OVA	↑	↑	↔	Medoff, 2002
TGF-β2 (ΔKTβRII)	FVB/N	CD2	OVA	↑	↑	NA	Schramm, 2003
hCysLT1R	BALB/c	VSM α-actin	AF	↑[a]	↔	↔	Yang, 2004

[a]Only to LTD$_4$; ↓, Reduced AHR or Eosinophilia compared with the wildtype animals; ↔, No difference in AHR or Eosinophilia compared with the wildtype group; ↑, Increased AHR or Eosinophilia compared with the wildtype animals; NA, Not assessed.
Abbreviations: AHR, airway hyperresponsiveness; IL, interleukin; OVA, ovalbumin; AF, *Aspergillus fumigatus*.

Table 2 Cytokine and Cytokine Receptor Deficient Mice

Cytokine	Mouse strain	Inflammation model	AHR	Eosinophilia	Airway remodeling	References
IL-1α	BALB/c	OVA	→	→	NA	Nakae, 2003
IL-1β	BALB/c	OVA	→	→	NA	Nakae, 2003
IL-1α/β	BALB/c	OVA	↕	→	NA	Nakae, 2003
IL-1R1[a]	Mixed	OVA	NA	→	→	Broide, 2000
IL-1R1[a]	BALB/c	OVA	NA	←	NA	Schmitz, 2003
IL-1Ra	BALB/c	OVA	←	NA	NA	Nakae, 2003
IL-1RI[a]	BALB/c	AF	NA	→	←	Kurup, 1999
IL-4[a]	C57BL/6	OVA	→	→	→	Herrick, 2000
IL-4[a]	BALB/c	OVA	→	→	NA	Leigh, 2004
IL-4[a]	C57BL/6	OVA	NA	NA	→	Hamelmann, 2000
IL-4Rα	BALB/c	OVA	→	→	NA	Whittaker, 2002
IL-5	C57BL/6	OVA	→	→	→	Hamelmann, 2000
IL-5	C57BL/6	OVA	NA	→	↕	Foster, 1996
IL-5	C57BL/6	IL-13	NA	→	→	Cho, 2004
IL-5	C57BL/6	OVA	NA	→	↕	Pope, 2001
IL-5Rα	BALB/c	OVA	NA	→	NA	Tanaka, 2004
IL-5Rα	Mixed	OVA	NA	←	NA	Tanaka, 2000
IL-6	C57BL/6	OVA	→	←	→	Wang, 2000
IL-6	BALB/c	OVA	←	↕	→	Qiu, 2004
IL-8R	BALB/c	OVA	↕	↕	↕	De Sanctis, 1999
IL-9	BALB/c	OVA	→	←	↕	McMillan, 2002
IL-10[a]	C57BL/6	RW	↕	←	NA	Justice, 2001
IL-10[a]	C57BL/6	OVA	NA	↕	NA	Ameredes, 2001

(Continued)

Table 2 Cytokine and Cytokine Receptor Deficient Mice (*Continued*)

Cytokine	Mouse strain	Inflammation model	AHR	Eosinophilia	Airway remodeling	References
IL-10[a]	Mixed	AF	↔	↑	NA	Grunig, 1997
IL-10[a]	C57BL/6	OVA	↔	↑	NA	Tournoy, 2000
IL-12	C57BL/6	OVA	NA	↑	NA	Zhao, 2000
IL-12p35	C57BL/6	OVA	NA	→	NA	Wang, 2001
IL-12p40 (homodimer)	C57BL/6	OVA	NA	→	NA	Wang, 2001
IL-13[a]	BALB/c	OVA	↑	↔	→	Webb, 2000
IL-13[a]	BALB/c	OVA	→	↔	→	Walter, 2001
IL-13[a]	BALB/c	OVA	NA	NA	→	Whittaker, 2002
IL-13[a]	Mixed	OVA	NA	→	NA	Herrick, 2003
IL-4/IL-13	BALB/c	OVA	→	→	→	Walter, 2001
IL-17	BALB/c	OVA	↔	↔	NA	Nakae, 2002

[a]Conflicting Data; ↓, Reduced airway hyperresponsiveness (AHR) or Eosinophilia compared with the wildtype animals; ↔, No difference in AHR or Eosinophilia compared with the wildtype group; ↑, Increased AHR or Eosinophilia compared with the wildtype animals; NA, not assessed.
Abbreviations: AHR, airway hyperresponsiveness; IL, interleukin; OVA, ovalbumin; AF, *Aspergillus fumigatus*; RW, Ragweed antigen.

Table 3 Chemokine and Chemokine Receptor Deficient Mice

Chemokine	Mouse strain	Inflammation model	AHR	Eosinophilia	Airway remodeling	References
TNF-α	C57BL/6	OVA	↑	↑	NA	Kanehiro, 2001
TNFR1 (p55)	C57BL/6	OVA	→	→	NA	Kanehiro, 2002
TNFR2 (p75)	C57BL/6	OVA	↔	→	NA	Kanehiro, 2002
TNFR1/TNFR2	C57BL/6	OVA	↔	↔	↑	Rudman, 2000
INF-γ	BALB/c	OVA	↔	→	NA	Hofstra, 1998
FCεRIα	Mixed	OVA	↔	→	NA	Mayr, 2002
CCR1	Mixed	AF	↔	↔	→	Blease, 2000
CCR2	Mixed	OVA	↔	↔	NA	MacLean, 2000
CCR2	Mixed	OVA	←	←	↑	Kim, 2001
CCR2	Mixed	AF	←	↑	↑	Blease, 2000
CXCR2 (IL-8r)	Not listed	AF	→	→	↔	Schuh, 2002
CXCR2 (IL-8r)	BALB/c	OVA	↔	↔	↔	DeSanctis, 1999
CXCL10	129/SV	OVA	→	→	NA	Medoff, 2002
CCR5	Mixed	AF	→	→	→	Schuh, 2002
CCR6	C57BL/6	CR	→	→	NA	Lukacs, 2001
Eotaxin	BALB/c	IL-13	NA	↔	↔	Pope, 2001
Eotaxin	Not listed	AF	→	→	NA	Schuh, 2002
IL-5/eotaxin	BALB/c	IL-13	NA	→	↔	Pope, 2001

↓, Reduced airway hyperresponsiveness (AHR) or Eosinophilia compared with the wildtype animals; ↔, No difference in AHR or Eosinophilia compared with the wildtype group; ↑, Increased AHR or Eosinophilia compared with the wildtype animals; NA, Not assessed.
Abbreviations: AHR, airway hyperresponsiveness; IL, interleukin; OVA, ovalbumin; AF, *Aspergillus fumigatus*; CR, Cockroach antigen.

Table 4 Th2 Cytokine Signaling Pathway Deficient Mice

Th2 cytokine signaling pathway	Mouse strain	Inflammation model	AHR	Eosinophilia	Airway remodeling	References
Fgr	C57BL/6	OVA	NA	↓	NA	Vicentini, 2002
Hck	C57BL/6	OVA	NA	↕	NA	Vicentini, 2002
PKCζ	129/SVJ	OVA	NA	↓	NA	Martin, 2005
Jak3	Mixed	OVA	NA	↓	NA	Verbsky, 2002
Stat 5α	BALB/c	OVA	NA	↓	NA	Kagami, 2000
Stat 5β	BALB/c	OVA	NA	↓	NA	Kagami, 2000
Stat 6	C57BL/6	OVA	↓	↓	NA	Miyata, 1999
Stat 6	C57BL/6	OVA	↓	↓	NA	Akimoto, 1998
Stat 6	Mixed	OVA	NA	↓	↓	Herrick, 2000
Stat 4	BALB/c	CR	↓	↓	↓	Raman, 2003
T-Bet (Tbx21)	Not listed	OVA	↑	↑	↑	Finotto, 2002
TGF-βl	C57BL/6 (HET)	OVA	↕	↑	↑	Scherf, 2005

↓, Reduced airway hyperresponsiveness (AHR) or Eosinophilia compared with the wildtype animals; ↕, No difference in AHR or Eosinophilia compared with the wildtype group; ↑, Increased AHR or Eosinophilia compared with the wildtype animals; NA, Not assessed.

Abbreviations: AHR, airway hyperresponsiveness; OVA, ovalbumin; CR, Cockroach antigen.

Table 5 Prostaglandin and Leukotriene Deficient Mice

Prostaglandin/leukotriene	Mouse strain	Inflammation model	AHR	Eosinophilia	Airway remodeling	References
PGHS 1 (Cox-1)	Mixed	OVA	↑	↑	↑	Gavett, 1999
PGHS 1 (Cox-1)	Mixed	OVA	↑	↑	NA	Carey, 2003
PGHS 2 (Cox-2)	Mixed	OVA	→	↑	↑	Gavett, 1999
PGHS 2 (Cox-2)	Mixed	OVA	↔	↑	NA	Carey, 2003
PGHS 2 (Cox-2)	C57BL/6	OVA	→	↑	↔	Nakata, 2005
Dp	C57BL/6	OVA	→	→	↓	Matsuoka, 2000
Ip	C57BL/6	OVA	NA	↑	NA	Takahashi, 2002
BLT1	BALB/c	OVA	→	↔	→	Miyahara, 2005
5-LO	Mixed	OVA	→	→	NA	Irvin, 1997

↓, Reduced AHR or Eosinophilia compared with the wildtype animals; ↑, Increased AHR or Eosinophilia compared with the wildtype group; ↔, No difference in AHR or Eosinophilia compared with the wildtype animals; NA, Not assessed.
Abbreviations: AHR, airway hyperresponsiveness; OVA, ovalbumin.

A) Transgenic

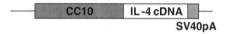

B) Lung Specific Transgenic

C) Temporal Specific Transgenic

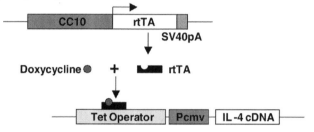

D) Temporal Specific tTS"on/off" Transgenic

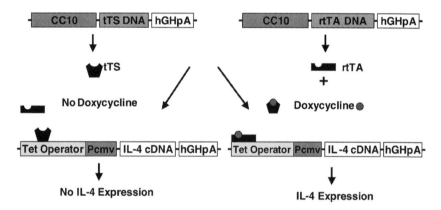

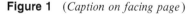

Figure 1   (*Caption on facing page*)

IL-5 transgenic mice exhibited eosinophilia in the bone marrow, bloodstream, spleen, lymphoid organs, gut, and lung. While these experiments demonstrated an in vivo role for these cytokines in IgE production and eosinophilia, two classic phenotypic features of asthma, it was the development of lung-specific tissue expression systems that has helped elucidate the effects of IL-4, IL-5, and other inflammatory mediators on the lung itself.

B. Lung-Specific Expression Systems

The tissues in which transgenes are expressed are generally determined by the characteristics of the promoter. Thus, the definition of promoters that drive gene expression in the lung has greatly expanded the ability of researchers to use this technology for studying lung diseases. Two different promoters are commonly used to drive gene expression in the lung. The promoter of the Clara cell secretory protein (CCSP, also called CC10 for Clara cell 10 kDa protein) or the surfactant apoprotein-C (SPC) promoter can be used to selectively target genes of interest to the lung parenchyma and/or airways (Fig. 1B). It is important to note that the most commonly used promoters are not of mouse origin; most experiments utilize the rat CCSP promoter and the human SPC promoter. Thus, the pattern of expression driven by these genes does not mimic that of the endogenous mouse genes. However both promoters result in expression of the genes in only the lung. Each has a unique expression pattern, both temporally and spatially in the developing lung and in the adult mouse. In the adult mouse, CCSP expression does not parallel the mouse counterpart whose expression is generally limited to the Clara cells for which the protein was named. Rather, the rat CCSP drives gene expression in a subset of alveolar type II cells as well as a subset but not all Clara cells in the airways (25). In the adult mouse, the human SPC promoter is expressed primarily in type II alveolar cells and in the respiratory epithelia in the adult mouse.

The details regarding the expression pattern of these promoters are less important when the aim is simply to observe and characterize

---

Figure 1 (*Figure on facing page*) Common strategies for the creation of transgenic mice. (**A**) Schematic illustration of an IL-4 transgene construct. The *plck* promoter drives expression of the IL-4 *cDNA*. Intronic regions and the 3′ UTR from the hGH gene is included to augment transgene expression. (**B**) Schematic illustration of a lung-specific IL-4 transgene construct. The CC10 promoter facilitates lung-specific constitutive expression of IL-4. The SV40 polyadenylation sequence is added to confer transcript stability. (**C**) Schematic illustration of a temporal specific IL-4 transgene construct. The CC10 promoter facilitates lung-specific constitutive expression of the rtTA. rtTA requires the tetracycline derivative, doxycycline, for specific *DNA* binding to the tet operator. Once bound, this initiates the expression of IL-4 by the pCMV promoter. (**D**) Schematic illustration of a temporal lung-specific tTS "on/off" transgene construct. The CC10 promoter facilitates lung-specific constitutive expression of both the rtTA and the tTS. In this situation, tTS binds to the tet operator in the absence of doxycycline. When doxycycline is administered, the silencer releases, allowing the rtTA to facilitate IL-4 expression. This system was designed to control for leaky transgene expression commonly encountered during the use of rtTA alone. *Abbreviations*: rtTA, reverse tetracycline transactivator; tet, tetracycline; pCMV, cytomegalovirus promoter; tTS, tetracycline-controlled transcriptional silencer; IL, interleukin.

the sequence of events that follow enhanced production of cytokines in the mouse lung. If the goal is to express a channel or receptor in a specific population of cells in the lung, the expression pattern of the promoter can dramatically impact the phenotype of the transgenic and consequently the information that can be gleaned from the study of the animals. As discussed later, the expression pattern is also critical when these promoters are incorporated into schemes utilized for the generation of mice with temporal and/or tissue-specific ablation of gene expression.

C. Transgenic Mice that Spontaneously Develop Asthmatic Phenotypes

Overexpression of Th2-associated cytokines results in pathognomonic mice with regards to asthma. The lung-specific rat CC10 promoter has been utilized to drive IL-4, IL-5, IL-9, and IL-13 expression in the lung. In all cases, overexpression of a single Th2 cytokine resulted in the induction of a number of phenotypes characteristic of asthma, and in all cases, this did not require exposure of the animals to antigen. While detailed comparisons are difficult because the parameters addressed did not overlap completely, all four mouse lines displayed an inflammatory response characterized by the enhanced eosinophilic airway inflammation and goblet cell metaplasia/ hyperplasia. However, differences were also noted between the lines. For example, IL-9 transgenics were the only mouse line in which an increase in the number of mast cells was observed (26). Charcot-Leyden–like crystals and extremely high levels of mucus were observed in the IL-13– overexpressing mice. Changes consistent with some aspect of airway remodeling were reported for some of the lines (27), IL-13, IL-9 and the IL-5 mice, but not for the IL-4 overexpressing lines. AHR to methacholine was noted in all the lines except the IL-4 mice, despite high levels of inflammation. Perhaps not surprisingly these elevated levels of cytokines can also lead to phenotypes not characteristic of asthma. For example, in the IL-9 mice, hypertrophy of the media of small arteries was noted (26).

When evaluating studies utilizing transgenic mice, it is important to note that mice generated with the same transgene can vary dramatically in the amount of cytokine produced and secreted. For example, sampling of the BAL from the various IL-9 founder transgenic lines revealed 10-fold differences between lines in the level of protein (26). If transgenic mice that express high levels of a given cytokine or chemokine are difficult to obtain, perhaps because these mice die in utero, misleading conclusions could arise regarding the relative potency of this mediator and its ability to induce asthma-like phenotypes. Another difficulty arises from the fact that not all investigators utilize inbred mice for the generation of their transgenic lines. Many transgenics have been made using F1 (filia generation 1) embryos, that is embryos generated by the intercross of two inbred lines such as C3H and C57BL/6. As is discussed in previous chapters, mouse lines can differ dramatically in both their naive airway reactivity to methacholine and the development of AHR after induction of allergic airway disease with antigens such as OVA. Differences in the genetic background and the alleles of the C3H and C57BL/6 in linkage with the insertion site during breeding could be responsible for phenotypic differences observed between transgenic animals and controls, rather than the transgene itself.

D. Transgenes Under Temporal Control

The expression pattern of these early transgenics was largely defined by the promoter utilized in their assembly. The identification of lung-specific promoters allowed high levels of expression in the lung while limiting complex phenotypes that might arise in other tissues as a result of overexpression of the inflammatory mediator. More recently, the ability to control expression of transgenes has been extended: it is now possible not only to have tissue-specific control of the transgene but also to turn the expression of transgene on and off during the lifetime of the animal (Fig. 1C). Such temporal control permits the study of genes whose enhanced expression during organogenesis may adversely impact normal lung development. This is particularly relevant to asthma where there is no evidence that the asthmatic lung at birth differs from individuals who will never develop the disease during their lifetime. The ability to regulate the transgenes expression in a temporal manner depends on the use of an inducible system- and tissue-specific mode of regulating tissue expression. The most common scheme utilized is a tetracycline-controlled expression system where the exposure of the mice to tetracycline or the stable analogue doxycycline turns on gene expression. This system is commonly referred to as a Tet-on system.

Tet-On Tet-Off System

This technology is the outgrowth of the discovery of the mechanism by which tetracycline resistance is conferred in *Escherichia coli*. The tetracycline resistance operon is carried by the *E. coli* transposon, Tn10. This operon has a negative mode of operation, where the interaction between a repressor protein, the Tet repressor (TetR) and the tet operator (*tet*O), a DNA sequence next to or juxtaposed with the promoter, prevents transcription of the genes—namely the TetR itself and a membrane protein that is capable of pumping the tetracycline from the cell. Tetracycline acts as an inducer by switching on the transcription system. It binds to the TetR, changing its conformation, so it can no longer remain attached to the operator. The ability of tetracycline to alter the DNA binding of this protein to the tet operator has been manipulated to generate both systems where exposure of the mice to tetracycline inhibits gene expression and systems where the exposure results in induction of gene expression. Because eukaryotic promoters cannot be directly regulated by the TetR, the development of both of these systems required the development of fusion proteins that possess both the DNA binding and tetracycline sensitivity of the TetR and the ability to activate a eukaryotic promoter. This was accomplished by fusing the TetR to the VP16 activation domain of herpes simplex virus. This fusion protein is often referred to as tet-controlled transcriptional activator (tTA). The promoter designed to be regulated by this fusion protein needed to be sensitive to the activation domain of VP16 after TetR binding mediates the binding of the fusion protein 5' of the transcriptional start site. A promoter with the appropriate characteristics was created by fusing multiple copies of the *tet*O with the minimal cytomegalovirus promoter. In the absence of tetracycline, the fusion protein, similar to the native TetR, binds to *tet*O, placing the VP16 domain in a position to activate gene expression. When tetracycline is added, the protein cannot bind and no expression is observed (28).

While this system provided a powerful means of regulating gene expression, it was not convenient for most transgenic experiments where, in general, the investigator would like to turn on gene expression at a specific time. As initially designed, mice would have to be fed tetracycline or doxycycline continually to prevent gene expression. This would be both costly and labor intensive. The induction of expression would take place slowly with the clearance of tetracycline from the system. The answer to these problems came with the development of a mutant form of the TetR protein, which differs from the wild-type TetR by four amino acid changes. When fused to the VP16 activator domain, this mutant protein creates a "reverse" tTA (rtTA) that activates transcription in the presence of tetracycline. This allows the gene to be turned on with the addition of tetracycline or doxycycline to the feed or water (28).

However, some inherent leakiness is expected in a system such as the Tet-on system, with low levels of transcription from the minimal CMV promoter observed even in the absence of tetracycline/deoxycycline. The extent to which this is a problem varies and is likely related to copy number of the transgene and the insertion site, as discussed later. To tighten control of transgene expression, some investigators have recently added an additional component to the system (Fig. 1D). This modification utilizes a eukaryotic silencer, a domain of the Kid-1 protein (kidney, ischemia developmentally regulated gene). A fusion protein is made, which consists of the KRAB-AB silencing domain of the Kid-1 protein and the wild type TetR protein (called tTS) (29). Because the fusion protein utilizes the wild type TetR, it binds to the promoter in the absence of tetracycline. The attached KRAB-AB acts as a potent suppressor of transcription from any promoter downstream of the *tet*O sequences. The use of this system requires generation of mice carrying three transgenes. In the lung, the lung-specific promoter will produce the rtTet and the tTS. In the absence of tetracycline, the tTS will bind to the promoter and prevent low-level leaky transcription from the minimal tetOCMV promoter. The rtTA will be produced but will be unable to bind in the absence of tet. The situation reverses when the animals are fed tetracycline, with the wild type TetR fusion protein (tTS) moving off the promoter to be replaced by the activation fusion protein rtTA (Fig. 1D) (30).

E. Temporal and Tissue-Specific Approach

Combining the tet-on tet-off system with the available lung-specific promoters has allowed the generation of mice in which cytokine expression can be regulated in both a temporal-specific and tissue-specific manner. In general, the transgene of interest is placed under control of the *tet*O minimal CMV promoter, a promoter, which, as discussed above, is dependent on the expression of the TetR VP16 fusion protein. If the gene encoding this fusion protein is also carried as a transgene and this transgene is under the control of a tissue-specific promoter, CC10 or CCSP, the expression of the gene becomes regulated by tetracycline, but only in the tissues expressing the tetRVIP protein. This "bitransgenic" system is not quite as complex as one might suppose. This technique takes advantage of the long-known fact that multiple DNA sequences introduced together into the pronucleus of the fertilized eggs form concatamers prior to integration. Because of this phenomenon, if two different DNAs are injected, they will generally reside at the same integration site, and as a result complex breeding issues are generally avoided. A general advantage of the inducible models is that they allow the investigator to manipulate the expression of the transgene throughout the lifetime of the animal.

A good comparison of the use of this method versus the generation of mice in which the transgene is driven directly by the tissue-specific promoter is afforded by the studies of IL-9. As discussed above, a transgenic mouse in which IL-9 expression was driven directly by the IL-9 gene was generated and this mouse developed a number of phenotypes relevant to asthma (26). With the development of the Tet-on technology, the same group generated a new mouse line in which the IL-9 gene was under the regulation of the tetOCMV promoter, while the TetRVIP fusion protein was under the regulation of the CC10 promoter (31). Adult mice were exposed to doxycycline for either 7 or 14 days and the change in inflammation compared to wild type mice and mice with the transgene that had not received the drug. Although levels of IL-9 were below detection in transgenic mice that received no drug, a small increase in inflammation and mucus production was noted, indicating that some low level production of IL-9 was likely occurring. However, changes in the lung after exposure for one to two weeks to the drug were dramatic and mimicked closely those findings observed in the animals in which IL-9 was constitutively produced under the direct control of CC10.

The ability to induce these changes facilitated a series of further experiments with these animals designed to determine the relationship between IL-9 and the other Th2 cytokines in the development of asthma (31). Using antibodies to inhibit various cytokines, the investigators were able to show the dependence of various aspects of the phenotype of the IL-9 mice on specific cytokines. For example, the eosinophilia observed in these mice could be abolished by inhibition of both IL-4 and IL-13, while goblet cell hyperplasia was only diminished when IL-13 was neutralized.

In the case of IL-9, the study of the inducible transgenics clearly demonstrated that chronic exposure to this cytokine was required for the development of asthma-like phenotypes. Furthermore, it facilitated the studies aimed at determining the relationship between IL-9 and IL-13 and IL-4, allowing inhibition of these cytokines prior to and during the development of disease. In this case, it allowed the authors to conclude that the asthma-like phenotypes of the IL-9–overexpressing mice was largely dependent upon elevated levels of IL-4 , IL-5, and IL-13 in these animals.

Difficulties and Limitations in the Use of Transgenic Mouse Lines

Transgenics have provided investigators with a powerful tool for cataloging the potential of specific inflammatory mediators to the development of discrete phenotypes within the allergic lung, e.g., the critical role of IL-13 to goblet cell hyperplasia. However, this approach is not without its shortcomings, some related to the technology itself and some more specific to the use of this approach and the interpretation of the findings gleaned from the study of these animals vis-à-vis the disease in humans.

Transgenes are introduced into the pronucleus where they are believed to undergo rolling circle amplification prior to insertion into the DNA. Generally, multiple copies of the transgene are located in the mouse, most at one insertion site. The copy number and expression is not only influenced by the number of copies of the gene inserted at the site, but by the site itself. Thus, a founder is often unique.

The phenotype of a transgenic line can drift for a number of reasons. Because of the tandem insertion of many copies of the same sequence into the genome, intrachromosomal recombination can occur, resulting in loss of the number of copies of the transgene at the insertion site. The tandem alignment of relatively short similar sequences into the genome can also trigger attempts by the organism to silence the "invading" genes. This silencing is accomplished by methylation of the DNA, preventing transcription of the inserted sequences (32). Thus, over time, the expression of some transgenes can be dramatically altered. The methylation of a number of transgenes has been studied in great detail. Interestingly, the site of integration can alter the susceptibility of the gene to methylation. Furthermore, some very nice examples of the influence of modifier genes on methylation of transgenes are present in the literature. This methylation effect needs to be considered when moving transgenes to new genetic backgrounds, because modifier genes on the new mouse strain may alter the methylation of the transgene. Under such a circumstance, reductions in trangene expression may account for the changes in phenotype.

Related to the problem of methylation is the observation that the expression of the transgene is often variegated. That is the transgene expression might be shut down in one cell and all its progenitors while the expression remains in neighboring cells. This variegation has been well documented in the mammary gland where often one lobe might express the transgene, while no expression can be detected in a neighboring lobe (33). This variegation, if not severe, is generally not a problem when the transgene expresses a soluble secreted factor. It also has not been problematic for situations where the transgene drives a powerful oncogene. Usually, the expression of the oncogene in even a small percentage of cells is sufficient to lead to the formation of tumors. However, in studies of cell surface receptors and channels, which may be limited in distribution, this variegation can be more problematic and lead to difficulties in interpretation. The use of larger transgenes such as bacterial artificial chromosomes provides a new option in some cases to deal with such issues. Because of their larger size, lower copy number, and inclusion of extensive upstream regulatory elements as well as introns, these transgenes often faithfully reproduce the expression pattern of the endogenous gene while remaining relatively innocuous, failing to trigger the host methylation system.

Finally, it is estimated that in 1 of 10 transgenes, the insertion alters the expression of an endogenous mouse gene. Generally, this proves to be problematic only if the transgene is maintained in a homozygous state. However, it leaves open the possibility that the phenotype observed in the transgenic mouse is in part the result of altered expression of genes other than the transgene. The study and comparison of a number of founder animals generally establishes the phenotype as a direct consequence of the expression of the transgene.

While the transgenic mouse provides a unique insight into putative roles of specific gene products in the lung, it is easy to overinterpret these findings. For example, in many cases, the levels of cytokine produced in the lung by transgenes exceeds levels documented in the BALF of asthmatic patients, and even those levels that can be achieved by a robust induction of airway disease in the mouse with allergen. Also, the expression profile and timing of production might not mimic the expression in asthma, even if high levels are found. It is often difficult to determine how many steps removed the overexpression of the protein is from a given phenotype and whether such a pathway is present and contributes to asthma in humans. For example, the study of the IL-9 transgene seems to suggest that the goblet cell hyperplasia is not the direct result of IL-9 but rather the indirect consequence of increased IL-13 production (26). Certainly, while this is an interesting finding, the question still remains regarding the role of IL-9 in the induction of IL-13 in the human disease. However, if a similar role for IL-9 is also found to be operative in asthma, interest in IL-9 as a potential therapeutic target is heightened, and further studies into other biological roles of this cytokine may help determine its suitability as a target.

F. Testing the Role of a Gene in the Development of Allergic Airway Disease: Generation of Mice with Null Alleles

Gene-Targeting by Homologous Recombination

It is now a relatively straightforward process to generate a null allele for a gene of interest in mouse. Replacement of part of an endogenous gene with a marker gene to create a null allele can be accomplished using homologous recombination in mouse embryonic stem (ES) cells. Generally the process entails the generation of a targeting plasmid with three essential components (Fig. 2A). First, the plasmid must contain sequences that share homology with the gene to be mutated: these sequences drive the recombination of the plasmid with the corresponding endogenous locus. Second, the plasmids usually carry a selectable marker that allows killing of all the ES cells that do not take up any plasmid DNA. The most common method for introducing DNA into ES cells is by electroporation, and using this method only a very small fraction, less than 2%, of the cells are transformed. Third, this selectable marker usually performs an additional function; it generally replaces part of the endogenous gene. Thus, the outcome of the recombination event is an allele in which the structure of one of the endogenous copies is altered in such a way that it no longer encodes a functional protein product. By far, the majority of studies using mouse models of asthma have examined the response of mice generated from ES cells carrying a null allele generated in this manner. For example, mice carrying null alleles for IL-4, IL-5, IL-9, and IL-13 have been generated and tested. In the majority of cases, loss of expression of genes alone is not sufficient to bring about changes in the lung, and generally these mice are challenged with antigen and the severity of the allergic airway disease monitored. However, a few notable exceptions have been reported. One such case is mice deficient in adenosine deaminase, a catabolic enzyme essential for maintaining normal serum and tissue adenosine levels (34). These mice developed severe respiratory distress with eosinophilic inflammatory infiltrates and goblet cell metaplasia observed histologically. These mice were shown to have elevated levels of adenosine in the BAL, suggesting that high levels of adenosine were responsible for the observed phenotype. Thus, in this case, the removal of an enzyme involved in the metabolism of a important inflammatory mediator results in high levels of this mediator, not unlike the overexpressing mice described above, and a asthma-like phenotype develops.

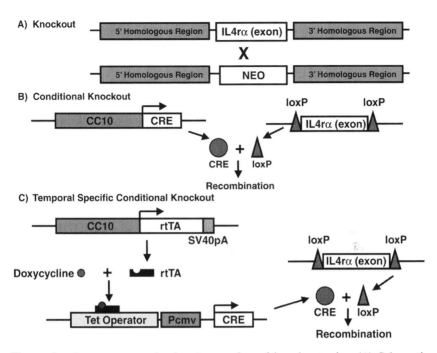

Figure 2 Common strategies for the creation of knockout mice. (**A**) Schematic illustration for the development of interleukin (IL)-4rα–deficient mice. A construct is designed, containing a neomycin resistance (Neo) cassette. Arms of homology are amplified from the endogenous locus from sites immediately 5′ and 3′ to a region critical to proper IL-4rα functioning. These amplification products are positioned adjacent to the Neo cassette. Following homologous recombination, the targeted IL-4rα region will be replaced with the Neo cassette. (**B**) Schematic illustration of the generation of a lung-specific IL-4rα–deficient mouse line. A transgene is designed containing the gene for Cre recombinase under the lung-specific CC10 promoter. A second mouse is generated in which critical regions of the IL-4Rα gene are flanked by *loxP* sites. In the presence of Cre recombinase, regions contained between *loxP* sites will be lost via recombination. (**C**) Schematic illustration of the generation of a temporal specific conditional IL-4rα–deficient mouse line. A construct is designed in which the CC10 promoter facilitates lung-specific constitutive expression of the reverse tetracycline transactivator (rtTA). rtTA requires the tetracycline derivative, doxycycline, for specific DNA binding to the tet operator. Once bound, this drives the expression of Cre recombinase. A second construct is designed in which loxP sites have been inserted into sequences flanking a region critical to proper IL-4rα functioning. In the presence of Cre recombinase, regions contained between loxP sites will be lost via recombination. *Abbreviations*: rtTA, reverse tetracycline transactivator; tet, tetracycline; IL, interleukin; NEO, gene for neomycin resistance.

Mice deficient in the T-box transcription factor T-bet, in the absence of allergen exposure, also develop a phenotype with similarities to asthma, including AHR measured indirectly by WBP (35). The role of this transcription factor in IFNγ expression in Th1 cells and its ability to redirect polarized Th2 cells to Th1 cells suggest that this phenotype is the result of altered balance in the activity of these two populations of T-cells.

In the majority of cases the mutations that have been studied in the allergic asthma models were introduced into ES cells derived from various substrains of 129 mice, with notable exceptions being the generation of the IL-4Rα null allele in BALB/c derived ES cells (36). The preeminence of 129 derived ES cells reflects the historical relationship between ES cells and 129 derived teratomas and the ease with which the pluripotency of these lines is maintained in culture. Remarkably, few mutations introduced into 129 mice have been maintained coisogenic (i.e., on the 129 background) and most studies have been conducted with populations generated after various numbers of backcrosses to either the C57BL/6 or the BALB/c genetic background. It is important to remember that even after 10 generations of backcrossing to a second strain, for example C57BL/6, it is estimated that around 20 cM of DNA will be of 129 origin. Thus, for example, IL-4 null mice will most certainly carry 129 alleles for the cluster of immunologically relevant genes clustered at 5q31 around the IL-4 gene. In contrast, control animals will be homozygous for the C57BL/6 alleles at all loci. Genes in epigenetic linkage with the 129 genes linked to the targeted locus may also be carried for many generations and can influence the outcome of complex experiments such as induction of allergic airway disease. In summary, considerable attention needs to be given to the origin of mutant mice generated by homologous recombination so that appropriate wild type controls can be anticipated.

The critical role of IL-4 in the maturation development of Th2 cells and in the isotype switching of B-cells to IgE production assured its place as one of the first genes mutated after establishment of the ES cell technology (36). Since the original description, these mice and mice lacking the alpha chain of the IL-4 receptor have been studied by a number of groups. Mice lacking the other TH2 cytokines followed behind and now these mice have been examined individually and in combination with other null alleles. For example, recently the IL-4-/-, IL-13-/- and mice homozygous for both mutations have been developed. Because of the close linkage of these two genes, mice were generated by a single recombination event that destroyed both genes (simultaneous disruption of interleukin, McKenzie) (37). In this study, mice were backcrossed to the BALB/c background, albeit for only six generations, and the AHR in response to methacholine examined by WBP. Naive mice lacking both IL-4 and IL-13 had essentially no inflammation in their lungs and thus, perhaps not surprisingly, had methacholine responsiveness that was indistinguishable from control animals. The attenuation of the inflammatory response was not the result of the loss of IL-13 as the inflammatory response was robust even in the absence of this cytokine. While, as described in the previous section, IL-13 overexpression results in a measurable increase in the number of eosinophils in the lung, the loss of this cytokine has little impact on recruitment of these cells in the OVA model. In contrast, the loss of IL-13 had a major impact on the production of mucus in this model. The transition of the airway epithelial Clara cells to periodic acid Schiff –positive mucus-producing goblet cells was attenuated. This finding is consistent with the high amounts of mucus produced in the transgenic IL-13 lines, and with findings discussed below in mice deficient in expression of an IL-13 receptor on airway epithelium in this same model. The mice that lacked IL-4 still developed AHR, suggesting that this change can occur independent of IL-4. Again, this is not surprising given that the transgenic mice with elevated IL-4 expression in the lung did not display AHR.

While overexpression of IL-9 resulted in a phenotype similar to that displayed by the other Th2 cytokine transgenics, the development of OVA-induced allergic airway disease was not greatly attenuated in mice lacking this cytokine (38). As discussed above, many of the asthma-like phenotypes of the IL-9 mice were shown to be dependant on IL-4, IL-5, and IL-13 expression in the lungs of these animals. The modest impact of the loss of this cytokine in the OVA model reflects this relationship; it is likely that IL-9–independent production of these Th2 cytokines drives the phenotypes in the IL9-/- animals.

Temporal-Specific and Tissue-Specific Removal of Gene Expression and Cell Types that Contribute to the Development of Asthma

Conditional Knockouts—Cre-Lox System

While mice carrying null mutations provided investigators with a powerful new tool for dissecting the role of a gene in complex pathways leading to allergic airway disease, these resources had their limitations. For example, it became apparent that many gene products are used in multiple ways, often by very different cell types, during the lifetime of an organism. If the gene under study plays an important role in embryonic development as well as in the development and/or function of the lung, studying the latter is not possible because of the early embryonic death of the animals homozygous for the null allele. New methods for circumventing this limitation in the new technology soon emerged. The methods for temporal and tissue-specific regulation of gene loss have their origins in the genetics of P1 phage and yeast, underscoring again the close interdependence of seemingly disparate lines or research. Research in the methods by which P1 bacteriophage excises from the bacterial chromosome and becomes a circular genome has led to the identification of Cre (cyclization recombination) recombinase and the DNA sequences to which it binds. These binding sites are 34 bp in length and are composed of an 8 bp core flanked by 13 bp inverted repeats. Cre recombinase recognizes a pair of *loxP* sites, and when two *loxP* sites are present in a segment of DNA, the spatial relationship of the two core sequences determines the nature of the recombination event mediated by the recombinase (Fig. 2A and C). Relevant to the discussion here, when the two sequences are orientated in the same direction, that is the *loxP* sites are in cis, the Cre will excise and circularize the DNA between the sites. When this occurs in mammalian cells, this recircularized DNA is usually quickly lost or degraded before the reverse event—integration back into the genome—can take place.

A second recombination system was identified in the yeast, *Saccharomyces cerevisiae*. The recombinase, termed "FLP," recognizes a pair of FLP recombinase target sequences termed "FLP recognition target" (FRT) sequences that are placed on each side of the genomic region of interest. As with *loxP* sites, orientation of the FRT sequences determines whether the recombination event leads to simply an inversion of these segments of DNA or a deletion event.

It was quickly realized that the P1 and yeast enzymes could carry out this recombination event in mammalian cells. For example, if the *loxP* sites are placed on either side of exon(s) essential for the function of a gene, then expression of Cre in the cell can be used to destroy the gene. Homologous recombination in ES cells provides a means of placing *loxP* sites around the exons of a particular gene in a live organism. Genes in which *loxP* sites flank critical exons are often referred to as "floxed" alleles or genes. If judiciously placed in intronic sequences upstream or downstream of a gene, the *loxP* sites can be added without interfering with the gene's expression. However, in cells in which the Cre protein is present, the *loxP* sites signal the destruction of the gene. Recombination removes the critical exons, and the normal function of the gene is lost. Which cells lose gene expression is dictated solely by the expression pattern of the Cre, which in turn is dictated by the promoter/induction systems used to drive the Cre transgene expression.

With Cre transgenics, the importance of obtaining a mouse in which the protein is expressed in a predicated pattern is amplified. It is essential that a very high percentage of the cell types under study express the protein at sufficient levels to ensure recombination between the two *loxP* sites. In addition, it is essential that rogue expression of the Cre in other cells does not occur because of the leaky expression of the promoter, perhaps due to the particular insertion site of the transgene. In addition, if Cre is expressed at a certain point in development in a broader spectrum of cells than in the adult, expression of the gene under study will be altered in all progenitors, even if these cells no longer express Cre. For, example, the human SPC promoter will drive Cre expression in the embryonic lung before formation of definite lung buds and therefore mediates recombination throughout the entire intrapulmonary respiratory epithelium (Perl PNAS) (39), even though in the adult lung, studies have shown that expression is restricted to specific subpopulations of lung epithelium cells. A detailed study of the expression throughout development of two promoters, CCSP and SPC, commonly utilized to regulate Cre expression in the lung has recently been published. In these systems, the Cre expression is placed under the control of the rtTA-regulated promoter. The rtTA expression in turn is regulated by either the rat CCSP protomer or the human surfactant C (SPC) promoter (Fig. 2C). The usefulness of both of these systems to generate mice in which loss of expression of a "floxed" gene is limited to the lung is detailed. One of these systems, the CCSPtTA transgenic, has since been used to examine the contribution of IL-4Rα expressed by the lung epithelium to the development of inflammation, goblet cell hyperplasia, and mucin gene expression in the OVA model (39).

IL-4Rα, a common subunit of the IL-4 and IL-13 receptor, is expressed by hematopoetic cells as well as cells in the lung—Clara cells and smooth muscle cells. Mice homozygous for the null IL-4Rα allele fail to develop allergic airway disease. However, because of the failure of these mice to develop inflamed lungs, the contribution of IL-4Rα activation on ASM and airway epithelia to development of AHR, goblet cell hyperplasia, and induction of mucin gene expression could not be addressed. To address this specific question, mice were generated, in which the loss of IL-4R was limited to airway cells. Mice carrying a floxed allele of IL-4R were mated to mice in which Cre expression required both expression of the CCSP-driven rtTA gene and dosing of the mice with tetracycline. Using this method, investigators found that while loss of IL-4Rα expression by the epithelial cells had no effect on the recruitment of mononuclear cells or eosinophils to the lung, it was required for goblet cell metaplasia and induction of mucin gene expression. The loss of IL-4Rα expression by airway epithelium had no affect on the development of AHR (40).

VI. Future Directions

Since the first establishment of laboratory strains of inbred mice originally derived from fancy mice that entertained the inhabitants of Victorian parlors, the laboratory mouse has provided the research community an invaluable resource for the study of mechanisms of human disease. With the development of a number of methods for the manipulation of the murine genome, the mouse has emerged as a model organism for the study of disease pathogenesis, drug discovery, and target validation. Despite the challenge of size, protocols for inducing allergic lung disease in mice more closely mimicking human asthma are continuing to be developed and refined. In the future, it is possible that strains will be engineered to carry multiple human alleles conferring genetic risk for asthma. While it is unlikely that such lines will spontaneously develop asthma in the absence of allergen, disease produced by allergen exposure models may more closely mirror the human disease. Combining routine and novel genetic approaches with better models of human disease will undoubtedly improve our understanding of the cellular and molecular events critical to asthma pathogenesis and suggest new targets for the prevention and treatment of this disease.

References

1. Campbell EM, Kunkel SL, Strieter RM, Lukacs NW. Temporal role of chemokines in a murine model of cockroach allergen-induced airway hyperreactivity and eosinophilia. J Immunol 1998; 161(12):7047–7053.
2. Coyle AJ, Wagner K, Bertrand C, Tsuyuki S, Bews J, Heusser C. Central role of immunoglobulin (Ig)E in the induction of lung eosinophil infiltration and T helper 2 cell cytokine production: inhibition by a non-anaphylactogenic anti-IgE antibody. J Exp Med 1996; 183(4):1303–1310.
3. Yu CK, Lee SC, Wang JY, Hsiue TR, Lei HY. Early-type hypersensitivity-associated airway inflammation and eosinophilia induced by dermatophagoides farinae in sensitized mice. J Immunol 1996; 156(5):1923–1930.
4. Taube C, Dakhama A, Gelfand EW. Insights into the pathogenesis of asthma utilizing murine models. Int Arch Allergy Immunol 2004; 135(2):173–186.
5. Kumar RK, Foster PS. Modeling allergic asthma in mice: pitfalls and opportunities. Am J Respir Cell Mol Biol 2002; 27(3):267–272.
6. Temelkovski J, Hogan SP, Shepherd DP, Foster PS, Kumar RK. An improved murine model of asthma: selective airway inflammation, epithelial lesions and increased methacholine responsiveness following chronic exposure to aerosolised allergen. Thorax 1998; 53(10):849–856.
7. Wegmann M, Fehrenbach H, Fehrenbach A, et al. Involvement of distal airways in a chronic model of experimental asthma. Clin Exp Allergy 2005; 35(10):1263–1271.
8. Hamelmann E, Schwarze J, Takeda K, et al. Noninvasive measurement of airway responsiveness in allergic mice using barometric plethysmography. Am J Respir Crit Care Med 1997; 156(3 Pt 1):766–775.
9. Petak F, Habre W, Donati YR, Hantos Z, Barazzone-Argiroffo C. Hyperoxia-induced changes in mouse lung mechanics: forced oscillations vs. barometric plethysmography. J Appl Physiol 2001; 90(6):2221–2230.
10. Bates JH, Irvin CG. Measuring lung function in mice: the phenotyping uncertainty principle. J Appl Physiol 2003; 94(4):1297–1306.
11. Tilley SL, Tsai M, Williams CM, et al. Identification of A3 receptor- and mast cell-dependent and -independent components of adenosine-mediated airway responsiveness in mice. J Immunol 2003; 171(1):331–337.
12. Levitt RC, Mitzner W. Expression of airway hyperreactivity to acetylcholine as a simple autosomal recessive trait in mice. Faseb J 1988; 2(10):2605–2608.
13. Martin TR, Gerard NP, Galli SJ, Drazen JM. Pulmonary responses to bronchoconstrictor agonists in the mouse. J Appl Physiol 1988; 64(6):2318–2323.

14. Hantos Z, Daroczy B, Suki B, Nagy S, Fredberg JJ. Input impedance and peripheral inhomogeneity of dog lungs. J Appl Physiol 1992; 72(1):168–178.
15. Schuessler TF, Bates JH. A computer-controlled research ventilator for small animals: design and evaluation. IEEE Trans Biomed Eng 1995; 42(9):860–866.
16. Poole JA, Matangkasombut P, Rosenwasser LJ. Targeting the IgE molecule in allergic and asthmatic diseases: review of the IgE molecule and clinical efficacy. J Allergy Clin Immunol 2005; 115(3):S376–S385.
17. Takeda K, Hamelmann E, Joetham A, et al. Development of eosinophilic airway inflammation and airway hyperresponsiveness in mast cell-deficient mice. J Exp Med 1997; 186(3):449–454.
18. Mehlhop PD, van de Rijn M, Goldberg AB, et al. Allergen-induced bronchial hyperreactivity and eosinophilic inflammation occur in the absence of IgE in a mouse model of asthma. Proc Natl Acad Sci USA 1997; 94(4):1344–1349.
19. Hamelmann E, Takeda K, Schwarze J, Vella AT, Irvin CG, Gelfand EW. Development of eosinophilic airway inflammation and airway hyperresponsiveness requires interleukin-5 but not immunoglobulin E or B lymphocytes. Am J Respir Cell Mol Biol 1999; 21(4):480–489.
20. Williams CM, Galli SJ. Mast cells can amplify airway reactivity and features of chronic inflammation in an asthma model in mice. J Exp Med 2000; 192(3): 455–462.
21. Ramos-Barbon D, Ludwig MS, Martin JG. Airway remodeling: lessons from animal models. Clin Rev Allergy Immunol 2004; 27(1):3–21.
22. Tepper RI, Levinson DA, Stanger BZ, Campos-Torres J, Abbas AK, Leder P. IL-4 induces allergic-like inflammatory disease and alters T cell development in transgenic mice. Cell 1990; 62(3):457–467.
23. Burstein HJ, Tepper RI, Leder P, Abbas AK. Humoral immune functions in IL-4 transgenic mice. J Immunol 1991; 147(9):2950–2956.
24. Dent LA, Strath M, Mellor AL, Sanderson CJ. Eosinophilia in transgenic mice expressing interleukin 5. J Exp Med 1990; 172(5):1425–1431.
25. Perl AK, Wert SE, Loudy DE, Shan Z, Blair PA, Whitsett JA. Conditional recombination reveals distinct subset of epithelial cells in trachea, bronchi, and alveoli. Am J Respir Cell Mol Biol 2005; 33(5):455–462.
26. Temann UA, Geba GP, Rankin JA, Flavell RA. Expression of interleukin 9 in the lungs of transgenic mice causes airway inflammation, mast cell hyperplasia, and bronchial hyperresponsiveness. J Exp Med 1998; 188(7):1307–1320.
27. Zhou Z, Homer RJ, Wang ZD, et al. Pulmonary expression of interleukin-13 causes inflammation, mucus hypersecretion, subepithelial fibrosis, physiologic abnomalities, and eotaxin production. J Clin Invest. 1999; 103(6):779–788.
28. Gossen M, Freundlieb S, Bender G, Muller G, Hillen W, Bujard H. Transcriptional activation by tetracyclines in mammalian cells. Science 1995; 268(5218): 1766–1769.
29. Freundlieb S, Schirra-Muller C, Bujard H. A tetracycline controlled activation/ repression system with increased potential for gene transfer into mammalian cells. J Gene Med 1999; 1(1):4–12.
30. Zhu Z, Ma B, Homer RJ, Zheng T, Elias JA. Use of the tetracycline-controlled transcriptional silencer (tTS) to eliminate transgene leak in inducible overexpression transgenic mice. J Biol Chem 2001; 276(27):25222–25229.

31. Temann UA, Ray P, Flavell RA. Pulmonary overexpression of IL-9 induces Th2 cytokine expression, leading to immune pathology. J Clin Invest. 2002; 109(1): 29–39.
32. Padjen K, Ratnam S, Storb U. DNA methylation precedes chromatin modifications under the influence of the strain-specific modifier Ssml. Mol Cell Biol 2005; 25(11):4782–4791.
33. Dobie KW, Lee M, Fantes JA, et al. Variegated transgene expression in mouse mammary gland is determined by the transgene integration locus. Proc Natl Acad Sci 1996; 93(13): 6659–6664.
34. Blackburn MR, Volmer JB, Thrasher JL, et al. Metabolic consequences of adenosine deaminase deficiency in mice are associated with defects in alveogenesis, pulmonary inflammation, and airway obstruction. J Exp Med 2000; 192(2): 159–170.
35. Finotto S, Neurath MF, Glickman JN, et al. Development of spontaneous airway changes consistent with human asthma in mice lacking T-bet. Science 2002; 295(5553):336–338.
36. Noben-Trauth N, Shultz LD, Brombacher F, Urban JF Jr., Gu H, Paul WE. An interleukin 4 (IL-4)-independent pathway for CD4+ T cell IL-4 production is revealed in IL-4 receptor-deficient mice. Proc Natl Acad Sci USA 1997; 94:10838–10843.
37. McKenzie GJ, Fallon PG, Emson CL, Grencis RK, McKenzie AN. Simultaneous disruption of interleukin (IL)-4 and IL-13 defines individual rules in T helper cells type 2-mediated responses. J Exp Med 1999; 189(10):1565–1572.
38. McMillan S, Bishop B, Townsend MJ, MeKenzie AN, Lloyd CM. The absence of interleukin 9 dose not affect the developement of allergen-induced pulmonary inflammation nor airway hyperreactivity. J Exp Med 2002; 195(1):51–57.
39. Perl AK, Wert SE, Nagy A, Lobe CG, Whitsett JA. Early restriction of peripheral and proximal cell lineages during formation of the lung. Proc Natl Acad Sci 2002; 99(16):10482–10487.
40. Kuperman DA, Huang X, Nguyenvu L, Holscher C, Brombacher F, Erle DJ. IL-4 receptor signaling in Clara cells is required for allergen-induced mucus production. J Immunol 2005; 175(6):3746–3752.

8

Comparative Genomics of Asthma

**IOANNIS M. STYLIANOU and
BEVERLY PAIGEN**

The Jackson Laboratory,
Bar Harbor, Maine, U.S.A.

JASPAL SINGH

Duke University Medical Center
and National Institute of
Environmental Health Sciences,
Durham, North Carolina, U.S.A.

DAVID A. SCHWARTZ

National Institute of Environmental
Health Sciences,
Durham, North Carolina, U.S.A.

I. Introduction

In this chapter, we briefly review the quantitative trait loci (QTL) that have been found for asthma and airway hyperresponsiveness (AHR) in mouse and human and show that many of these QTL map to homologous locations in both species. Whenever QTL for asthma are concordant in both species, we illustrate how comparative genomics can be used to narrow the QTL regions, thus reducing the potential number of candidate genes to be evaluated. We also review the progress that has been made in other fields using bioinformatics to find QTL genes and suggest that a systematic survey of AHR in multiple inbred mouse strains followed by several QTL crosses in the mouse could increase the usefulness of such bioinformatics tools for the field of asthma. Other chapters in this volume have reviewed the mouse as a model for asthma (1) and the asthma linkages found by whole genome scans in humans (2,3).

Because the primary trait measured in the mouse is AHR and as this chapter is focused on comparative genomics, we limited our review to human QTLs of AHR and clinically defined asthma, thus eliminating QTLs for atopy, IgE, eosinophilia, and other features of asthmatic disease. Each of these traits share QTLs with asthma, but each also has its own unique QTLs as well (2). AHR does not constitute clinical asthma; however, it is recognized as a critical phenotypic trait in humans, and individuals exhibiting AHR are more likely to display clinical asthma (4).

II. Concordance of Quantitative Trait Loci Across Species

Concordance refers to the observation that QTLs for the same trait map to homologous locations in different species. This was first shown for hypertension QTLs in rat, mouse, and human (5,6), but was subsequently extended to a variety of other diseases including kidney disease (7), plasma lipids (8), atherosclerosis (9), bone density (10), and asthma (shown below). This relationship has been quantified for a few traits; using human QTLs as the benchmark, 93% of high density lipoprotein cholesterol, 100% of low density lipoprotein cholesterol, 80% of triglyceride, and 63% of atherosclerosis QTLs are concordant with mouse QTLs for the same trait (8,9). Concordance facilitates the search for QTL genes because it can be used to narrow QTL regions and to test candidate genes as discussed below.

III. Asthma Quantitative Trait Loci in Humans and the Mouse

The 16 genome-wide scans and linkage studies for human asthma and its related phenotypes have been reviewed recently both in this volume (2,3) and elsewhere (11,12). Because we are focusing on comparative genomics, we limited the QTLs we discuss to asthma and AHR studies; the QTL from these 14 studies are listed in Table 1 and the locations depicted in the human-centric genomic map (Fig. 1). Each separate report of a QTL is shown as a bar in Figure 1. Human QTLs are to the left of each chromosome (Chr); mouse QTLs that map to homologous positions are shown to the right of the Chr (only those portions of the mouse QTL homologous to the human QTL are depicted). Figure 1 shows that some QTL have been found multiple times in diverse human populations and many of these QTL have also been found in homologous regions in the mouse. These QTL can be regarded with considerable confidence even though individual studies may not have reached statistical significance. Figure 1 also indicates the location of genes that have been reported to underlie certain QTL although a discussion of the evidence for these genes is beyond the scope of this chapter.

Inbred mouse lines are powerful tools for locating disease loci because an individual mouse is genetically homogenous to members of its strain and the environment can be rigorously controlled. In spite of these considerable advantages, only six asthma QTL studies have been performed

Table 1 Human Asthma and Bronchial Hyperresponsiveness QTL

Phenotype	Nearest marker	Chr	Peak	Upper boundary +15 Mb	Lower boundary +15 Mb	Band	p-Value	References
Clinical asthma	5p15	5	20,000,000	45,000,000	0	5p15	0.0008	(13)
Clinical asthma	17p11.1–17q11.2	17	19,500,000	44,500,000	0	17p11.1–17q11.2	0.0015	(13)
Clinical asthma	11p15	11	20,000,000	45,000,000	0	11p15	0.0089	(13)
Clinical asthma	2q33	2	198,000,000	223,000,000	173,000,000	2q33	0.0005	(13)
Clinical asthma	21q21	21	25,000,000	50,000,000	0	21q21	0.004	(13)
Clinical asthma	D14S1069–D14S289	14	69,046,450	84,046,450	52,457,943	14q24	0.0001	(14)
Clinical asthma	GATA31A10	7	37,908,040	52,908,040	22,908,040	7p14–7p15	0.005	(15)
Asthma, BHR	D20S482	20	4,454,279	19,454,279	0	20p13	0.001	(16)
Asthma	D1S255	1	37,318,810	52,318,810	22,318,810	1p34.3	0.005	(17)
Asthma	D1S197	1	50,462,529	65,462,529	35,462,529	1p33	0.007	(17)
Asthma	D5S426	5	34,798,707	49,798,707	19,798,707	5p13.2	0.006	(17)
Asthma	D11S968	11	133,323,661	134,452,384	118,323,661	11q25	0.003	(17)
Asthma	D4S2924	4	186,827,156	201,827,156	171,827,156	4q35.1	0.007	(17)
Asthma	D9S1786	9	96,119,566	111,119,566	81,119,566	9q22.32	0.006	(17)
Asthma	D12S1716	12	95,447,645	110,447,645	80,447,645	12q23.1	0.005	(17)
Asthma	D11S1337	11	67,888,234	82,888,234	52,888,234	11q13	0.0001	(18)
Asthma	FCERB	11	59,612,713	74,612,713	44,612,713	11q12	0.003	(19)
Asthma	D16S289	16	78,510,030	88,827,254	63,510,030	16q23.4	0.003	(19)
Asthma, BHR	D2S2298	2	44,053,930	59,053,930	29,053,930	2p21	0.0073	(20)
Asthma	D6S309	6	8,169,997	23,169,997	0	6p24.3	0.0134	(20)
Asthma	D6S291	6	36,373,494	51,373,494	21,373,494	6p21.31	0.0081	(20)
Asthma, BHR	D9S156	9	16,234,181	31,234,181	1,234,181	9p22.3	0.0073	(20)
Asthma	D9S283	9	89,643,900	104,643,900	74,643,900	9q22.2	0.0081	(20)
Asthma	D9S1784	9	105,118,300	120,118,300	90,118,300	9q31.1	0.0073	(20)
Asthma	D12S327	12	93,272,830	108,272,830	78,272,830	12q22	0.0177	(20)
Asthma	D17S250	17	34,405,618	49,405,618	19,405,618	17q12–q21	0.005	(21)
Asthma	D1S209	1	61,684,257	76,684,257	46,684,257	1p31	0.0006	(21)

(Continued)

Table 1 Human Asthma and Bronchial Hyperresponsiveness QTL (*Continued*)

Phenotype	Nearest marker	Chr	Peak	Upper boundary +15 Mb	Lower boundary +15 Mb	Band	p-Value	References
BHR	D19S180	19	58,441,514	63,859,143	43,441,514	19q13	0.05	(21)
Strict asthma	D1S468	1	3,608,114	18,608,114	0	1p36.32	0.0002	(11)
Strict asthma	D1S3669	1	17,528,974	32,528,974	2,528,974	1p36.13	0.0005	(11)
Loose asthma	D3S3564	3	42,393,981	57,393,981	27,393,981	3p22.1	0.0004	(11)
BHR	D5S1470	5	32,528,047	47,528,047	17,528,047	5p13.3	0.001	(11)
Loose asthma	D5S1462	5	96,406,286	111,406,286	81,406,286	5q15	0.0007	(11)
Strict asthma	D8S1477	8	32,186,709	47,186,709	17,186,709	8p12	0.0004	(11)
Strict asthma	D8S1110	8	53,343,525	68,343,525	38,343,525	8q11.23	0.0006	(11)
Strict asthma	D8S1136	8	65,753,949	80,753,949	50,753,949	8q13	0.0009	(11)
Loose asthma	GATA193A07[a]	14	88,000,000	103,000,000	73,000,000	14q24	0.0001	(11)
BHR	D19S900	19	48,859,247	63,859,247	33,859,247	19q13.31	0.001	(11)
BHR	D19S540	19	47,493,024	62,493,024	32,493,024	19q13.1	0.0004	(11)
Allergic asthma	D1S1646–D1S2667	1	9,244,643	22,244,643	0	1p36	2.02[b]	(22)
Allergic asthma	D5S1466	5	109,047,452	124,047,452	94,047,462	5q31	2.03[b]	(22)
Allergic asthma	D6S1006	6	12,968,137	27,968,137	0	6p24–22	2.37[b]	(22)
BHR	D3S1766	3	58,956,715	73,956,715	43,956,715	3p14.2	2.44[b]	(23)
Asthma	D3S2409	3	49,393,088	64,393,088	34,393,088	3p21.31	2.57[b]	(23)
Asthma, BHR	D5S816	5	135,329,409	150329,409	120,329,409	5q31.1	2.87[b]	(23)
Asthma	D19S714	19	15,589,159	30,589,159	589,159	19p13.12	2.17[b]	(23)
Allergic asthma	D4S2417–D4S408	4	183,034,937	191,411,208	168,034,937	4q35	0.0002	(24)
Allergic asthma	D5S820	5	156,054,978	171,054,978	141,054,978	5q33.3	0.00013	(24)
Allergic asthma	D5S1471	5	166,809,050	181,809,050	151,809,050	5q34	0.00017	(24)
Allergic asthma	D13S175–D13S217	13	24,008,193	39,008,193	9,0008,193	13q11	0.0004	(24)
BHR	D2S1780	2	3,238,478	18,238,478	0	2p25.3	0.00002	(25)
BHR	D16S412	16	23,070,122	38,070,122	8,070,122	16p12.1	0.02	(25)
BHR	D19S433	19	35,108,867	50,108,867	20,108,867	19q12	0.002	(25)

[a]Positions estimated from neighboring Marshfield markers.

[b]LOD scores.

Abbreviations: Chr, chromosome; BHR, bronchial hyperresponsiveness; LOD, logarithm of odds.

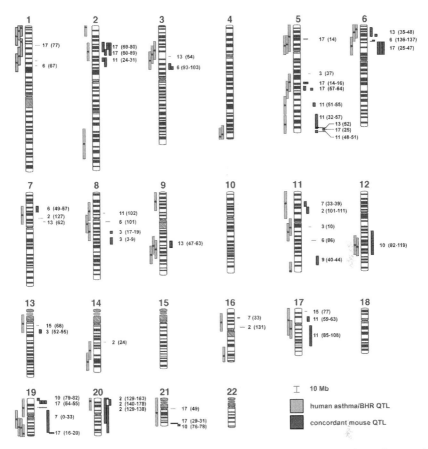

Figure 1 Chromosome map of human quantitative trait loci (QTL) for asthma and bronchial hyperresponsiveness and mouse concordant regions. The 95% confidence intervals (CIs) of human QTL are shown as gray bars to left of their respective chromosome, with the peaks indicated by a black line. This data are also given in Table 1. Mouse asthma QTL that are concordant to human QTL are shown to the right of each chromosome with the mouse chromosome and the position given in parentheses. Chromosomes are drawn to scale, based on the length of each chromosome from the Human Genome Browser. As many of the human studies do not report CIs or names of the markers that flank the intervals, determining accurate CIs is difficult. Here (and in Table 1) we generated a conservative CI by including a region of 15 million base pairs both up and downstream of the peak. *Abbreviations*: BHR, bronchial hyperresponsiveness; CI, confidence intervals; QTL, quantitative trait loci.

in the mouse using AHR as the phenotype (27–32) and two additional studies examined associated markers for asthma, such as the response to lipopolysaccharide (LPS) (33) and interleukin (IL)-4 and γδ-cells (34). These QTL are listed in Table 2 with the location of the QTL and the

Table 2 Summary of Quantitative Trait Loci Found for Airway Hyperresponsiveness and Related Phenotypes in the Mouse[a]

Cross	Naive/sensitized	Chr	Genetic marker	cM (95% CI)	Mb (95% CI)	Human syntenic region	LOD sign	Locus name	References
(B6×A) B6	Naive	2	D2Mit409	74.3 (69–105)	158.5 (122.5–163.3)	20q11/12	3[b]	*Bhr1*	(27)
	Naive	15	D15Mit107	49 (34.2–61.7)	84.7 (64.7–104.0)	22q12	3.7[b]	*Bhr2*	
	Naive	17	D17Mit26	11.7 (4.1–24)	23.9 (3.9–46.7)	16p13	2.8[c]	*Bhr3*	
(C3H×A) C3H	Naive	6	D6Mit366	42 (55–95)	115.6 (72.5–146.0)	3p24	3.3[b]	*Bhr5*	(28)
	Naive	7	D7Mit247	16 (0–30)	25.6 (0–54)	19q12/13	3.8[b]	*Bhr4*	
	Naive	17	D17Mit215	23 (0–43)	41.8 (0–80)	3p12/21	1.7[c]		
(C3H×A) C3H	Naive	6	D6Mit62	51 (26.4–63.3)	116.1 (53.2–132.6)	3p24	3.1[b]		(29)
A (C3H×A)	Ova	2	D2Mit39	5 (0–10)	9.3 (9.3–21.9)	11p11	4.2[b]	*Abhr1*	(30)
		2	D2Mit298	30 (10–31.7)	48.6 (23.0–55.3)	2q22	3.7[b]	*Abhr2*	
		7	D7Mit56	2.5 (0–22.5)	8.6 (0–28.6)	19q13	1.9[c]	*Abhr3*	
(B6×A) B6	Naive	2	Nr	Nr (80–105)	Nr (142.5–178.5)	20q12	1.1[c]		(35)
		6	Nr	Nr (0.5–36.5)	Nr (4.2–87.8)	7p15	1.4[c]		
(BP2×BALB/c) F2	Ova	9	D9Mit142	18 (7.1–27.2)	56.5 (40.5–61.7)	15q24/25	2.5[c]		(31)
	Ova	10	D10Mit70	44 (24–64)	102.8 (75–119)	12q23	3.8[c]		
	Ova	11	D11Mit19	7 (5.4–33.1)	25.3 (12.2–63)	2p16	3.4[b]		
	Ova	11	D11Mit99	52 (41.1–61.3)	99.3 (81.4–108.2)	17q21	3.7[b]		
	Ova	17	D17Mit32	10 (6.5–21.2)	33.2 (29–55.6)	6p21/22	2.1[b]		

(B6×DBA/2) F2 and RI	Naive	13	D13Ncvs44	30 (7.5–40)	50 (44–70)	6p22	2.5^b		(32)
BALB/c×B6 RC	Ova	17	Nr	Nr (7.6–55.7)	Nr (9.3–55.2)	6p21	Nr		(1)
BALB/c/DBA/2 congenic	Ova	11	D11Mit271–22	Nr (21–25)	Nr (45.5–47.5)	6p21/22	Nr	*Tapr*	(36)
(B6×DBA/2) F2	Naive	3	D3Mit63	22 (0–100)	40.8 (0–80)	4q27/28	5.3^b	*LadT1*	(34)
	Naive	17	D17Mit41	53 (42–57)	82.9 (60–93)	2q21	3.6^b	*LadT2*	
(B6×DBA/2) F2 and RI	LPS	11	Nr	50 (35–65)	87.4 (72–102)	17q23	5Nr	*Lppl1*	(33)
	LPS	11	Nr	40 (25–55)	65 (53–83)	17p13	6Nr	*Lptl1*	
	LPS	2	Nr	65 (50–80)	117.9 (97.9–137.9)	15q14	2Nr	*Lptl2*	

[a] 95% CI or 1.5 LOD drop; cM position as reported by the authors or based on the MGD map; Mb is megabase position based on NCBI 33 ensemble build 31; LOD score reported or converted to an equivalent value; Nr, not reported or could not be deduced from the publication.

[b] Genome wide significant.

[c] Genome wide suggestive.

Abbreviations: Chr, chromosome; CI, confidence interval; cM, centimorgans; Mb, millions of base pairs; LPS, lipopolysaccharide; LOD, logarithm of odds.

95% confidence intervals (CI) in centimorgans (cM) and in millions of base pairs (Mb) from the centromere. The locations are depicted in the mouse-centric genomic map (Fig. 2) with each bar representing a QTL from a separate cross. Mouse QTL are to the left of the Chr and human QTL that map to homologous locations are to the right of the Chr. Some human homologous regions are very small and consist of only one to two genes; these may be true homologies or they may be genes that have not been mapped correctly. We place greater weight on those homologous regions that are larger in size. Some murine QTL are consistent across multiple crosses such as the locus on Chr 17, which appears in three independent crosses (27,28,31). Further evidence for an asthma locus on Chr 17 originates from studies using recombinant congenic strains with BALB/c and STS backgrounds (1) and a QTL in this location for change in $\gamma\delta$ cells from a C57BL/6 (B6)×DBA/2 F2 intercross (34). Finding a QTL in multiple crosses not only indicates that the mutation causing it is likely to be an ancestral mutation shared by many strains, but also greatly enhances the probability of finding the causal gene because the QTL region can be narrowed by haplotype analysis as explained below.

In addition to the loci for main effects, four occurrences of epistasis are reported, that is, loci that interact to affect the asthma phenotype (Table 3); these are indicated by arrows in Figure 2. De Sanctis et al. (27) identified one interaction between Chr 2 and Chr 17, and a second interaction between Chr 15 and Chr 17. Ackermam et al. (35) reported another interaction between Chr 2 and Chr 6; however, it is difficult to determine whether this is the same as the Chr 2 loci in the DeSanctis study because the confidence intervals of interacting loci include the uncertainty of both loci and therefore are large. Ewart et al. (30) reported an interaction between two closely linked QTL on proximal Chr 2, which are different from the previously reported Chr 2 interacting loci.

Table 3 summarizes the major features of these QTLs for asthma. For human asthma, at least 31 genomic regions contain asthma QTL, although that number may increase if some of these regions contain multiple closely linked QTLs. Of these, 14 (45%) have been replicated at least twice, increasing the confidence in their validity. Moreover, 19 (61%) have strong homology to mouse QTL, defined as a homologous region that is at least a megabase in size, and 26 (84%) have some homology to a mouse QTL (including those homologous regions that are very small and may include only one or two genes) indicating that asthma QTL are concordant as are the QTL for other diseases. For mouse QTL, at least 16 genomic regions contain AHR QTL. Of these, 9 (56%) have been replicated at least twice; moreover, 12 (75%) have strong homology to human QTL, and all 16 have homology to human QTL if the very small homology regions are included (Table 4).

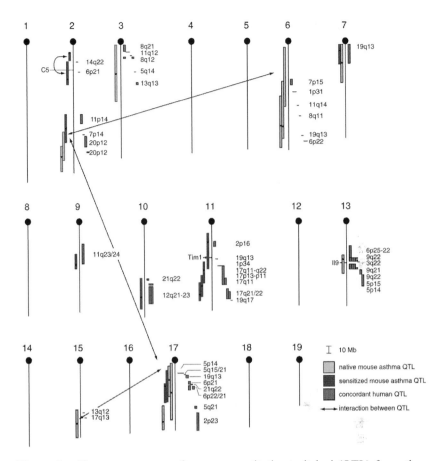

Figure 2 Chromosome map of mouse quantitative trait loci (QTL) for asthma, human concordant regions and QTL candidate genes. The 95% confidence intervals (CI) of mouse QTL are shown as bars to left of their respective chromosome, with the peaks indicated by a black line. Bars are light gray if the QTL is derived from a naïve, and black if derived from a sensitized mouse study. This data is also given in Table 2. Human asthma QTLs that are concordant to mouse QTL are shown to the right of each chromosome along with the human chromosomal region. Interactions between loci (as listed in Table 3) are indicated by the arrows. Chromosomes are drawn to scale with the centromere at the top, based on the length of each chromosome from Mouse Genome Browser. If CIs were not reported or could not be elucidated from the data, a conservative region was created here (and in Table 2) covering 20 million base pairs up and downstream of the peak of the QTL. Candidate genes are to the left of the chromosomes. *Abbreviations*: CI, confidence intervals; QTL, quantitative trait loci.

Table 3 Mouse Quantitative Trait Loci Interactions

Cross	Chr a	Chr b	Locus interaction	References
(C57BL/6×A/J) C57BL/6	2	17	*Bhr1xBhr3*	(27)
	15	17	*Brh2xBhr3*	
(C57BL/6×A/J) C57BL/6	2	6		(35)
AJ (C3H/HeJ×A/J)	2	2	*Abhr1xAbhr2*	(30)

Abbreviation: Chr, chromosome.

IV. Comparative Genomics

Comparative genomics is a powerful tool in the search for QTL genes in multiple ways. First, finding QTLs in homologous regions in different species is essentially a replication of that QTL and thus, it adds to the confidence that a gene affecting the phenotype maps to that region. Second, comparative genomics can be used to narrow the QTL region for both species. When a mouse and human QTL are found in homologous locations, we make the assumption that the same gene underlies the QTL in both species. The narrowing of QTL regions can occur because many chromosomal breaks and rearrangements have happened during mammalian evolution. Currently, there are about 340 known conserved segments between mouse and human (38). A typical mouse QTL may be homologous to three to five human Chrs; if one of these is homologous to a QTL for the same trait in humans, this immediately narrows the region to that homologous segment, thus reducing the size of the QTL in both species. This assumption could be incorrect if a cluster of related genes map to the same location on the chromosome and one gene underlies the QTL in the mouse and a different one in the human; and if this is the case, it will become apparent when individual candidate genes are tested further. Finally, comparative

Table 4 Summary of QTL Trait Loci in Human and Mouse and the Degree of Concordance

	Number	Percentage
Number of human QTL regions	31	—
Number replicated	14	45
Number with strong homology to mouse	19	61
Number with any homology to mouse	19	84
Number of mouse QTL regions	16	—
Number replicated	9	56
Number with strong homology to human	12	75
Number with any homology to human	16	100

Abbreviation: QTL, quantitative trait loci.

genomics can be used to help identify or prove the correct candidate gene when the number of candidate genes has been reduced to only one or a few genes. These candidates can be tested in humans in a case-control association study, but because of the prior knowledge derived from the animal model, such a hypothesis-driven association study has greater statistical power. This strategy of identifying a limited number of candidate genes in the mouse, testing them in a case-control association study in humans, and finally returning to the mouse for additional studies on gene function or for final gene proof using genetically engineered models has been used successfully to find QTL genes in a number of studies including *Ox40l* for atherosclerosis (39), complement factor 5 for liver fibrosis (40), and *Csnk1e* for amphetamine sensitivity (41,42). This finding of the same gene underlying a QTL in two different species is one of the multiple lines of proof for a candidate gene being the causal gene as outlined by the Complex Trait Consortium (43).

Here we illustrate two examples of how comparative genomics and another bioinformatics tool, haplotype analysis, can be used to narrow QTL. The mouse Chr 7 QTL was reported in two separate studies, both using the same parental strains, A/J and C3H. This chromosomal region is homologous to human 19q13, which also contains a QTL associated with asthma and BHR. The location of the two mouse QTLs is shown in Figures 2 and 3 in more detail showing the position of the homologous region of the human Chr 19 QTL. If one narrows the mouse QTL to only that portion homologous to the human Chr 19 QTL, the region is narrowed from 54 to 28.5 Mb. Next, the QTL region can be narrowed by haplotype analysis. This is based on the observation that common inbred mouse strains share regions of DNA that are identical by descent (IBD) due to common progenitors about 100 years ago (44). QTL genes are unlikely to be in these IBD regions, because 97% of mutations are ancestral (45). Thus, these IBD regions, which are inferred by single nucleotide polymorphism (SNP) haplotypes, can be eliminated from consideration in the QTL [explained more fully in a recent review by DiPetrillo et al. (46)]. The results of the SNP haplotype analysis, shown in Figure 3, reduced the QTL region to 18.5 Mb. The reduction of QTL by haplotyping becomes more powerful as more strains are involved. Thus, these two bioinformatics tools of comparative genomics and haplotype analysis narrowed the QTL from 54 Mb containing 710 transcripts to 18.5 Mb containing 304 transcripts, which greatly reduces the region that must be searched for candidate genes.

Another example is shown for mouse Chr 13. By reanalyzing the phenotypic data of the BxD recombinant inbred lines in the original paper (32) in combination with the new SNP genotyping data from Oxford (47), we found that this QTL has two distinct peaks, which are indicated in Figure 3 by black lines in the QTL. The first is homologous to human 6p21, and the second is homologous to 9q22. Narrowing the QTL to the regions with human homology narrows the QTL from 26.5 to 21 Mb; further narrowing by

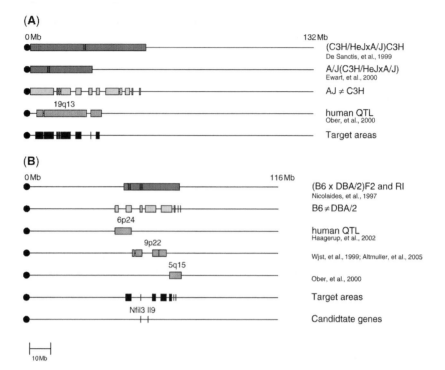

Figure 3   Fine detailed maps of mouse chromosomes 7 (**A**) and 13 (**B**). Maps are generated with three sets of data leading to "target areas" that satisfy the best conditions for containing candidate genes of interest. First each map shows the mouse chromosomes with 95% confidence interval of the QTL, given in dark gray horizontal bars, and within these intervals the peaks are given by vertical dark bars in the 95% CI. Second, the regions that should be further considered are the regions that are not homologous by descent between the strains of mice that generated the QTL, e.g., for Chr 7 the regions that are of further interest are the regions that differ between A/J and C3H—indicated by the light gray bars in (**A**). Finally, the regions that are of additional interest are the regions that contain concordant human QTL as indicated for each study by the medium gray bars, leading to finalized regions satisfying all three optimal conditions indicated by black bars. *Abbreviations*: QTL, quantitative trait loci; CI, confidence intervals.

haplotype analysis reduces the QTL to several distinct regions that together total 10.5 Mb. Most importantly, a small 3.6 Mb region containing 10 genes surrounds the first QTL peak, and a smaller 0.7 Mb region containing four genes surrounds the second QTL peak. This considerably focuses the search for asthma genes. For example, the second region of four genes contains *E4bp4*/*Nfil3*, which is a transcription factor that transactivates Il3 (48), a cytokine known to be important in asthma (49). Previous reports have suggested that *Il9* might account for this QTL, but the *Nfil3* gene should be tested as well.

These examples illustrate why it is so important that additional QTL crosses be carried out for asthma in the mouse; the assumption that QTL genes represent ancestral mutations and that regions of DNA IBD can be eliminated are best made when the QTL has been replicated in two crosses rather than relying on a single cross as we have done in both examples. QTLs found in a single cross could result from recent mutations, although these are estimated to represent only 3% of all mutations, and haplotype analysis, which is based on the assumption that the mutation is ancestral, would then be based on a false assumption and lead to an incorrect gene.

V. Steps that Would Enhance Asthma Research

Several new bioinformatics tools that enhance the search for the identity of QTL genes have been developed recently and are explained in a recent review (46). We illustrated the use of two of these tools, comparative genomics and haplotype analysis, for Chrs 7 and 13. However, the use of some of the other tools, those of combining crosses and haplotype association mapping, cannot be readily applied to the field of asthma research at this time due to the lack of appropriate infrastructure. To move the field forward rapidly and to make full use of the power of the mouse model in identifying human asthma genes, several steps need to be taken. These are (i) a comprehensive survey of asthma susceptibility among mouse strains, (ii) a number of additional QTL crosses, and (iii) a commitment to place the raw data for QTL crosses into a public database beginning with the crosses that are already published and adding new ones as they are published.

A. Comprehensive Survey of Asthma Susceptibility Among Inbred Strains

An extended strain survey of a set of 30 to 40 inbred strains should be carried out following the general principles set out in the Mouse Phenome Project (50), testing at least 10 males and 10 females of each strain at two to three months of age under standard conditions. Such a strain survey would set the stage for additional QTL crosses between susceptible and resistant strains, because it would allow an investigator to choose parents that differ in the trait. Although six QTL crosses for asthma (AHR) have been carried out previously, most used A/J as the hyperresponsive parent, and we need to have a wider sampling of the genetic diversity available among inbred mouse strains. At least five strain surveys of AHR have been carried out (51,52), but they used six to nine strains, a variety of different challenges, and different methods of measuring AHR. In general, they agree that certain strains such as A/J and AKR/J are highly responsive whilst other strains, C57BL/6J, SJL/J, and C3H/HeJ, are the least responsive, but to be effective, the strain survey must be carried out for many more strains with constant conditions.

In addition to being useful for choosing parents for additional QTL crosses, an extensive survey of strains for AHR could be used for in silico QTL mapping (53), a technique that we prefer to call haplotype association mapping (46). Genome-wide association of haplotype with strain phenotype predicts the location of QTL, and when these predicted QTL fall within an experimental QTL, they serve to narrow the QTL region. QTLs found by haplotype association mapping are very small, on the order of a few megabases, compared to cross QTLs, which can be 40 Mb in size. Thus, the number of candidate genes is reduced considerably, making the QTL gene identification easier. This powerful tool cannot be used in asthma research until an extensive strain survey is carried out. An additional benefit from the strain survey followed by haplotype association mapping would be that predicted QTLs not already found in the mouse could be used as a guide to choosing the parents for future crosses in a hypothesis-driven QTL study. Currently, one chooses the parents of a QTL cross primarily by maximizing the phenotypic difference between the parents and perhaps also taking into account the genetic diversity between the parental strains. However, a computational QTL analysis would indicate which parental strains could be intercrossed with the expectation that new QTLs would be found. Such an exercise would be particularly useful for a trait such as chronic obstructive pulmonary disease, a trait for which no QTL crosses exist. By doing a strain survey followed by haplotype association mapping to find the computation QTLs, one could select the parents for QTL crosses efficiently.

B. Additional QTL Crosses

It is important to carry out enough QTL crosses for a trait so that the QTL map approaches saturation; that is new crosses using different parental strains detect primarily QTL that have been previously found. This has occurred for HDL cholesterol QTL in the mouse (54) and indicates that most major QTL have been found. The fact that QTL are replicated in many different strains enhances the power of haplotype analysis for reducing QTL regions. Although six crosses have been carried out for asthma in the mouse, three of these use the same parental strains (A and C3H), so this is equivalent to only four samplings of the genetic information of inbred strains. Based on the number of QTL crosses for other traits needed before significant replication of QTLs occurred and the fact that 40% of asthma QTLs have already been replicated with the limited crosses done, we estimate that at least six additional crosses are needed using parental strains that differ from the limited set used so far (B6, DBA/2, BALB/c, C3H, A/J, BP2, and STS).

C. Placing Data for QTL Crosses into a Public Database

Another powerful bioinformatics tool for narrowing QTL regions is the ability to statistically combine data from existing QTL crosses. This method is usually done on a chromosome by chromosome basis but can be done for an entire cross (55). The assumption is that the same gene underlies a QTL that maps to the same place, so combining the data increases the number of recombination events and results in better resolution of the QTL interval. If this assumption is incorrect, then the combining of crosses will lead to a broadening of the QTL peak or even a splitting of the peak into two peaks, providing evidence for two closely linked QTLs. Combined cross analysis provides increased power to detect QTLs, to narrow QTL regions, and to resolve closely linked QTLs as compared to individual crosses. The drawback is that the statistician must have access to the raw data from the crosses; the published information is not sufficient. To facilitate this bioinformatics tool, a public database has been created by Dr. Churchill at The Jackson Laboratory where investigators can deposit their raw QTL cross data after it has been published (56). This archive now contains data from over 30 QTL crosses although no asthma crosses are there. For example, in Figure 3, two crosses for a QTL on Chr 7 are shown. If these data were combined, the QTL region could be narrowed considerably at the cost of a few days of statistical effort. QTL data is often lost over time and this archive is a safe place to store it. Furthermore, as advances are made in QTL mapping, such as the ability to search for gene interaction, to calculate 95% CI, or to combine crosses, these advances can be applied to previously made crosses. Asthma research would benefit if there was a commitment of investigators to place the raw data from each QTL cross into a public database after the results are published beginning with the already published crosses.

VI. Concluding Remarks

In conclusion, we see that the QTLs for asthma and AHR in human and mouse are concordant, that is they map to homologous regions, as they do for many other diseases. Using human QTLs as the benchmark, the degree of concordance is 61%, which is somewhat lower than for plasma lipids, which are 93% for HDL cholesterol, and 100% for LDL cholesterol. This lower degree of concordance for asthma does not represent a difference between diseases, but rather a paucity of mouse studies for asthma because only six QTL crosses have been done and three used the same set of parents, so a very limited sampling of the mouse genome has occurred. The fact of concordance facilitates QTL gene finding because the mouse model and human studies can be used to complement each other.

Comparative genomics and haplotype analysis are two bioinformatics tools that can be used to narrow QTL regions, and thus reduce the effort in search for QTL genes. Other bioinformatics tools such as combined crosses and haplotype association mapping cannot be used in the field of asthma or chronic obstructive pulmonary disease until certain infrastructure is built. These include an extensive strain survey of the phenotype, a number of QTL crosses, and a commitment by the community to deposit raw QTL cross data in a common archive. These steps could accelerate the pace of gene finding for asthma and chronic obstructive pulmonary disease research.

Acknowledgments

We thank Jesse Hammer from the multimedia services of the Jackson Laboratory for graphical assistance.

References

1. Piavaux B, van Osterhout AM, Hylkema MN. Mouse models for asthma and mouse asthma genetics. In: Potsma DS, Weiss ST, eds. Genetics of Asthma and COPD, 2006; 6:103–124.
2. Howard TD, Celedon J. Linkage for asthma and intermediate phenotype. In: Potsma DS, Weiss ST, eds. Genetics of Asthma and COPD, 2006; 10:197–203.
3. Moffatt MF, Cookson WO. Fine mapping strategies in asthma and COPD and whole genome association studies. In: Potsma DS, Weiss ST, eds. Genetics of Asthma and COPD, 2006; 12:221–236.
4. Laprise C, Boulet LP. Asymptomatic airway hyperresponsiveness: a three-year follow-up. Am J Respir Crit Care Med 1997; 156(2 Pt 1):403–409.
5. Stoll M, Kwitek-Black AE, Cowley AW Jr., et al. New target regions for human hypertension via comparative genomics. Genome Res 2000; 10(4):473–482.
6. Sugiyama F, Churchill GA, Higgins DC, et al. Concordance of murine quantitative trait loci for salt-induced hypertension with rat and human loci. Genomics 2001; 71(1):70–77.
7. Korstanje R, DiPetrillo K. Unraveling the genetics of chronic kidney disease using animal models. Am J Physiol Renal Physiol 2004; 287(3):F347–F352.
8. Wang X, Paigen B. Genome-wide search for new genes controlling plasma lipid concentrations in mice and humans. Curr Opin Lipidol 2005; 16(2):127–137.
9. Wang X, Ishimori N, Korstanje R, et al. Identifying novel genes for atherosclerosis through mouse-human comparative genetics. Am J Hum Genet 2005; 77(1):1–15.
10. Klein RF. Genetic regulation of bone mineral density in mice. J Musculoskelet Neuronal Interact 2002; 2(3):232–236.
11. Ober C, Leavitt SA, Tsalenko A, et al. Variation in the interleukin 4-receptor alpha gene confers susceptibility to asthma and atopy in ethnically diverse populations. Am J Hum Genet 2000; 66(2):517–526.
12. Wills-Karp M, Ewart SL. The genetics of allergen-induced airway hyperresponsiveness in mice. Am J Respir Crit Care Med 1997; 156(4 Pt 2):S89–S96.

13. CSGA, The Collaborative Study on the Genetic of Asthma. A genome-wide search fot asthma susceptibility loci in ethnic diverse populations. Nat Genet 1997; 15:389–392.

14. Hakonarson H, Bjornsdottir US, Halapi E, et al. A major susceptibility gene for asthma maps to chromosome 14q24. Am J Hum Genet 2002; 71(3):483–491.

15. Laitinen T, Daly MJ, Rioux JD, et al. A susceptibility locus for asthma-related traits on chromosome 7 revealed by genome-wide scan in a founder population. Nat Genet 2001; 28(1):87–91.

16. Van Eerdewegh P, Little RD, Dupuis J, et al. Association of the ADAM33 gene with asthma and bronchial hyperresponsiveness. Nature 2002; 418(6896): 426–430.

17. Altmuller J, Seidel C, Lee YA, et al. Phenotypic and genetic heterogeneity in a genome-wide linkage study of asthma families. BMC Pulm Med 2005; 5(1):1.

18. Huang SK, Mathias RA, Ehrlich E, et al. Evidence for asthma susceptibility genes on chromosome 11 in an African–American population. Hum Genet 2003; 113(1):71–75.

19. Daniels SE, Bhattacharrya S, James A, et al. A genome-wide search for quantitative trait loci underlying asthma. Nature 1996; 383(6597):247–250.

20. Wjst M, Fischer G, Immervoll T, et al. A genome-wide search for linkage to asthma. German Asthma Genetics Group. Genomics 1999; 58(1):1–8.

21. Dizier MH, Besse-Schmittler C, Guilloud-Bataille M, et al. Genome screen for asthma and related phenotypes in the French EGEA study. Am J Respir Crit Care Med 2000; 162(5):1812–1818.

22. Haagerup A, Bjerke T, Schiotz PO, et al. Asthma and atopy—a total genome scan for susceptibility genes. Allergy 2002; 57(8):680–686.

23. Meyers DA, Postma DS, Stine OC, et al. Genome screen for asthma and bronchial hyperresponsiveness: interactions with passive smoke exposure. J Allergy Clin Immunol 2005; 115(6):1169–1175.

24. Yokouchi Y, Nukaga Y, Shibasaki M, et al. Significant evidence for linkage of mite-sensitive childhood asthma to chromosome 5q31-q33 near the interleukin 12 B locus by a genome-wide search in Japanese families. Genomics 2000; 66(2): 152–160.

25. Xu X, Fang Z, Wang B, et al. A genomewide search for quantitative-trait loci underlying asthma. Am J Hum Genet 2001; 69(6):1271–1277.

26. www.ensembl.org/Homo_sapiens.

27. De Sanctis GT, Merchant M, Beier DR, et al. Quantitative locus analysis of airway hyperresponsiveness in A/J and C57BL/6J mice. Nat Genet 1995; 11(2): 150–154.

28. De Sanctis GT, Singer JB, Jiao A, et al. Quantitative trait locus mapping of airway responsiveness to chromosomes 6 and 7 in inbred mice. Am J Physiol 1999; 277(6 Pt 1):L1118–L1123.

29. Ewart SL, Mitzner W, DiSilvestre DA, et al. Airway hyperresponsiveness to acetylcholine: segregation analysis and evidence for linkage to murine chromosome 6. Am J Respir Cell Mol Biol 1996; 14(5):487–495.

30. Ewart SL, Kuperman D, Schadt E, et al. Quantitative trait loci controlling allergen-induced airway hyperresponsiveness in inbred mice. Am J Respir Cell Mol Biol 2000; 23(4):537–545.

31. Zhang Y, Lefort J, Kearsey V, et al. A genome-wide screen for asthma-associated quantitative trait loci in a mouse model of allergic asthma. Hum Mol Genet 1999; 8(4):601–605.
32. Nicolaides NC, Holroyd KJ, Ewart SL, et al. Interleukin 9: a candidate gene for asthma. Proc Natl Acad Sci USA 1997; 94(24):13,175–13,180.
33. Cook DN, Wang S, Wang Y, et al. Genetic regulation of endotoxin-induced airway disease. Genomics 2004; 83(6):961–969.
34. Azuara V, Pereira P. Genetic mapping of two murine loci that influence the development of IL-4-producing Thy-1dull gamma delta thymocytes. J Immunol 2000; 165(1):42–48.
35. Ackermam KG, Huang H, Grasemann H, et al. Interacting genetic loci cause airway hyperresponsiveness. Physiol Genomics 2005; 21(1):105–111.
36. McIntire JJ, Umetsu SE, Akbari O, et al. Identification of Tapr (an airway hyperreactivity regulatory locus) and the linked Tim gene family. Nat Immunol 2001; 2(12):1109–1116.
37. www.ensembl.org/Mus_musculus.
38. Pennacchio LA. Insights from human/mouse genome comparisons. Mamm Genome 2003; 14(7):429–436.
39. Wang X, Ria M, Kelmenson PM, et al. Positional identification of TNFSF4, encoding OX40 ligand, as a gene that influences atherosclerosis susceptibility. Nat Genet 2005; 37(4):365–372.
40. Hillebrandt S, Wasmuth HE, Weiskirchen R, et al. Complement factor 5 is a quantitative trait gene that modifies liver fibrogenesis in mice and humans. Nat Genet 2005; 37(8):835–843.
41. Palmer AA, Verbitsky M, Suresh R, et al. Gene expression differences in mice divergently selected for methamphetamine sensitivity. Mamm Genome 2005; 16(5):291–305.
42. Veenstra-Vanderweele J, Qaadir A, Palmer AA, et al. Association between the Casein Kinase 1 Epsilon gene region and subjective response to D-amphetamine. Neuropsychopharmacology 2005:1–8.
43. Abiola O, Angel JM, Avner P, et al. The nature and identification of quantitative trait loci: a community's view. Nat Rev Genet 2003; 4(11):911–916.
44. Wade CM, Kulbokas EJ III, Kirby AW, et al. The mosaic structure of variation in the laboratory mouse genome. Nature 2002; 420(6915):574–578.
45. Frazer KA, Wade CM, Hinds DA, et al. Segmental phylogenetic relationships of inbred mouse strains revealed by fine-scale analysis of sequence variation across 4.6 Mb of mouse genome. Genome Res 2004; 14(8):1493–1500.
46. DiPetrillo K, Wang X, Stylianou IM, et al. Bioinformatics toolbox for narrowing rodent quantitative trait loci. Trends Genet 2005; 21(12):683–692.
47. Wellcome—CTC Mouse Strain SNP Genotype Set. http://www.well.ox.ac.uk/mouse/INBREDS.
48. Zhang W, Zhang J, Kornuc M, et al. Molecular cloning and characterization of NF-IL3A, a transcriptional activator of the human interleukin-3 promoter. Mol Cell Biol 1995; 15(11):6055–6063.
49. Park BL, Kim LH, Choi YH, et al. Interleukin 3 (IL3) polymorphisms associated with decreased risk of asthma and atopy. J Hum Genet 2004; 49(10):517–527.

50. www.jax.org/phenome.
51. Schwartz DA, Berman KG, Whitehead GS, et al. Lung response to environmental stress: ovalbumin. Mouse Phenome Database (MPD:98), 2001.
52. DeSanctis GT, Drazen JM. Genetics of native airway responsiveness in mice. Am J Respir Crit Care Med 1997; 156:82S–88S.
53. Pletcher MT, McClurg P, Batalov S, et al. Use of a dense single nucleotide polymorphism map for in silico mapping in the mouse. PLoS Biol 2004; 2(12): 2159–2169.
54. Wang X, Paigen B. Genetics of variation in HDL cholesterol in humans and mice. Circ Res 2005; 96(1):27–42.
55. Li R, Lyons MA, Wittenburg H, et al. Combining data from multiple inbred line crosses improves the power and resolution of QTL mapping. Genetics 2005; 169(3):1699–1709.
56. htpp://www.jax.org/staff/Churchill/labsite/datasets/qtl/qtlarchive.

9

Proteomic Techniques for Asthma and Chronic Obstructive Pulmonary Disease Research

MEGAN S. LIM and KOJO S. J. ELENITOBA-JOHNSON

Department of Pathology, Associated Regional and
  University Pathologists Institute for Clinical and Experimental Pathology,
  University of Utah Health Sciences Center,
Salt Lake City, Utah, U.S.A.

I. Introduction

Proteomics is defined as the study of the proteome. The proteome is defined as the total protein complement of an organelle, cell, tissue, or an entire organism (1). Proteomics entails multifaceted approaches to study protein expression and posttranslational modification and protein interactions, organization, and function at a global level. While the cause of a disease aberration may be at the genetic level, the functional consequences of such an aberration are often expressed at the protein level. Thus, disruption of protein structure, function, or interaction is the underlying mechanism of the majority of diseases. Further, several questions relating to the fundamental basis of diseases are best addressed at the protein level because they occur as posttranslational events or relate to abnormal regulation of protein function or aberrant protein–protein or protein–DNA interactions. Mass spectrometry (MS)-based proteomic studies have led to large-scale information datasets and high-throughput analyses of diseases. The application of MS to the study of asthma/chronic obstructive pulmonary disease (COPD) will ultimately lead to identification of biomarkers that are critical for the detection, diagnosis, monitoring, prognosis, and treatment of these disorders. The development of a proteomic strategy to study the asthma and COPD must take into consideration the complex pathophysiology and cellular makeup of the disease. In this chapter, we provide an overview of the technical aspects involved in MS-based proteomics and their potential applications to asthma and COPD. The challenges to the study of complex multigenic diseases such as asthma and COPD are discussed.

II. Tools for Proteomics

A. Sample Preparation

Most proteomic studies require proteins extracted from fresh or snap frozen cells, frozen tissue biopsies, or biological fluids, such as serum, urine, or effusions. Cellular proteins have to be isolated from samples containing other biological molecules including carbohydrates, lipids, and nucleic acids. Thus protein extraction protocols involve the homogenization of cells and tissues followed by application of detergents such as 3-(dimethylammonio)-1 pro-pane sulfate (2), Tween, and sodium dodecyl sulfate (SDS), which help to dissolve the proteins and separate them from the lipid components, reducing agents such as dithiothreitol, denaturing agents such as urea, which disrupt the bonds that are responsible for the formation of secondary and tertiary conformational structure, and enzymes that degrade nucleic acids, such as DNAses and RNAses. Tissues obtained from laser capture microdissection of human cancer (3) have been successfully used for two dimentional gel electrophoresis (2D-GE) followed by matrix-assisted laser desorption/ionization-time of flight (MALDI-TOF) MS analysis and 2D liquid chromatography (LC) tandem MS (4). Due to cross-linking and degradation of proteins, paraffin-embedded formalin-fixed tissues have not been ideal sources for proteomic studies until recently. Proteins extracted from ethanol-fixed paraffin-embedded tissues can be utilized for 2D-GE–MS analysis (5) and proteins extracted from formalin-fixed paraffin-embedded tissues have been shown to be amenable to high-throughput mass spectrometric analysis (6). More recently, the mass spectrometric identification of hundreds of proteins has been successfully carried using tissues obtained from a variety of sources including laser capture microdissection–derived material (7).

B. General Strategy for Proteomic Experiments

Proteomic studies require the simplification of a complex mixture of proteins into less complex components that are more amenable for analysis. In this regard, intact proteins with different biophysical characteristics such as molecular weight, hydrophobicity, and posttranslational modifications may be present within a complex mixture intended for analysis.

In "top-down" proteomics, intact proteins are analyzed. In "bottom-up" proteomics, the proteins are proteolytically cleaved using enzymes such as trypsin with specific cleavage sites (at the carboxy terminal of lysines or arginines) or those with nonspecific cleavage specificity such as elastase or subtilisin (8,9). Several techniques are utilized for the analytical separation of proteins. Figure 1 illustrates different modalities commonly used for the separation of proteins from complex mixtures. These include 1D-GE, which achieves resolution of cellular proteins based on molecular weight, 2D-GE, which involves initial separation of proteins based on isoelectric point (pI) followed by subsequent separation based on size, high-performance liquid chromatography (HPLC), ion exchange, and different types of affinity chromatography (10). The most powerful strategy entails the integration of the different protein and peptide separation methods as multidimensional combinations. In this regard, ion exchange LC in tandem with reverse phase (RP)-HPLC is a powerful tool for resolving complex peptide mixtures and has been automated to maximize efficiency (11). When used with a 100 µm 2D strong cationic exchange-RP packed microcapillary HPLC, the MS system is capable of achieving a detection limit

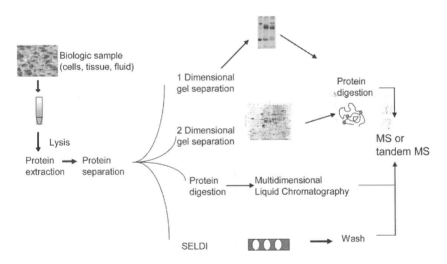

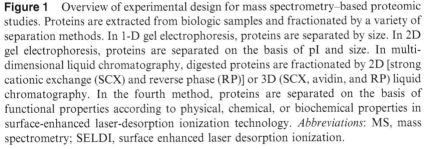

Figure 1   Overview of experimental design for mass spectrometry–based proteomic studies. Proteins are extracted from biologic samples and fractionated by a variety of separation methods. In 1-D gel electrophoresis, proteins are separated by size. In 2D gel electrophoresis, proteins are separated on the basis of pI and size. In multidimensional liquid chromatography, digested proteins are fractionated by 2D [strong cationic exchange (SCX) and reverse phase (RP)] or 3D (SCX, avidin, and RP) liquid chromatography. In the fourth method, proteins are separated on the basis of functional properties according to physical, chemical, or biochemical properties in surface-enhanced laser-desorption ionization technology. *Abbreviations*: MS, mass spectrometry; SELDI, surface enhanced laser desorption ionization.

of 10 fmol for identifying a single tryptically digested protein (12). The sensitivity of multidimensional protein identification technology (MudPIT) is very attractive for the study of complex proteomes such as mammalian cellular samples. MudPIT has been applied to large-scale protein characterization and identification of up to 1484 proteins from yeast in a single experiment (11). Furthermore, cellular subfractionation into cytosolic, membrane, and nuclear compartments and subsequent LC–MS/MS enhances the identification of proteins (13).

C. Mass Spectrometers

A mass spectrometer is a highly sensitive and accurate weighing scale and is typically composed of three components: an ionization source, a mass analyzer, and a detector. The ionization source creates ions from the sample to be analyzed. The mass analyzer resolves the ions by their mass-to-charge ratio (m/z). The detector determines the mass of the ions. The most frequently utilized ionization sources and mass analyzers are discussed below. Mass spectrometers measure the mass of the smallest of molecules with very high accuracy, and hence MS can be considered as the smallest weighing scale. In parallel with the technological advancements in MS, improvements in ionization methods have also enhanced the ability to analyze complex biologic molecules by MS (14,15). The final component that has greatly facilitated the ability to conduct proteomic studies is the development of translated genomic databases and specialized software algorithms such SEQUEST (15) or MASCOT, which rapidly search experimental mass spectrometric data against predicted spectra of proteins within genomic databases.

In general, the measurement of fragmented peptide masses by MS is more accurate than measuring the mass of intact proteins. Thus in "bottom-up" proteomics, the typical workflow involves initial simplification of a complex protein mixture followed by digestion into peptides, which are subjected to mass spectrometric analysis. The mass spectrometric data is then analyzed using specialized software algorithms that identify the proteins from which the peptide sequences are derived. The ability to accurately determine the mass of a unique peptide that originates from a particular protein greatly facilitates the identification of that protein. In essence, protein identification centers on the fact that a peptide sequence, composed of six amino acid residues or greater, provides a unique opportunity for the identification of the parent protein. This is because the probability that any one amino acid would occupy a particular position within a peptide sequence is 1 in 20. Thus, for a sequence of six amino acid residues, the theoretical probability of identification of a peptide with that sequence can be as high as 1 in $20^6 = 1$ in 64,000,000. In practice, however, the quality of the mass spectra may be insufficient to permit unequivocal identification of a protein from peptide tandem mass spectra. Identification of overlapping or longer peptide sequences with multiple "hits" to a particular protein provides an even greater degree of certainty in the identification of the protein. It is thus possible in many cases to utilize database searches to identify a protein from only a few peptides.

D. Challenges of Proteomics Research for Asthma and COPD

There are several goals for proteomic analyses of asthma and COPD. The first is to discover markers that would be helpful for early diagnosis. The second would be to identify signaling pathways that are deregulated in the cells responsible for disease manifestation of asthma and COPD. The outcome of these types of research should be for the development of innovative therapeutic agents. As proteomics can provide a global perspective to deregulated proteins in asthma and COPD, a systematic study of the disease-affected tissues is warranted. Several challenges are expected, however. One is the limited availability of tissues that are involved by asthma and COPD. As a consequence, many of the studies have been limited to the analysis of the bronchoalveolar lavage (BAL) fluid. BAL fluid contains cells, cellular secretions, inhaled particles, and microorganisms that reside in the terminal bronchi. Another source of disease sample is the bronchial brushing, which contains the bronchial epithelial cells. Secondly, due to the intimate interplay between the immune-mediated inflammatory cells and the host tissues that respond to these insults, the origin versus the consequence of disease pathogenesis is unclear. Inherent in the complex pathophysiology of asthma and COPD are the contributions by inflammatory cells, including eosinophils, mucus production, plasma infiltration, airway remodeling, and tissue damage and repair (16). Cellular heterogeneity of the bronchial tissues contributing to asthma and COPD imposes difficulties in accurate determination of the contribution of proteins. Bronchial tissues are composed of different cell types including epithelial glandular cells, fibroblasts, myoepithelial cells, endothelial cells, infiltrating inflammatory cells that are dependent on the activity of the disease, adipocytes, and nerve fibers. Furthermore, many of these cells are influenced by the complex interplay of cytokines and growth factors, which can induce autocrine and paracrine stimuli, which ultimately will affect the proteome of the tissues.

III. Application of Proteomic Techniques to the Study of Asthma and COPD

There are two major types of applications of proteomics to the study of human disease. One is "expression proteomics," which deals with the identification/quantification of proteins expressed and the levels of proteins expressed in a given sample such as body fluids, normal or disease tissues. This protein expression "signature" is conceptually similar to that obtained by genomic microarray analyses and would allow investigators to identify biomarkers or disease-specific proteins that may represent therapeutic targets. The second application is "functional proteomics," which encompasses the study of protein in their functional environment. This includes the analysis of protein interactions with other proteins, interactions with DNA or RNA, and posttranslational modifications such as phosphorylation and glycosylation. The latter approach allows investigators to obtain information regarding function of a protein, e.g., identifying networks of signaling pathways that are characteristic of physiologic and pathologic states.

A. Protein Expression Profiling

The application of proteomics to the identification of disease markers from body fluids and tissue has received significant attention. The potential of obtaining mass spectral profiles of peptides and proteins without the need to carry out protein separation is highly suitable for biomarker discovery, especially as it would have reduced sample requirements and represent a high-throughput approach. Surface enhanced laser desorption ionization-time of flight (SELDI-TOF) (17–19) MS has been a popular platform with distinct features that make it attractive for biomarker discovery. One of the advantages of this method is that only small quantities of biological fluid or tissue material are needed. The mass spectral patterns generated reflect the protein and peptide content of the interrogated samples. In this regard, artificial intelligence–based bioinformatics analyses of mass spectral patterns have been proposed to distinguish serum of normal patients with that of a number of neoplastic conditions (17,20). Such analyses require extensive pre- and postacquisition procedures including mass calibration, baseline correction, and noise subtraction to facilitate identification of bona fide features that are robust and biologically relevant discriminators of the normal, benign, and malignant states (21,22). Proteomic patterns of nipple aspirate fluids (23), cytologic specimens (24), and tissue biopsies (25) using SELDI-TOF have also revealed a potential for utility in discovery of novel biomarkers that aid in diagnosis. To date, serum profiling of patients with asthma/COPD using SELDI-TOF has not been performed, but represents a potential area of investigation.

Using multiple experimental approaches including gel-based high-resolution 2D gels, three-dimensional HPLC, and a combination of MALDI and electrospray MS, a large-scale protein expression profiling and annotation of the proteome of the human pulmonary fibroblast at the resting and activated states has been curated (26). Based on approximately 2000 protein identifications, the 2DDB database (27) has been built, which also allows interactive query bioinformatics analysis.

B. Proteomic Analysis of Bronchoalveolar Lavage

BAL obtained by fiber-optic bronchoscopy has diagnostic utility and provides information about the cellular composition of the extraluminar spaces of airways during episodes of asthma/COPD. Initial studies optimizing sample preparation using BAL for proteomic analysis demonstrated that the high salt concentration in BAL [from the phosphate buffered saline (PBS) used in the lavage] interferes with 2D gel analyses. A combination of dialysis and ultra-membrane centrifugation is required to remove salt from the BAL samples for adequate 2D gel analysis. Furthermore, the high concentrations of albumin present in BAL also limit detection of many low-abundance proteins.

Proteomic analysis of BAL fluid obtained by fiber-optic bronchoscopy has been obtained after optimizing sample preparation using dialysis, ultramembrane filtration, precipitation, and gel filtration and the effect of albumin in the annotation (28). The major soluble proteins present in BAL fluid were determined by 2D-GE in 1979 (29), and comprehensive proteomic maps of BAL fluid in various respiratory diseases such as cystic fibrosis (30), pulmonary fibrosis (31), and hypersensitivity pneumonitis (32) have been generated. More recently, a comprehensive differential proteomic analysis of BAL fluid from asthmatic patients and healthy subjects before and 24 hours after segmental allergen challenge was performed (33). In contrast to 2D–GE, automated multidimensional HPLC in combination with MS is capable of detecting low-abundance proteins with the ability for large-scale analysis of complex protein mixtures (11). After immunoaffinity depletion of highly abundant serum proteins BAL fluid, SDS-polyacrylamide gel electrophoresis (PAGE) fractionation, protein in-gel digestion and subsequence nanoLC/MS/MS, more than 1500 distinct proteins were identified. The proteins were annotated based on protein cellular localization and biologic function using gene ontology (GO) terms (34). Moreover, the relative abundance of proteins were estimated on the basis of the peak areas of the extracted ion chromatograms for each peptide precursor ion in the full scan more using commercially available software (33). These analyses indicated that approximately 10% of the proteins exhibited significant upregulation in asthmatic patients after segmental allergic challenge. The differentially expressed proteins presented a wide spectrum of functional categories such as complement factors, acute phase proteins, monocyte-specific granule proteins, local matrix proteins, chemokines, cytokines, and proteases.

C. Proteomic Analysis of Mouse Models of Asthma and COPD

Because the immune system is a key player in the pathogenesis of asthma and COPD, the study of the molecular pathways regulating the inflammatory infiltrate such as cytokines and chemokines may be fruitful avenues for proteomic investigation. To study these low-abundance proteins, however, effective strategies must be employed to enrich and concentrate the samples of interest. Alternatively, mouse models of asthma or COPD could alleviate the limited sample availability. Indeed analysis of total mouse lung tissue revealed significant up- and downregulation of proteins following antigen challenge (35). Many were identified by MS, which were linked to asthma-related symptoms such as stress, inflammation, lung detoxification, plasma exudation and tissue remodeling. More recent developments in 2D-GE methods using overlapping pH gradients and creation of composite zoom gels built *in silico* have led to increased visualization of proteins to 8000, which would ultimately lead to enhanced identification of candidate proteins.

Laser capture microdissection (36) can be used to enrich for specific cell types. Epithelial mucosal cells from control and allergen challenged mouse lungs were enriched using laser capture microdissection and evaluated by 2D–GE (37). Although 7000 laser shots of 30 μm diameter were required for identification of approximately 500 protein spots on a 2D SDS-PAGE and labor-intensive manipulation by histopathologists was involved, such analyses can lead to useful identifications. Recognizing that a minimum of 100,000 cells are required for 2D gel analysis, non–gel-based methods such as isotope-coded affinity tagging and endoproteinase catalyzed ^{18}O isotope labeling methods would allow comparable data with 100 to 10,000 cells (37).

D. Imaging Mass Spectrometry

MS has been used for the in situ analyses of proteins in tissue sections and those obtained by laser capture microdissection (38), thereby allowing imaging and comparison of protein expression between normal and disease tissues (39). In this strategy, frozen tissue sections are applied to a MALDI plate and analyzed at regular spatial intervals. The mass spectral data obtained at different intervals are compared to yield a spatial distribution of masses (proteins) across the tissue section. Analyses using this approach have revealed up to 1600 protein peaks from histologically selected 1 mm diameter regions of single frozen sections (40). Using this approach, investigators have been able to distinguish glial neoplasms from benign brain tissues and differentiate tumors of different histological grades (41). Imaging mass spectrometric analysis of tissues involved by asthma and COPD would lead to the identification of proteins that are specifically expressed by cellular constituents associated with disease and contribute to elucidation of the underlying complex cellular pathophysiology of the disease.

E. Array-Based Proteomic Studies of Asthma and COPD

Microarrays composed of protein, antibodies, and peptides allow for high-throughput large-scale analysis with the advantage of less analyte consumption and enhanced sensitivities. Protein microarrays have been created to evaluate antibody–antigen, protein–protein, protein–nucleic acid, protein–small molecules, and ligand–receptor interactions and analysis of enzymatic activities (42). Protein microarrays have great potential but to date have not been utilized for the analyses of asthma and COPD.

F. Quantitative Proteomic Analysis of Asthma and COPD

Two-Dimensional Gel Electrophoresis

Most quantitative proteomic studies are designed to determine the proteomic differences between one cellular state and another, and these are "relative." In this regard, 2D–GE has been extensively utilized, with great success (43). Two-dimensional GE, although a traditionally popular method for determining relative protein expression between two cellular states, is limited by its requirement for a large amount of starting material (on the order of 50 μg) with low sensitivity for detection of low-abundance proteins such as cytokines and signaling molecules. Furthermore, proteins at both extremes of pI and molecular weight and those associated with the membrane fractions are not well represented by 2D–GE (10). Despite these limitations, due to highly automated and robotized spot picking technologies, numerous reports have successfully used 2D–GE followed by MALDI-TOF analysis to determine differential expression of protein profiles in asthma and COPD.

The contribution of tissue remodeling of the bronchial airway by myofibroblast formation, smooth muscle hyperplasia, and deposition of the extracellular matrix is a well-established feature of asthma (44). Platelet-derived growth factor has been implicated in the initiation of peribronchial fibrosis (45). Two dimensional gel electrophoretic analysis of mesenchymal cells stimulated with platelet derived growth factor (PDGF) affected the synthesis of proteins involved in remodeling such as collagen VI, FK506-binding protein, which is involved in smooth muscle differentiation, and proteins involved in cytoskeletal reorganization (actin-related protein ARP3, T-complex protein, and heat shock protein 60). Additional studies to determine the effect of other growth factors important in pathophysiology of asthma such as transforming growth factor β (45) and epidermal growth factor will aid in understanding the contribution of these proteins to the pathophysiology of asthma and COPD.

Stable Isotope Labeling in Cell Culture

Stable isotope labeling with amino acids in cell culture (SILAC) is another useful global quantification strategy for the evaluation of differential expression of proteins from two distinct cellular populations (46,47). In essence, the SILAC procedure entails culturing of cells from two different bio-logic conditions in parallel culture media that are deficient in a natural amino acid, but supplemented with monoisotopically labeled amino acid (e.g., ^{12}C, ^{13}C; ^{14}N, ^{15}N, respectively). The two cell populations metabolically incorporate the corresponding "light" or "heavy" isotopes in the synthesis of their respective cellular proteins. The proteins from each sample can thus be isolated, mixed at a 1:1 ratio, and subjected to proteolytic digestion and mass spectrometric analysis. Corresponding peptides from each sample coelute during LC and relative quantification of a particular peptide repre-sented in both samples can be performed by measuring the ratios of the peptide mass peak intensities from matching isotopic peak pairs. The sequence of the peptide is subsequently obtained from tandem mass spec-trometric analysis greatly facilitating identification proteins with differential expression in the two conditions. Of necessity, isolated cells must be capable of protein synthesis in vitro.

Isotope-Coded Affinity Tag Method

The isotope-coded affinity tags (ICAT) strategy is a relatively new tech-nology for relative protein quantification, relying on postharvested, stable isotope labeling. The ICAT method uses the ICAT^{TM} reagent to differen-tially label protein samples on their cysteine residues. The ICAT method is advantageous in that it permits the evaluation of low-abundance pro-teins and proteins at both extremes of molecular weight and Ip (48). The ICAT reagent is composed of (i) a thiol-reactive group that reacts with the cysteine residues, (ii) a linker in which stable isotopes have been incorporated, and (iii) a biotin tag that enables affinity isolation and detec-tion of peptides labeled with either the heavy or light versions of the ICAT reagent. In this system, one sample is labeled with a tag containing a light isotope, and the other sample to which it is being compared is labeled with a heavy isotope tag. The two samples are combined, proteolytically digested, and analyzed by MS (Fig. 2). Because ICAT-labeled peptides coelute as pairs through the chromatography stages, calculating the ratio of the areas under the curve for identical peptide peaks labeled with the light and heavy ICAT reagent allows the determination of the relative abundance of that peptide in each sample. Advantages of the ICAT strat-egy include internal quantitation, automation, and reduced complexity of the peptide mixture. The original ICAT reagents featured either eight deuterium or hydrogen atoms at particular positions in the linker. The recently improved cleavable ICAT reagent contains nine ^{13}C in the heavy version of the linker and nine ^{12}C in the light version of the linker. The resultant database search is constrained by requiring a cysteinyl group, is compatible with analysis of low-abundance proteins, and can be performed from proteins obtained from snap-frozen archival tissues.

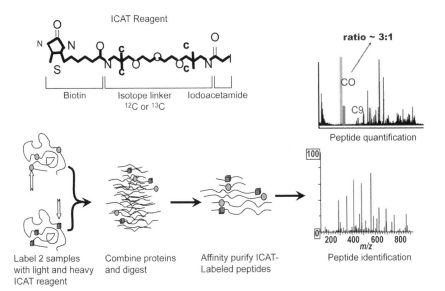

Figure 2 Outline of experimental protocol used for differential protein expression profiling by isotope-coded affinity tage (ICAT)^{TM}. Protein mixtures obtained from two cell populations are either labeled with light or heavy isotopic versions of the cleavable ICAT reagent. Labeled proteins are combined, subjected to multidimensional separation by strong cationic exchange, reverse phase, and avidin affinity chromatography, and analyzed by tandem mass spectrometry for peptide and protein identification. Based on the relative ratio of the two isotopically labeled peptides, a relative abundance of protein expression can be determined.

More recently, ^{18}O has been used for stable isotopic labeling for identification and quantitation of peptides (49). The ^{18}O labeling approach is nonproprietary and relatively inexpensive but needs to be utilized in concert with specialized software programs. Table 1 compares the differential methods of quantitative differential protein profiling.

To identify potential small-molecular-weight peptide biomarker profiles of asthma, Yeo et al. (50) used a combination of LC and quantitative MS to analyze plasma samples from control and asthmatic mice. Peptide mass fingerprinting from MALDI-TOF/MS identified a fragment of complement (C3f) to be present at much higher levels in controls than in chronic asthmatic mice.

G. Posttranslational Modifications

Proteins are modified to their mature functional form through a highly regulated and complex sequence of posttranslational processing. Most modifications are reversible and play important roles in regulating the biologic function of the protein. There are more than 200 reported modes of

Table 1 Comparison of Methods for Quantitative Protein Expression Profiling

Parameters	2D gel	ICAT	^{16}O and ^{18}O labeling	SILAC
Time	1 to 2 days for 2D gel, followed by spot identification and MS	Up to 1 wk for labeling, multidimensional separation followed by MS	Up to 1 wk for labeling, multidimensional separation followed by MS	1 to 2 wk to grow cells in special media
Samples	One sample analyzed per gel	Pairs of samples analyzed	Pairs of samples analyzed	Pairs of samples analyzed
Amount of protein required	50–100 μg	$10\ \mu g$–1 mg	$10\ \mu g$–1 mg	1 mg
Potential for automation	Yes	Yes	Yes	Limited
Type of samples	Cell lines, biopsy tissues	Cell lines, biopsy tissues	Cell lines, biopsy tissues	Viable cells grown in culture
Sensitivity	Moderate	High	High	High
Average number of proteins identified and quantitated per experiment	50–70	300–500	300–500	300–500
Limitations	Poor sensitivity for proteins with extremes of pI and size. Membrane proteins are poorly detected	ICAT reagent is costly	Although inexpensive, requires specialized software (ZoomQuant) for analysis	Direct quantitative comparisons are most feasibly done using viable cells

Abbreviations: MS, mass spectrometry; ICAT, Isotope-coded affinity tag; pI, isoelectric point; 2D, two-dimensional; SILAC, stable isotope labeling in cell culture.

posttranslational modification of proteins such as phosphorylation, glycosylation, and ubiquitination to mention a few. Of these, methods to determine the type and sites of protein phosphorylation have received significant attention. Reversible phosphorylation of proteins is a key event in signal transduction from extracellular stimulus via a transmembrane receptor to the nucleus (51). Phosphorylation occurs mainly on serine, threonine, and tyrosine residues, with the ratio being 1800:200:1 in vertebrates (52). Although the phosphorylation of tyrosine residues is much less frequent in the proteome, it has been most extensively studied.

More recently, attempts have been made to define the phosphorylation status of proteins at a global scale (53). Most approaches involve the use of phospho-specific antibodies to enrich for proteins with phosphorylated residues. Due to the availability of excellent antibodies that react with phospho-tyrosines, the analysis of tyrosine phosphoproteins far outnumbers those for serine and threonine phosphoproteins. Using phospho-specific antibodies, serine/threonine-phosphorylated proteins were enriched by immunoprecipitation and identified by MS. Functional studies led to the identification of a novel protein, which was demonstrated to be a substrate of protein kinase A (54). Similarly, a novel phosphotyrosine protein was identified and characterized to be an immune receptor tyrosine-based activation motif–containing signal transduction protein induced by epidermal growth factor stimulation (55). Using 2D-GE and MS, Lim et al. (56) identified over 50 distinct tyrosine phosphoproteins induced by epidermal growth factor in a human epidermoid carcinoma cell line, which may represent novel targets for therapy. Similarly, phosphotyrosine proteomes have been characterized from thrombin-activated platelets (57) and in response to heat shock (58). More large-scale studies of phosphoproteins have taken advantage of commercially available immobilized metal-ion affinity chromatography, which allows enrichment of phosphopeptides (59) and also allows identification of several phosphorylation sites on single proteins (60).

The induction of phosphoproteins and intracellular signaling cascades that may play a role in diesel exhaust particle (DEP), an air pollutant known to lead to exacerbation of asthma through excitation of allergic inflammation, has been analyzed using a new phosphosensor fluorescent dye, Pro-Q Diamond (61). In this study, SYPRO Ruby dye was used to stain the control reference 2D gel while the that containing the DEP-treated proteins were stained with Pro-Q Diamond. Staining of the Pro-Q diamond and SYPRO Ruby gels were detected using different wavelengths and computer-generated differential display maps were generated using commercially available software. Many proteins that belong to a number of signaling pathways including mitogen-activated protein kinases (ERK-1, ERK-2, MAPKAPK-2, p38 MAPK, JNK1,2) and oxidative stress pathways [HSP27, TNFa convertase, TNF ligand, proteosome α(20S), and protein disulfide isomerase precursor] were induced by DEP exposure in human bronchial epithelial cells.

H. Cellular Subproteomics

One of the major initiatives of the Human Proteome Organization is the comprehensive characterization of the complete subproteome of each cell type. Defining the global fingerprint of proteins expressed in a given cell type will aid in the identification of deregulated proteins that are characteristic of certain disease states and aid in diagnostics and prognostication.

Protein secretion by diseased cell types contributing to asthma and COPD may provide a means for earlier detection of the diseases. Systematic approaches to purify and identify secreted proteins from a variety of cell types have been reported. Martin et al. (62) have used a combination of ICAT and tandem MS to identify and quantitate a comprehensive list of over 500 proteins, which were secreted from a neoplastic prostate cancer cell line (LNCaP) in the presence or absence of androgen receptor stimulation. Similar studies have identified numerous secreted proteins during differentiation of 3T3-L1 preadipocytes to adipocytes (63), during osteoclast differentiation (64), and astrocytes (65).

Proteomic approaches for the comprehensive profiling and identification of proteins on cell surface or membranes have been reported. Cell surface membranes may be subjected to biotinylation, affinity-captured, and purified on avidin columns. Biotinylated intact proteins, which were eluted, can be separated by 2D–GE and protein spots from matching gels analyzed by MS. Alternatively, plasma membrane fractions can be purified by sucrose gradient centrifugation and analyzed by MS. Using these approaches, cell surface membrane proteins of human leukemia cells have been characterized (66). Analysis of the cell surface proteome of cancer cells of a variety of histologies has revealed an abundance of proteins with chaperone function such as GRP78, HSP70 and protein disulfide isomerase (67).

Systematic analysis of the proteins expressed by specific intracellular organelles such as the cancer-cell mitochondria (68), lymphocyte-derived exosomes (2), the lipofuscin in human retinal pigment epithelial cells (69), the phagosome (70), microsomes (71), lipid rafts (72), and human nucleolus (73) have provided extensive insights into the organellar proteomes, which were previously impossible to obtain. These studies also demonstrate that even intracellular organelles as small as nucleoli are much more complicated in their protein expression profiles and express hundreds of proteins, some of which are not previously associated with their function. They also show that the protein composition of organelles is not static and can respond significantly to changes in the states of the cells.

I. Bioinformatics Analyses

Due to the large amount of data that is typically generated by high-throughput large-scale mass spectrometric analyses, a key component of data analysis is efficient data processing software and informatics database.

Once a list of proteins is generated, a template for the workflow of data processing usually encompasses the following. All proteins are categorized on the basis of their biologic function and location within the cell using the GO project (74). The determination of biologically relevant information can be obtained using pathway analysis software programs such as Ingenuity (75).

IV. Summary

The recent advances in protein separation techniques, MS, and completion of the genome sequences of several organisms are all critical developments that facilitate proteomic studies. At present, substantial progress has been made in the development of high-throughput technologies for analysis of proteins including protein and antibody arrays. The challenges for the future lie in the archiving and integration of the vast amounts of data derived from MS experiments into cohesive information relevant to physiologic and disease processes. Bioinformatic tools for MS-based proteomic studies are being developed, such as GOminer, pathway analysis tools, and interaction analysis tools (HPRD). It will be critical to integrate the various aspects of proteomics such as diagnostic proteomics, high-throughput analyses of posttranslational modifications, imaging MS, protein–protein interaction mapping, and quantitative protein expression profiling to formulate coherent hypotheses regarding the pathogenesis of disease entities. These studies will have to occur in concert with large-scale validation studies on clinical samples obtained from well-controlled patient populations with asthma/ COPD before they can be considered for potential diagnostic, prognostic, or therapeutic biomarkers.

References

1. Wasinger VC, Cordwell SJ, Cerpa-Poljak A, et al. Progress with gene-product mapping of the Mollicutes: Mycoplasma genitalium. Electrophoresis 1995; 16:1090–1094.
2. Wubbolts R, Leckie RS, Veenhuizen PT, et al. Proteomic and biochemical analyses of human B cell-derived exosomes. Potential implications for their function and multivesicular body formation. J Biol Chem 2003; 278: 10,963–10,972.
3. Lawrie LC, Curran S, McLeod HL, Fothergill JE, Murray GI. Application of laser capture microdissection and proteomics in colon cancer. Mol Pathol 2001; 54:253–258.
4. Li C, Hong Y, Tan YX, et al. Accurate qualitative and quantitative proteomic analysis of clinical hepatocellular carcinoma using laser capture microdissection coupled with isotope-coded affinity tag and two-dimensional liquid chromatography mass spectrometry. Mol Cell Proteomics 2004; 3:399–409.

5. Ahram M, Flaig MJ, Gillespie JW, et al. Evaluation of ethanol-fixed, paraffin-embedded tissues for proteomic applications. Proteomics 2003; 3:413–421.

6. Crockett DK, Lin Z, Vaughn CP, Lim MS, Elenitoba-Johnson KS. Identification of proteins from formalin-fixed paraffin-embedded cells by LC-MS/MS. Lab Invest 2005; 85:1405–1415.

7. Hood BL, Darfler MM, Guiel TG, et al. Proteomic analysis of formalin fixed prostate cancer tissue. Mol Cell Proteomics 2006. In press.

8. Blackstock WP, Weir MP. Proteomics: quantitative and physical mapping of cellular proteins. Trends Biotechnol 1999; 17:121–127.

9. MacCoss MJ, McDonald WH, Saraf A, et al. Shotgun identification of protein modifications from protein complexes and lens tissue. Proc Natl Acad Sci USA 2002; 99:7900–7905.

10. Gygi SP, Corthals GL, Zhang Y, Rochon Y, Aebersold R. Evaluation of two-dimensional gel electrophoresis-based proteome analysis technology. Proc Natl Acad Sci USA 2000; 97:9390–9395.

11. Washburn MP, Wolters D, Yates JR III. Large-scale analysis of the yeast proteome by multidimensional protein identification technology. Nat Biotechnol 2001; 19:242–247.

12. Gatlin CL, Kleemann GR, Hays LG, Link AJ, Yates JR III. Protein identification at the low femtomole level from silver-stained gels using a new fritless electrospray interface for liquid chromatography-microspray and nanospray mass spectrometry. Anal Biochem 1998; 263:93–101.

13. Guillemin I, Becker M, Ociepka K, Friauf E, Nothwang HG. A subcellular prefractionation protocol for minute amounts of mammalian cell cultures and tissue. Proteomics 2005; 5:35–45.

14. Fenn JB, Mann M, Meng CK, Wong SF, Whitehouse CM. Electrospray ionization for mass spectrometry of large biomolecules. Science 1989; 246: 64–71.

15. Yates JR III. Mass spectrometry and the age of the proteome. J Mass Spectrom 1998; 33:1–19.

16. Cohn L, Elias JA, Chupp GL. Asthma: mechanisms of disease persistence and progression. Annu Rev Immunol 2004; 22:789–815.

17. Petricoin EF, Zoon KC, Kohn EC, Barrett JC, Liotta LA. Clinical proteomics: translating benchside promise into bedside reality. Nat Rev Drug Discov 2002; 1:683–695.

18. Rosenblatt KP, Bryant-Greenwood P, Killian JK, et al. Serum proteomics in cancer diagnosis and management. Annu Rev Med 2004; 55:97–112.

19. Rui Z, Jian-Guo J, Yuan-Peng T, Hai P, Bing-Gen R. Use of serological proteomic methods to find biomarkers associated with breast cancer. Proteomics 2003; 3:433–439.

20. Adam BL, Qu Y, Davis JW, et al. Serum protein fingerprinting coupled with a pattern-matching algorithm distinguishes prostate cancer from benign prostate hyperplasia and healthy men. Cancer Res 2002; 62:3609–3614.

21. Coombes KR, Fritsche HA, Jr., Clarke C, et al. Quality control and peak finding for proteomics data collected from nipple aspirate fluid by surface-enhanced laser desorption and ionization. Clin Chem 2003; 49:1615–1623.

22. Baggerly KA, Morris JS, Coombes KR. Reproducibility of SELDI-TOF protein patterns in serum: comparing datasets from different experiments. Bioinformatics 2004; 20:777–785.
23. Paweletz CP, Trock B, Pennanen M, et al. Proteomic patterns of nipple aspirate fluids obtained by SELDI-TOF: potential for new biomarkers to aid in the diagnosis of breast cancer. Dis Markers 2001; 17:301–307.
24. Fetsch PA, Simone NL, Bryant-Greenwood PK, et al. Proteomic evaluation of archival cytologic material using SELDI affinity mass spectrometry: potential for diagnostic applications. Am J Clin Pathol 2002; 118:870–876.
25. Lin Z, Jenson S, Lim M, Elenitoba-Johnson K. Application of SELDI-TOF mass spectrometry for the identification of differentially expressed proteins in transformed follicular lymphoma. Mod Pathol 2004; 17:670–678.
26. Malmstrom J, Larsen K, Malmstrom L, et al. Proteome annotations and identifications of the human pulmonary fibroblast. J Proteome Res 2004; 3:525–537.
27. www.2DDB.org
28. Plymoth A, Lofdahl CG, Ekberg-Jansson A, et al. Human bronchoalveolar lavage: biofluid analysis with special emphasis on sample preparation. Proteomics 2003; 3:962–972.
29. Bell DY, Hook GE. Pulmonary alveolar proteinosis: analysis of airway and alveolar proteins. Am Rev Respir Dis 1979; 119:979–990.
30. von Bredow C, Birrer P, Griese M. Surfactant protein A and other bronchoalveolar lavage fluid proteins are altered in cystic fibrosis. Eur Respir J 2001; 17:716–722.
31. Lenz AG, Meyer B, Costabel U, Maier K. Bronchoalveolar lavage fluid proteins in human lung disease: analysis by two-dimensional electrophoresis. Electrophoresis 1993; 14:242–244.
32. Wattiez R, Hermans C, Cruyt C, Bernard A, Falmagne P. Human bronchoalveolar lavage fluid protein two-dimensional database: study of interstitial lung diseases. Electrophoresis 2000; 21:2703–2712.
33. Wu J, Kobayashi M, Sousa EA, et al. Differential Proteomic Analysis of Bronchoalveolar Lavage Fluid in Asthmatics following Segmental Antigen Challenge. Mol Cell Proteomics 2005; 4:1251–1264.
34. Ashburner M, Ball CA, Blake JA, et al. Gene ontology: tool for the unification of biology. The Gene Ontology Consortium. Nat Genet 2000; 25:25–29.
35. Houtman R, Krijgsveld J, Kool M, et al. Lung proteome alterations in a mouse model for nonallergic asthma. Proteomics 2003; 3:2008–2018.
36. Bonner RF, Emmert-Buck M, Cole K, et al. Laser capture microdissection: molecular analysis of tissue. Science 1997; 278:1481,1483.
37. Fehniger TE, Sato-Folatre JG, Malmstrom J, et al. Exploring the context of the lung proteome within the airway mucosa following allergen challenge. J Proteome Res 2004; 3:307–320.
38. Xu BJ, Caprioli RM, Sanders ME, Jensen RA. Direct analysis of laser capture microdissected cells by MALDI mass spectrometry. J Am Soc Mass Spectrom 2002; 13:1292–1297.
39. Stoeckli M, Chaurand P, Hallahan DE, Caprioli RM. Imaging mass spectrometry: a new technology for the analysis of protein expression in mammalian tissues. Nat Med 2001; 7:493–496.

40. Yanagisawa K, Shyr Y, Xu BJ, et al. Proteomic patterns of tumour subsets in non-small-cell lung cancer. Lancet 2003; 362:433–439.
41. Schwartz SA, Weil RJ, Johnson MD, Toms SA, Caprioli RM. Protein profiling in brain tumors using mass spectrometry: feasibility of a new technique for the analysis of protein expression. Clin Cancer Res 2004; 10:981–987.
42. Lueking A, Cahill DJ, Mullner S. Protein biochips: A new and versatile platform technology for molecular medicine. Drug Discov Today 2005; 10:789–794.
43. Rabilloud T. Detecting proteins separated by 2D gel electrophoresis. Anal Chem 2000; 72:48A–55A.
44. Holgate S. Mechanisms of allergy and adult asthma. Curr Opin Allergy Clin Immunol 2001; 1:47–50.
45. Tiedemann K, Malmstrom A, Westergren-Thorsson G. Cytokine regulation of proteoglycan production in fibroblasts: separate and synergistic effects. Matrix Biol 1997; 15:469–478.
46. Ong SE, Blagoev B, Kratchmarova I, et al. Stable isotope labeling by amino acids in cell culture, SILAC, as a simple and accurate approach to expression proteomics. Mol Cell Proteomics 2002; 1:376–386.
47. Ong SE, Kratchmarova I, Mann M. Properties of 13C-substituted arginine in stable isotope labeling by amino acids in cell culture (SILAC). J Proteome Res 2003; 2:173–181.
48. Gygi SP, Rist B, Gerber SA, Turecek F, Gelb MH, Aebersold R. Quantitative analysis of complex protein mixtures using isotope-coded affinity tags. Nat Biotechnol 1999; 17:994–999.
49. Hicks WA, Halligan BD, Slyper RY, Twigger SN, Greene AS, Olivier M. Simultaneous quantification and identification using 18O labeling with an ion trap mass spectrometer and the analysis software application "ZoomQuant" J Am Soc Mass Spectrom 2005; 16:916–925.
50. Yeo S, Roh GS, Kim DH, et al. Quantitative profiling of plasma peptides in asthmatic mice using liquid chromatography and mass spectrometry. Proteomics 2004; 4:3308–3317.
51. Pawson T, Scott JD. Signaling through scaffold, anchoring, and adaptor proteins. Science 1997; 278:2075–2080.
52. Hunter T. The Croonian Lecture 1997. The phosphorylation of proteins on tyrosine: its role in cell growth and disease. Philos Trans R Soc Lond B Biol Sci 1998; 353:583–605.
53. Mann M, Ong SE, Gronborg M, Steen H, Jensen ON, Pandey A. Analysis of protein phosphorylation using mass spectrometry: deciphering the phosphoproteome. Trends Biotechnol 2002; 20:261–268.
54. Gronborg M, Kristiansen TZ, Stensballe A, et al. A mass spectrometry-based proteomic approach for identification of serine/threonine-phosphorylated proteins by enrichment with phospho-specific antibodies: identification of a novel protein, Frigg, as a protein kinase A substrate. Mol Cell Proteomics 2002; 1:517–527.
55. Pandey A, Fernandez MM, Steen H, et al. Identification of a novel immunoreceptor tyrosine-based activation motif-containing molecule, STAM2, by mass spectrometry and its involvement in growth factor and cytokine receptor signaling pathways. J Biol Chem 2000; 275:38,633–38,639.

56. Lim YP, Diong LS, Qi R, Druker BJ, Epstein RJ. Phosphoproteomic finger-printing of epidermal growth factor signaling and anticancer drug action in human tumor cells. Mol Cancer Ther 2003; 2:1369–1377.
57. Maguire PB, Wynne KJ, Harney DF, O'Donoghue NM, Stephens G, Fitzgerald DJ. Identification of the phosphotyrosine proteome from thrombin activated platelets. Proteomics 2002; 2:642–648.
58. Kim HJ, Song EJ, Lee KJ. Proteomic analysis of protein phosphorylations in heat shock response and thermotolerance. J Biol Chem 2002; 277: 23,193–23,207.
59. Ficarro SB, McCleland ML, Stukenberg PT, et al. Phosphoproteome analysis by mass spectrometry and its application to *Saccharomyces cerevisiae*. Nat Biotechnol 2002; 20:301–305.
60. Fuglsang AT, Visconti S, Drumm K, et al. Binding of 14-3-3 protein to the plasma membrane H(+)-ATPase AHA2 involves the three C-terminal residues Tyr(946)-Thr-Val and requires phosphorylation of Thr(947). J Biol Chem 1999; 274:36,774–36,780.
61. Wang M, Xiao GG, Li N, Xie Y, Loo JA, Nel AE. Use of a fluorescent phosphoprotein dye to characterize oxidative stress-induced signaling pathway components in macrophage and epithelial cultures exposed to diesel exhaust particle chemicals. Electrophoresis 2005; 26:2092–2108.
62. Martin DB, Gifford DR, Wright ME, et al. Quantitative proteomic analysis of proteins released by neoplastic prostate epithelium. Cancer Res 2004; 64: 347–355.
63. Kratchmarova I, Kalume DE, Blagoev B, et al. A proteomic approach for iden-tification of secreted proteins during the differentiation of 3T3-L1 preadipocytes to adipocytes. Mol Cell Proteomics 2002; 1:213–222.
64. Kubota K, Wakabayashi K, Matsuoka T. Proteome analysis of secreted proteins during osteoclast differentiation using two different methods: two-dimensional electrophoresis and isotope-coded affinity tags analysis with two-dimensional chromatography. Proteomics 2003; 3:616–626.
65. Lafon-Cazal M, Adjali O, Galeotti N, et al. Proteomic analysis of astrocytic secretion in the mouse. Comparison with the cerebrospinal fluid proteome. J Biol Chem 2003; 278:24,438–24,448.
66. Boyd RS, Adam PJ, Patel S, et al. Proteomic analysis of the cell-surface mem-brane in chronic lymphocytic leukemia: identification of two novel proteins, BCNP1 and MIG2B. Leukemia 2003; 17:1605–1612.
67. Shin BK, Wang H, Yim AM, et al. Global profiling of the cell surface proteome of cancer cells uncovers an abundance of proteins with chaperone function. J Biol Chem 2003; 278:7607–7616.
68. Verma M, Kagan J, Sidransky D, Srivastava S. Proteomic analysis of cancer-cell mitochondria. Nat Rev Cancer 2003; 3:789–795.
69. Schutt F, Ueberle B, Schnolzer M, Holz FG, Kopitz J. Proteome analysis of lipofuscin in human retinal pigment epithelial cells. FEBS Lett 2002; 528: 217–221.
70. Garin J, Diez R, Kieffer S, et al. The phagosome proteome: insight into phago-some functions. J Cell Biol 2001; 152:165–180.

71. Wright ME, Eng J, Sherman J, et al. Identification of androgen-coregulated protein networks from the microsomes of human prostate cancer cells. Genome Biol 2003; 5:R4.
72. Foster LJ, De Hoog CL, Mann M. Unbiased quantitative proteomics of lipid rafts reveals high specificity for signaling factors. Proc Natl Acad Sci USA 2003; 100:5813–5818.
73. Andersen JS, Lyon CE, Fox AH, et al. Directed proteomic analysis of the human nucleolus. Curr Biol 2002; 12:1–11.
74. www.geneontology.org
75. http://www.ingenuity.com/

10

Linkage to Asthma and Its Intermediate Phenotypes

TIMOTHY D. HOWARD

Center for Human Genomics and
Department of Pediatrics, Wake Forest
University School of Medicine,
Winston-Salem, North Carolina, U.S.A.

JUAN C. CELEDÓN

Channing Laboratory and Respiratory
Disorders Program, Brigham and
Women's Hospital,
Harvard Medical School,
Boston, Massachusetts, U.S.A.

I. Introduction

Asthma is a common respiratory disease characterized by chronic inflammation of the airways, airflow obstruction that is often reversible either spontaneously or with treatment, and increased airway responsiveness to a variety of stimuli (1). A significant proportion of individuals with asthma are sensitized to at least one allergen (atopic). Although potential environmental causes of asthma and its intermediate phenotypes have been studied for years, only recently has significant progress been made in identifying genes responsible for susceptibility to asthma.

In this chapter, we review findings from genome-wide linkage analyses of asthma and its intermediate phenotypes (except lung function phenotypes, which are reviewed in another chapters of this book) in human populations. These studies have shown that multiple chromosomal regions are likely to contain asthma-susceptibility genes, further suggesting that asthma is a complex disease influenced by the interaction among variants in multiple genes (acting alone or in combination) and environmental exposures. As asthma-susceptibility genes within linked genomic regions are identified and characterized, their relationships to each other and to various environmental stimuli will become important topics of research.

II. Common Approaches to Genetic Studies of Asthma

Two strategies have been primarily used for genetic studies of complex diseases such as asthma: studies of candidate genes and positional cloning. The goal of candidate-gene studies is to evaluate genes that are believed to influence the pathogenesis of a disease of interest. There are several advantages to this approach, including relatively low cost and feasibility (few polymorphisms are needed to thoroughly screen a candidate gene). On the other hand, the list of potential candidate genes can quickly grow into the thousands, and genes that do not fit into known pathways for asthma will not be identified by candidate-gene studies. This approach is discussed in detail in another chapter of this book.

A second approach to genetic studies of asthma is positional cloning, in which disease-susceptibility genes are identified on the basis of their chromosomal location. In positional cloning, data from families are used to identify chromosomal regions that contain disease-susceptibility genes by examining cosegregation between the phenotype(s) of interest and DNA markers. Positional cloning thus identifies genes by first locating regions of the genome that are consistently inherited by affected offspring or consistently shared between affected siblings. The primary advantage of this approach is that it is not biased by any prior knowledge of disease pathogenesis and thus novel disease-susceptibility genes may be identified. On the other hand, genes with weak to moderate effects on a disease or trait may not be identified by this approach because of limited statistical power with sample sizes typically used for positional cloning studies.

The initial step of positional cloning is to perform a genome scan with highly polymorphic genetic markers (e.g., short-tandem repeats) evenly spaced throughout the genome. The typical resolution of these markers is approximately 10 centiMorgans (cM), which yields a reasonable amount of information in a cost-efficient manner. After a genomic region has been linked to a phenotype of interest, additional markers are usually genotyped to narrow the candidate genomic region and eventually localize the disease-susceptibility gene(s). This overall approach is straightforward but labor-intensive, as it requires ascertainment and recruitment of individuals with asthma and their relatives, collection of genotypic data, and analysis and interpretation of results.

Genome scans involve testing for linkage between hundreds of DNA markers and a phenotype(s) of interest. Lander and Kruglyak have proposed stringent criteria for suggestive and significant evidence of linkage in genome scans for complex diseases (2). For commonly used analyses, these authors consider a logarithm of odds ratio (LOD) score (base$_{10}$ logarithm of the likelihood of the odds ratio for linkage) greater than or equal to 1.9 but less than 3.3 (equivalent to p values 0.0017 but > 0.000049) as suggestive evidence of linkage, and a LOD score greater than or equal to 3.3 (equivalent to p value 0.000049) as significant evidence of linkage.

The positional cloning approach has been very effective in identifying causal genes for monogenic diseases. While the ability of positional cloning to identify susceptibility genes for complex diseases such as asthma was previously questioned, recent successes have provided support for this approach (3–7). To date, 15 genome scans for asthma and/or asthma-related phenotypes have been performed in 17 distinct populations. Follow-up studies of these populations with recruitment of additional families, further genotyping, and/or modified analyses have been conducted.

Positional cloning has identified five candidate genes for asthma susceptibility—*ADAM33* (3), *PHF11* (4), *DPP10* (5), *GPR154* (6), and *HLAG* (7). Variants in two of these genes (*ADAM33* and *GPR154*) have been associated with asthma and/or its intermediate phenotypes in at least six distinct populations, and functional data in rodents and humans further support a significant role of GPR154 in asthma pathogenesis (8). Because positional cloning generally disregards preconceived notions about the pathophysiology of the disease of interest, asthma-susceptibility genes identified by this approach could uncover new disease pathways and, ultimately, novel therapeutic applications.

III. Phenotypic Definition of Asthma

Asthma is truly a syndrome that can be divided into distinct categories (e.g., atopic vs. nonatopic, childhood vs. adult-onset). Because of this phenotypic complexity, the best clinical definition of asthma may not be the best definition for studies of asthma genetics. A common approach to the diagnosis of asthma for genetic studies is to categorize as asthmatics those subjects who have physician-diagnosed asthma, current respiratory symptoms, and airway responsiveness to bronchoconstrictors or a significant response to bronchodilator administration (9). Because of the lack of a standardized diagnosis of asthma, different asthma definitions have been used in genome-wide linkage analyses.

Intermediate phenotypes of asthma are objectively defined, quantitative, and may be influenced by a smaller number of genes than the disease itself. Intermediate phenotypes of asthma can be divided into three groups: (i) lung function phenotypes: airway responsiveness, spirometric measures, and bronchodilator responsiveness; (ii) factors influencing airway inflammation: skin test reactivity to aeroallergens, serum total and allergen-specific immunoglobulin (Ig)E, and eosinophil count; and (iii) factors indicating variable expression of asthma: asthma severity and lung function phenotypes.

IV. Genome-Wide Linkage Analyses of Asthma and Its Intermediate Phenotypes

To date, there have been genome scans for asthma and/or its intermediate phenotypes in 17 distinct human populations (Table 1). In spite of obvious differences among populations included in these scans (e.g., ethnicity, area of residence, environmental exposures), several genomic regions have shown suggestive and/or significant evidence of linkage (2) to asthma and/or its intermediate phenotypes in two or more studies.

Most human populations included in genome-wide linkage analysis of asthma and/or its intermediate phenotypes have been predominantly of European descent (6,10,15–19,21,22,25–30). A genome scan for quantitative and qualitative intermediate phenotypes of asthma was first conducted among sibling pairs in Busselton (Australia) (10). In that study, there was significant evidence of linkage (2) to a quantitative measure of atopy (skin test index, on chromosome 11q12) and suggestive evidence of linkage to total serum IgE (on chromosome 16q), eosinophil count (on chromosome 6p), airway responsiveness (on chromosomes 4q and 7p), and atopy (as a binary trait, on chromosomes 6p and 13q). Among 415 members of 97 families of siblings with asthma in Germany and Sweden, no chromosomal region showed suggestive or significant evidence of linkage to asthma or its intermediate phenotypes (16). However, there was modest evidence of linkage ($p < 0.01$) to asthma (on chromosomes 2pter, 6p, and 9q), total serum IgE (on chromosomes 1p, 2pter, 2q, 6p, 9q, 15q, and Xq), airway hyperresponsiveness (AHR) (on chromosomes 2pter and 9p), eosinophil count (on chromosomes 1p, 6p, 6q, 11q, and Xq), and atopy (on chromosomes 2p, 4q, 6p, 7p, and 9q). In a study of 107 nuclear families of French siblings with asthma, there was suggestive evidence of linkage to eosinophil count on chromosome 12q24 ($p = 0.0007$), and other chromosomal regions showed some evidence of linkage ($p < 0.01$) to total serum IgE (on chromosome 11p), asthma (on chromosome 17q), and atopy (on chromosome 17q) (21). In a follow-up study with 188 additional families, chromosome 1p31 showed suggestive evidence of linkage to asthma and allergic rhinitis (LOD = 2.8) and some evidence of linkage to asthma alone (LOD = 1.5) (22). In a study of 424 members of nuclear families of individuals with clinical atopy in Denmark, there was suggestive evidence of linkage to asthma (on chromosomes 1p, 5q, and 6p), total serum IgE (on chromosomes 3q, 5q, and 6p), and atopy (on chromosome 6p) (25). Van Eerdewegh et al. reported partial results of a genome-wide linkage analysis of asthma and AHR in 460 sibling pairs in the United States and the United Kingdom (3). In that study, there was significant evidence of linkage to asthma (defined as physician-diagnosed asthma and AHR) on chromosome 20p13 (LOD = 3.93).

Ferreira et al. recently conducted a genome-wide linkage analysis of asthma and its intermediate phenotypes in 591 members from families of

Table 1 Main Results of Genome-Wide Linkage Analyses of Asthma and/or Its Intermediate Phenotypes

Reference	Population	No. of families (subjects)	Linkage to asthma	Linkage to intermediate phenotypes of asthma
Daniels et al. (10)	Australian	80 (363)	Not assessed	Skin test index = $11q12$; AHR = 4q, 7p; eosinophil count = 6p; atopy = 6p, 13q; total serum IgE = 16q
Xu et al. (11); Huang et al. (12); Blumenthal et al. (13), (14)	North American (white, Hispanic, African-American)	266–287 (885–1931)	6p (whites); 1p (Hispanics); $11q13$ (African-Americans)	Dust-mite allergy = $19p13$ (whites); Atopy = 21q (Hispanics)
Ober et al. (15)	Hutterites	1 (693)[a]	1p, 3p, 5q, 8p	AHR = 5p, 19p; dust-mite allergy = 2q; mold allergy = 3q, 11p
Wjst et al. (16)	German and Swedish	97 (415)		
Xu et al. (17); Koppelman et al. (18); Meyers et al. (19)	Dutch	200 (1174)	3p, 5q	AHR = 3p, 5q; total serum IgE: 2q, 3q, 5q, $7q21$, 12q, 13q; eosinophil count: 2q, 15q, 17q
Yokouchi et al. (20)	Japanese	47 (197)	4q, $5q31–q33$, 6p, 12q, 13q	Not assessed
Dizier et al. (21); Dizier et al. (22)	French	107–295 (not available)	1p (asthma and allergic rhinitis)	Eosinophil count: 12q
Laitinen et al. (23)	Finnish	86 (443)	4q, 7p14–p15 (asthma and increased total serum IgE)	Total serum IgE = $7p14–p15$

(*Continued*)

Table 1 Main Results of Genome-Wide Linkage Analyses of Asthma and/or Its Intermediate Phenotypes (*Continued*)

Reference	Population	No. of families (subjects)	Linkage to asthma	Linkage to intermediate phenotypes of asthma
Xu et al. (24)	Chinese	533 (2551)	Not assessed	AHR = 2p25, 19q; total serum IgE: 1q; cockroach allergy = 4q
Haagerup et al. (25)	Danish	100 (424)	1p, 5q, 6p	Total serum IgE: 3q, 5q, 6p; atopy = 6p
Hakonarson et al. (26)	Icelandic	175 (1134)	14q24	Not assessed
Van Eerdewegh et al.[b] (3)	North American and British	460 (920)	20p13	Not assessed (results for AHR not presented separately from asthma)
Ferreira et al. (27)	Australian	202 (591)	1q, 4p, 11p, 17q, 18p, 19p	AHR = 6p, 20q; atopy = 2q, 3q, 6p, 17q, 20q; dust-mite allergy = 20q13; total serum IgE = 10q
Evans et al. (28)	Australian	539 (2360)	Not assessed	Eosinophil count = 2q33, 8q
Pillai et al. (29)	North American, European, Australian	414 (1555)		AHR = 2p16, 4p

Note: Only regions showing suggestive or significant evidence of linkage (as defined by Lander and Kruglyak) to asthma and/or its intermediate phenotypes (other than measures of lung function) are shown. Regions with significant evidence of linkage to asthma and/or its intermediate phenotypes are italicized.

[a]Large pedigree divided into 10 to 20 subpedigrees for data analysis.
[b]Complete linkage results for all chromosomes not published.
Abbreviations: AHR, airway hyperresponsiveness; IgE, immunoglobulin E.

Australian twins with and without asthma (27). In that study, there was significant evidence of linkage to dust-mite allergy on chromosome 20q13 (LOD = 4.93) and suggestive evidence of linkage to asthma (on chromosomes 1q, 4p, 11p, 17q, 18p, and 19p), AHR (on chromosomes 6p and 20q13), atopy (on chromosomes 2q, 3q, 6p, 17q, and 20q13), and total serum IgE (on chromosome 10q). Evans et al. conducted a genome-wide linkage analysis of eosinophil count in 738 pairs of Australians twins not ascertained on the basis of asthma or atopy (28). In that study, there was significant evidence of linkage to eosinophil count on chromosome 2q33 (LOD = 4.6) and suggestive evidence of linkage to eosinophil count on chromosome 8q.

Several genome-wide linkage analyses for intermediate phenotypes of asthma have been conducted in 200 families of individuals with asthma in The Netherlands (17–19). For the initial analysis of total serum IgE, there was significant evidence of linkage to chromosome 7q21 (LOD = 3.36) and suggestive evidence of linkage to chromosomes 5q31 (LOD = 2.73) and 12q24 (LOD = 2.46) (17). In a second analysis, there was suggestive evidence of linkage to eosinophil count (on chromosomes 2q, 15q, and 17q) and to total serum IgE (on chromosomes 2q, 3q, and 13q) (18). In the third and most recent analysis, there was suggestive evidence of linkage to asthma and AHR on chromosomes 3p and 5q (19). After stratification by passive exposure to cigarette smoking, there was significant evidence of linkage to AHR (LOD = 3.77) and suggestive evidence of linkage to asthma (LOD = 2.54) on chromosome 5q among individuals exposed to passive smoking. In contrast, there was no evidence of linkage to AHR or asthma in individuals who were not exposed to passive smoking, suggesting that a locus (or loci) on chromosome 5q interacts with passive smoking in the pathogenesis of AHR and asthma.

Multicenter studies have the potential advantage of accruing relatively large sample sizes, which may result in increased statistical power. The Collaborative Study on the Genetics of Asthma (CSGA) is unique in that it included members of three ethnic groups in the United States: whites, African-Americans, and Hispanics from New Mexico (31). At least one chromosomal region showed suggestive evidence of linkage to asthma within each ethnic group (chromosome 19q in whites, chromosome 2q in Hispanics, and chromosomes 5p and 17p in African-Americans), but no chromosomal region was linked to asthma in two of the three ethnic groups. When a follow-up study was conducted with an additional 126 families, none of the genomic regions that showed suggestive evidence of linkage to asthma in the original study had suggestive or significant evidence of linkage to asthma (11). However, there was at least one new genomic region with suggestive evidence of linkage to asthma within each ethnic group (chromosome 6p in whites, chromosome 11q in African-Americans, and chromosome 1p in Hispanics), and some evidence of linkage (LOD > 1) was reported for a few genomic regions within each ethnic group (including chromosome 19q in whites and chromosome 2q in Hispanics). In a follow-up study in African-Americans in the CSGA, a repeat analysis after genotyping additional markers revealed significant evidence of linkage to asthma on chromosome 11q13 (LOD = 4.38) (12). In other follow-up studies of the CSGA, there was significant evidence of linkage to dust-mite allergy on chromosome 19p13 in whites (LOD = 3.51) and suggestive evidence of linkage to atopy on chromosome 21q in Hispanics (13,14). More recently, a genome-wide linkage analysis of asthma and AHR in nuclear families of siblings with asthma from Europe, Australia, and the United States (29) showed suggestive evidence of linkage to AHR on chromosome 4p (LOD = 2.62) and some evidence of linkage to AHR on chromosome 2p (LOD = 1.82). After genotyping additional markers, a repeat analysis showed significant evidence of linkage to AHR on chromosome 2p16 (LOD = 4.58) and suggestive evidence of linkage to AHR on chromosome 4p (LOD = 3.07).

Because relatively few genes may influence a complex disease such as asthma in genetic isolates, several studies have attempted to identify genomic regions containing asthma-susceptibility genes in populations with significant founder and/or bottleneck effects. Ober et al. conducted genome-wide linkage analyses of asthma and its intermediate phenotypes in a European-American population with a strong founder effect (the Hutterites) (15,30). Among 693 members of families of Hutterite individuals with asthma, there was suggestive evidence of linkage to asthma (defined in several ways) (on chromosomes 1p, 3p, 5q, and 8p), AHR (on chromosomes 5p and 19p), dust-mite allergy (on chromosome 2q), and mold allergy (on chromosomes 3q and 11p) (15). Hakonarson et al. studied 175 families of 596 individuals with asthma in a relatively isolated population in Iceland (26) and found suggestive evidence of linkage to asthma on chromosome 14q24 (LOD = 2.66). A repeat analysis after genotyping additional markers revealed significant evidence of linkage to asthma on chromosome 14q24 (LOD = 4.0). In a genome-wide linkage analysis of asthma and its intermediate phenotypes among individuals in an isolated subpopulation of Finland (in Kainuu), there was suggestive evidence of linkage to asthma on chromosomes 4q (LOD = 2.5) and 7p (LOD = 2.0) (6). After genotyping additional markers on chromosome 7p, there was significant evidence of linkage to an increased total serum IgE level (LOD = 3.9) and suggestive evidence of linkage to asthma with an elevated total serum IgE level (LOD = 3.1). Linkage of chromosome 7p14–p15 to asthma and total serum IgE was then confirmed in two independent populations in Canada and Finland.

There have been two genome-wide linkage analyses of asthma and/or its intermediate phenotypes in Asian populations (20,24). In a study of 47 families of Japanese siblings with asthma who were sensitized to dust-mite allergen, there was significant evidence of linkage to mite-sensitive asthma on chromosome 5q31–q33 (LOD = 4.8) and suggestive evidence of linkage to asthma on several genomic regions (chromosomes 4q, 6p, 12q, and 13p) (20). Among 533 families of Chinese individuals with asthma, there was significant evidence of linkage to airway responsiveness on chromosome 2p25 and suggestive evidence of linkage to airway responsiveness (on chromosome 19p), total serum IgE (on chromosome 1q), and cockroach allergy (on chromosome 4q) (24).

V. Summary

Table 1 summarizes the main findings of published genome-wide linkage analyses of asthma and/or its intermediate phenotypes. Eleven genomic regions have shown significant evidence of linkage to asthma or its intermediate phenotypes: chromosomes 2p16 (to AHR, in families from Europe, Australia, and the United States) (29), 2p25 (to AHR, in Chinese families) (24), 2q33 (to eosinophil count in Australian twins) (28), 5q31–q33 (to mite-sensitive asthma in a Japanese population) (20), 7p14–p15 (to total serum IgE in a Finnish population) (23), 7q21 (to total serum IgE in a Dutch population) (17), 11q12–q13 (to atopy in Australians and asthma in African-Americans) (10,12), 14q24 (to asthma in an Icelandic population) (26), 19p13 (to dust-mite allergy in whites in the United States) (13), 20p13 (to asthma in families from the United States and United Kingdom) (3), and 20q13 (to dust-mite allergy in Australians) (27). Two potential asthma-susceptibility genes have already been identified in two of these genomic regions: *ADAM33* (on chromosome 20p13) (3) and *GPR154* (on chromosome 7p14) (6).

As shown in Table 1, several genomic regions have shown suggestive and/or significant evidence of linkage to the same (or very similar) asthma-related phenotype in at least two genome scans: chromosomes 1p, 3p, 4q, 5q, 6p, and 7p (to asthma); chromosome 2q (to eosinophil count); chromosomes 2q, 3q, 6p, 13q (to atopy and/or total serum IgE), and 2p (to AHR). Four potential asthma-susceptibility genes have been identified in these regions: *DPP10* (on chromosome 2q14) (5), *HLAG* (on chromosome 6p22) (7), *GPR154* (on chromosome 7p14) (6), and *PHF11* (on chromosome 13q14) (4). Other genomic regions such as chromosome 12q have shown suggestive evidence of linkage to at least one asthma-related phenotype in two or more genome scans and may also contain asthma-susceptibility genes (Table 1).

Results of published genome-wide linkage analyses of asthma and/or its intermediate phenotypes strongly suggest that certain genomic regions are likely to contain variants in genes that influence asthma pathogenesis across diverse ethnic groups. On the other hand, some genomic regions may be more relevant to asthma pathogenesis in certain populations than others. This is not surprising, as the relative influence of variants in a gene(s) on asthma pathogenesis likely depends on interactions with environmental exposures and/or genetic variants whose frequency is known to vary across ethnic groups.

There are explanations other than variation in genetic and environmental exposures for the discrepant findings of genome-wide linkage analyses of asthma and/or its intermediate phenotypes, including differences in phenotypic definition, statistical power, and data analysis among published studies. Differences in phenotypic definition are of particular importance for categorical phenotypes such as asthma, thus emphasizing the importance of including intermediate quantitative phenotypes of asthma in genome scans. Inadequate statistical power due to relatively small sample size may explain negative findings for certain genomic regions in some of the published genome scans. Finally, differences in analytical approach may explain some of the discrepant findings for genome scans for asthma and/or its intermediate phenotypes.

VI. Conclusions

Genome-wide linkage analyses of asthma and/or its intermediate phenotypes have greatly contributed to our understanding of asthma genetics. In particular, five potential asthma-susceptibility genes have been positionally cloned, and key candidate genomic regions for asthma-susceptibility genes have been identified. Fine-mapping studies of linkage and association in linked regions will likely lead to the discovery of novel asthma-susceptibility genes in the next few years.

Future genome-wide linkage analyses of asthma and/or its intermediate phenotypes should adequately assess the effects of gene-by-gene and gene-by-environment interactions on asthma susceptibility. Such studies will require novel analytic methods to incorporate existing data from genome scans and candidate-gene studies, as well as data from upcoming genome-wide association studies. Results from genome-wide linkage analyses may help prioritize findings and thus reduce the number of false-positive results of genome-wide association studies of asthma and/or its intermediate phenotypes. Because of their capacity to detect weak to moderate genetic effects, genome-wide association studies should help address the effects of complicated interactions among genetic and environmental exposures on asthma pathogenesis. Eventually, information from genome-wide studies of linkage and association should lead to a better understanding of the pathophysiology of asthma, which we hope will result in improved options for the prevention, diagnosis, and treatment of asthma.

References

1. National Asthma Education and Prevention Program. Expert panel report 2: guidelines for the diagnosis and management of asthma. Bethesda: National Institutes of Health Publication No. 97–4051, 1997.
2. Lander ES, Schork N. Genetic dissection of complex traits. Science 1994; 265: 2037–2048.

3. Van Eerdewegh P, Little RD, Dupuis J, et al. Association of the ADAM33 gene with asthma and bronchial hyperresponsiveness. Nature 2002; 418(6896):426–430.

4. Zhang Y, Leaves NI, Anderson GG, et al. Positional cloning of a quantitative trait locus on chromosome 13q14 that influences immunoglobulin E levels and asthma. Nat Genet 2003; 34(2):181–186.

5. Allen M, Heinzmann A, Noguchi E, et al. Positional cloning of a novel gene influencing asthma from chromosome 2q14. Nat Genet 2003; 35(3):258–263.

6. Laitinen T, Polvi A, Rydman P, et al. Characterization of a common susceptibility locus for asthma-related traits. Science 2004; 304(5668):300–304.

7. Nicolae D, Cox NJ, Lester LA, et al. Fine mapping and positional candidate studies identify HLA-G as an asthma susceptibility gene on chromosome 6p21. Am J Hum Genet 2005; 76(2):349–357.

8. Ober C, Hoffjan S. Asthma genetics 2006: the long and winding road to gene discovery. Genes Immun 2006; 7:95–100.

9. Celedon JC, Silverman EK, Weiss ST, Wang B, Fang Z, Xu X. Application of an algorithm for the diagnosis of asthma in Chinese families: limitations and alternatives for the phenotypic assessment of asthma in family-based genetic studies. Am J Respir Crit Care Med 2000; 162(5):1679–1684.

10. Daniels SE, Bhattacharrya S, James A, et al. A genome-wide search for quantitative trait loci underlying asthma. Nature 1996; 383:247–250.

11. Xu J, Meyers DA, Ober C, et al. Genomewide screen and identification of gene-gene interactions for asthma-susceptibility loci in three U.S. populations: collaborative study on the genetics of asthma. Am J Hum Genet 2001; 68(6): 1437–1446.

12. Huang SK, Mathias RA, Ehrlich E, et al. Evidence for asthma susceptibility genes on chromosome 11 in an African-American population. Hum Genet 2003; 113(1):71–75.

13. Blumenthal MN, Ober C, Beaty TH, et al. Genome scan for loci linked to mite sensitivity: the Collaborative Study on the Genetics of Asthma (CSGA). Genes Immun 2004; 5:226–231.

14. Blumenthal MN, Langefeld CD, Beaty TH, et al. A genome-wide search for allergic response (atopy) genes in three ethnic groups: Collaborative Study on the Genetics of Asthma. Hum Genet 2004; 114(2):157–164.

15. Ober C, Tsalenko A, Parry R, Cox NJ. A second-generation genomewide screen for asthma-susceptibility alleles in a founder population. Am J Hum Genet 2000; 67(5):1154–1162.

16. Wjst M, Fischer G, Immervoll T, et al. A genome-wide search for linkage to asthma. German Asthma Genetics Group. Genomics 1999; 58(1):1–8.

17. Xu J, Postma DS, Howard TD, et al. Major genes regulating total serum immunoglobulin E levels in families with asthma. Am J Hum Genet 2000; 67(5): 1163–1173.

18. Koppelman GH, Stine OC, Xu J, et al. Genome-wide search for atopy susceptibility genes in Dutch families with asthma. J Allergy Clin Immunol 2002; 109(3):498–506.

19. Meyers DA, Postma DS, Stine OC, et al. Genome screen for asthma and bronchial hyperresponsiveness: interactions with passive smoke exposure. J Allergy Clin Immunol 2005; 115(6):1169–1175.

20. Yokouchi Y, Nukaga Y, Shibasaki M, et al. Significant evidence for linkage of mite-sensitive childhood asthma to chromosome 5q31-q33 near the interleukin 12 B locus by a genome-wide search in Japanese families. Genomics 2000; 66(2):152–160.
21. Dizier MH, Besse-Schmittler C, Guilloud-Bataille M, et al. Genome screen for asthma and related phenotypes in the French EGEA study. Am J Respir Crit Care Med 2000; 162(5):1812–1818.
22. Dizier MH, Bouzigon E, Guilloud-Bataille M, et al. Genome screen in the French EGEA study: detection of linked regions shared or not shared by allergic rhinitis and asthma. Genes Immun 2005; 6(2):95–102.
23. Laitinen T, Daly MJ, Rioux JD, et al. A susceptibility locus for asthma-related traits on chromosome 7 revealed by genome-wide scan in a founder population. Nat Genet 2001; 28(1):87–91.
24. Xu X, Fang Z, Wang B, et al. A genomewide search for quantitative-trait loci underlying asthma. Am J Hum Genet 2001; 69(6):1271–1277.
25. Haagerup A, Bjerke T, Schiotz PO, Binderup HG, Dahl R, Kruse TA. Asthma and atopy—a total genome scan for susceptibility genes. Allergy 2002; 57(8): 680–686.
26. Hakonarson H, Bjornsdottir US, Halapi E, et al. A major susceptibility gene for asthma maps to chromosome 14q24. Am J Hum Genet 2002; 71(3):483–491.
27. Ferreira MA, O'Gorman L, Le Souef P, et al. Robust estimation of experiment-wise P values applied to a genome scan of multiple asthma traits identifies a new region of significant linkage on chromosome 20q13. Am J Hum Genet 2005; 77(6):1075–1085.
28. Evans DM, Zhu G, Duffy DL, Montgomery GW, Frazer IH, Martin NG. Major quantitative trait locus for eosinophil count is located on chromosome 2q. J Allergy Clin Immunol 2004; 114(4):826–830.
29. Pillai SG, Chiano MN, White NJ, et al. A genome-wide search for linkage to asthma phenotypes in the genetics of asthma international network families: evidence for a major susceptibility locus on chromosome 2p. Eur J Hum Genet 2006; 14(3):307–316.
30. Ober C, Cox NJ, Abney M, et al. Genome-wide search for asthma susceptibility loci in a founder population. The Collaborative Study on the Genetics of Asthma. Hum Mol Genet 1998; 7(9):1393–1398.
31. A genome-wide search for asthma susceptibility loci in ethnically diverse populations. The Collaborative Study on the Genetics of Asthma (CSGA). Nat Genet 1997; 15(4):389–392.

11

Linkage Analysis of Spirometric Phenotypes and Chronic Obstructive Pulmonary Disease

DAWN L. DEMEO, CRAIG P. HERSH, and EDWIN K. SILVERMAN

Channing Laboratory and Division of Pulmonary and Critical Care Medicine,
Department of Medicine, Brigham and Women's Hospital, Harvard Medical School,
Boston, Massachusetts, U.S.A.

I. Linkage Analysis: General Description

Linkage analysis methods have facilitated successful mapping and identification of genes for many Mendelian diseases, but the utilization of linkage methods for mapping quantitative traits, such as lung function measurements, and complex diseases, such as chronic obstructive pulmonary disease (COPD), has proved more challenging. This chapter will provide a brief introduction to linkage analysis, followed by a discussion of linkage analysis of pulmonary function measures in the general population and in COPD families.

Before considering a quantitative trait, such as forced expiratory volume in one second (FEV_1) or the ratio of FEV_1 to forced vital capacity (FVC), as an intermediate phenotype of disease, one typically first determines that there is significant heritability of the trait. Heritability represents the proportion of the variance in the trait due to genetic effects, and a large heritability value typically increases the probability of observing a significant linkage result. Linkage analysis has often been performed using data generated by genotyping highly polymorphic short tandem repeat (STR) markers (usually two to four nucleotide repeats) generally spaced about 10 cM apart, across the entire human genome. More recently, panels of larger numbers of single nucleotide polymorphisms (SNPs) have also been used. The linkage markers are genotyped in families, with the goal of identifying which chromosomal regions cosegregate with traits or diseases of interest; these regions may harbor relevant genetic determinants. Linkage is often investigated through statistical genetics tools that allow for the calculation of the logarithm of odds (LOD) score. The LOD score is defined as the $\log_{10}$ of the odds for linkage, typically assessed between a postulated disease locus and a marker locus. For extended pedigree studies, LOD scores greater than 3.3 are considered to indicate genome-wide significance, and a LOD score of at least 1.9 is considered suggestive of linkage (1). However, lower LOD scores should not be summarily discounted, as linkage studies may be underpowered.

For common diseases, such as asthma and COPD, linkage analyses have lead to the identification of a limited number of confirmed genetic determinants. Although linkage methods have been quite successful at identifying genetic determinants of obviously Mendelian diseases (such as cystic fibrosis), linkage methods are less powerful for localizing genes with more modest effects. Newer methods of whole genome association may result in more rapid candidate gene localization by allowing for an efficient, high throughput evaluation of common genetic variation to test for association with common diseases or intermediate phenotypes. These methods may accelerate the identification of genes relevant to normal pulmonary function and COPD, thus overcoming some of the limitations of linkage methods.

II. Heritability of Spirometric Phenotypes in the General Population

Linkage analysis of lung function phenotypes such as FEV_1 and FEV_1/FVC in general population samples has identified genomic regions that may be relevant to normal lung development. An extensive review of the genetic epidemiology of pulmonary function is beyond the scope of this chapter; a summary has been published, detailing the extensive work that has been performed to understand the familial aggregation and correlation of lung function parameters in family and twin studies (2). One crucial step, prior to using spirometric phenotypes such as FEV_1 and FEV_1/FVC in linkage and association studies, is the demonstration of heritability of these quantitative phenotypes in families. As described in Chapter 1, assessment of heritability may be carried out using twin studies or using the techniques of path analysis or variance component analysis.

Heritability studies of pulmonary function have been performed in twin as well as nontwin family studies. Heritability estimates for quantitative phenotypes such as lung function may be overestimated in twin studies, due to the increased environmental sharing/similarity that begins in utero and proceeds throughout life for monozygotic twins. For FEV_1, heritability estimates in twins have ranged from zero (3) to 0.77 (4). A summary of heritability assessments for FEV_1 in family studies is presented in Table 1. These heritability estimates fall between the extremes observed in twin studies, and they suggest that FEV_1 is a heritable phenotype to consider in linkage studies of normal lung function as well as obstructive lung diseases including asthma and COPD. One important caveat in the comparison of heritability assessments across studies is that the variable inclusion of environmental exposures (such as cigarette smoking) may impact the heritability estimates, especially in the setting of a gene-by-smoking interaction. A comparison of heritability estimates across studies should be considered only after a full assessment of the models and covariates included in the calculations.

The heritability of cross-sectional spirometric parameters is important, but the evaluation of the longitudinal decline in lung function phenotypes within families likely also can provide important insights into lung health and disease. The Tucson Epidemiological Study of Airway Obstructive Diseases (17) and The Framingham Heart Study (18) both considered the familial correlation and heritability of lung function decline. In the Tucson Study, participants had at least three pulmonary function evaluations during a 5- to 20-year time frame. These data suggested a strong correlation of decline in FEV_1 within smoking concordant siblings, while smoking discordant pairs demonstrated no correlation (17). The Framingham Heart Study used a variance component approach for the calculation of the heritability in the longitudinal decline in FEV_1. These heritability estimates varied from 0.05 for FEV_1 decline in models that included all participants, to an estimate of 0.18 in models limited to individuals with concordant smoking status (18). Both the Tucson and Framingham studies demonstrate similarities in rates of lung function decline within families, which could relate to susceptibility to develop COPD. These studies also point to the importance of considering gene-by-smoking interactions in models of linkage.

III. Linkage Analysis of Pulmonary Function

Linkage analysis of pulmonary function phenotypes has been performed in general population samples, revealing several genomic regions of interest. The identification of genomic regions that contribute to quantitative pulmonary function phenotypes may provide insights into normal lung development, lung growth throughout childhood and adolescence, and lung function decline; identifying such genomic regions may also provide insights into various pulmonary diseases.

Table 1 Heritability of Forced Expiratory Volume in One Second

Year	Authors	Study population	Heritability of FEV$_1$	Comments
1984	Lewitter (5)	404 families in East Boston, Massachusetts, U.S.A.	0.470 ± 0.057 (yr 1) 0.467 ± 0.058 (yr 5)	Path analysis of FEV$_1$ at years one, four, and five of the study
1984	Devor and Crawford (6)	96 Mennonite families in Kansas and Nebraska ascertained for a study of aging	0.169	Path analysis
1985	Astemborski et al. (7)	108 families ascertained through controls in a COPD study, Baltimore, Maryland, U.S.A.	0.278	Variance component analysis of residuals
1987	Beaty et al. (8)	158 families ascertained through a COPD proband	0.087	Variance component model with ascertainment correction
1990	Cotch et al. (9)	384 families in Maryland ascertained through probands with lung cancer, pulmonary and nonpulmonary disease	0.396 ± 0.061	Path analysis
1991	Coultas et al. (10)	733 Hispanic "households" in New Mexico, U.S.A.	0.42 ± 0.05	Path analysis
1996	Chen et al. (11)	214 families in the Humboldt Family Study in Saskatchewan	0.264	Regressive models
2000	Wilk et al. (12)	455 families in the NHLBI Family Heart Study	0.515	Regressive models
2001	Palmer et al. (13)	468 families in an Australian population-based sample	0.389 ± 0.091	Variance component
2002	Silverman et al. (14)	72 families ascertained through a proband with severe early-onset COPD	0.353 + 0.063	Variance component with ascertainment correction
2002	Joost et al. (15)	330 families in the Framingham Study	0.35	Variance component
2003	Malhotra et al. (16)	26 Utah CEPH pedigrees	0.46	Segregation analysis

Abbreviations: COPD, chronic obstructive pulmonary disease; NHLBI, National Heart, Lung, and Blood Institute; CEPH, Centre d'Etude du Polymorphisme Humain; FEV$_1$, forced expiratory volume in one second.

Studies of lung function phenotypes have identified linkage to several regions across the human genome, suggesting that quantitative pulmonary function phenotypes are influenced by multiple genes. In a genome-wide scan of STR markers (approximately 10 cM apart) analyzed in 1578 members of 330 families in the Framingham Heart Study, variance component linkage models adjusted for age, height, body mass index, and smoking status revealed LOD scores greater than 1.0 on chromosomes 5, 6, 10, and 19 for FEV_1/FVC, and LOD scores greater than 1.0 on chromosomes 3, 4, 6, 10, and 21 for FEV_1. The highest LOD score for FEV_1 was 2.4 on chromosome 6q, with a maximum LOD equal to 1.4 for FEV_1/FVC in this region (15). Additional markers were genotyped in a subset of families in a follow-up analysis on chromosome 6q27, revealing an increase in LOD score to 5.0 for FEV_1. This finding suggests the presence of a putative gene influencing FEV_1 located at approximately 184.5 cM (near D6S503) (19), although no confirmed genetic determinant has been reported to date.

Linkage analysis for pulmonary function phenotypes was also performed in the National Heart, Lung, and Blood Institute Family Heart Study. This study consisted of 391 pedigrees; 12 pedigrees had individuals also included in the Framingham Heart Study described above. This genome scan revealed multipoint LOD scores greater than 1.5 for FEV_1 on chromosome 3, and for FEV_1/FVC on chromosomes 1, 4, 9, and 17. These investigators also observed a LOD score of 2.74 on chromosome 18 for FVC. When additional markers were genotyped on chromosomes 4 and 18, the maximum LOD score for FEV_1 increased to 2.37 on chromosome 18; the maximum LOD score for FEV_1/FVC increased to 3.51 on chromosome 4 (20).

Linkage of spirometric phenotypes to chromosomes 2 and 5 has also been demonstrated by Malhotra et al. who studied 264 members of 26 Utah Genetic Reference Pedigrees, collected as part of the Centre d'Etude du Polymorphisme Humain (CEPH) genetic mapping project. One of the important features of this study was the use of more than 1300 markers across the genome at average distance of 2.5 cM, closer than the more commonly used 10 cM marker spacing for STR markers. The highest LOD scores for linkage were observed for FEV_1/FVC on chromosome 2 (LOD = 2.36 for a dominant model), and chromosome 5 (LOD = 2.23 for a recessive model) (16). Importantly, the linkage region on chromosome 2 overlapped the linkage peak for FEV_1/FVC in the Boston Early-Onset COPD Study, as detailed below (14).

Studies of pulmonary function phenotypes have demonstrated limited replication of linked genomic regions. Across these human family studies, nonreplication may be due to phenotypic and genetic heterogeneity, as well as small sample size. One way to corroborate human linkage findings is to evaluate syntenic regions in murine models of lung function. A recent genome-wide linkage analysis of lung function in mice observed linkage for different lung function quantitative trait loci to murine chromosomes

5, 15, 17, and 19 (21). The intersection of murine and human linkage data can provide supportive evidence for the existence of a valid genetic determinant in that region. For example, the region of linkage on murine chromosome 17 is syntenic to human chromosome 6q27, demonstrated by Wilk et al. to be significantly linked to FEV_1, as described above. Although a candidate gene has yet to be reported, utilizing mouse models may provide important insights into genetic determinants of lung function in health and disease. Focusing investigation on syntenic regions that replicate in both murine and human linkage studies may speed the discovery of pulmonary function genetic determinants.

IV. Linkage Analysis in COPD Families

The only proven genetic cause of COPD is an inherited deficiency of alpha 1-antitrypsin (AAT); however, this deficiency accounts for a small minority of COPD in the general population. Even amongst individuals with severe AAT deficiency, there is heterogeneity of lung function and disease, suggesting a potential role for modifier genes. Segregation analysis in 44 families with AAT deficient members supports a role for additional genetic influences on the manifestations of lung disease (22). Large-scale linkage studies in AAT sibling pairs are currently underway to identify genomic regions that may harbor such modifier genes.

Most individuals with COPD do not inherit a severe deficiency of AAT. This has lead to the hypothesis that COPD is a complex human disease characterized by contributions from multiple genes, environmental factors, and gene-by-smoking (environment) interactions. Genetic factors may contribute to the development of COPD through influences on lung development, programmed responses to oxidative and protease stress, cytokine levels, and innate immunity. To date, only the Boston Early-Onset COPD Study has reported linkage results identifying genomic regions that may harbor susceptibility genes for the development of COPD.

COPD is a heterogeneous disease consisting of chronic bronchitis (CB), emphysema, and small airway disease. Spirometric features are used to classify both the presence of obstructive lung disease (FEV_1/FVC less than 70%) and the severity of lung disease (FEV_1 as a percent of predicted). Familial aggregation of COPD has been described, as detailed in Table 2. In the Boston Early-Onset COPD Study, probands were ascertained on the basis of a physician diagnosis of severe COPD (FEV_1 less than 40% predicted) at age younger than 53 and without severe AAT deficiency. When compared to community-based controls, current or exsmoking first-degree relatives of early-onset COPD probands were observed to have increased risks for FEV_1 less than 80% predicted (odds ratio $= 4.5$), and CB (odds ratio $= 3.6$) as well as increased bronchodilator responsiveness (27,29). The risk for lower FEV_1 was more pronounced in women, suggesting

Table 2 Familial Aggregation of Chronic Obstructive Pulmonary Disease

Year	Authors	Cohort	Phenotype	Comments
1975	Higgins and Keller (23)	9226 participants in the Tecumseh Community Health Study	CB	CB more common in offspring of parents with CB, when either one or both parents had CB
1976	Tager et al. (24)	148 households, East Boston, Massachusetts, U.S.A.	CB	Observed CB clustering within families ($p < 0.001$)
1978	Tager et al. (25)	430 probands and 1340 relatives	CB and obstructive lung disease defined as $FEV_1 < 65\%$ predicted	Increased risk for CB in first-degree relatives of probands with CB or obstructive lung disease ($RR > 1.41$ varying with model)
1985	Khoury et al. (26)	150 COPD patients, 325 first-degree relatives, 56 spouses, and 107 controls	CB, airflow obstruction ($FEV_1/FVC < 0.68$)	Relatives of COPD patients increased risk for CB (odds ratio = 1.9 for siblings and 2.1 for offspring), and airflow obstruction (odds ratio = 2.4 for siblings and 6.4 for offspring)
1998	Silverman et al. (27)	44 Probands with severe, early-onset COPD, 204 first-degree and 45 second-degree relatives, and 83 controls	CB, airflow limitation	Smoking first-degree relatives had increased risk for CB and reduced FEV_1 (see text)
2001	McCloskey et al. (28)	150 probands and 173 siblings and 419 controls from the EPIC-Norfolk cohort	Airflow obstruction ($FEV_1/FVC < 0.7$) and COPD ($FEV_1/FVC < 0.7$ with $FEV_1 < 80\%$ predicted)	Siblings of probands had higher prevalence of COPD (odds ratio = 4.70)

Abbreviations: COPD, chronic obstructive pulmonary disease; CB, chronic bronchitis; FEV_1, forced expiratory volume in one second; FVC, forced vital capacity; RR, relative risk.

potentially important roles for sex and gender as factors in COPD susceptibility (30). Although McCloskey et al. demonstrated a similar increased
risk for COPD in siblings of probands with a history of smoking, no female
predominance of COPD-related phenotypes was observed (28). In the Boston Early-Onset COPD Study, midflow measures (FEF_{25-75} and FEF_{25-75}/
FVC) were also demonstrated to be lower in first-degree relatives (both
smokers and nonsmokers) (31), suggesting that investigation of FEF_{25-75}
and FEF_{25-75}/FVC might elucidate genomic regions for COPD susceptibility, not necessarily influenced by gene-by-smoking interactions but perhaps
influenced by lung development.

Linkage analyses for qualitative and quantitative COPD-related phenotypes have been performed in the Boston Early-Onset COPD Study.
An autosomal 10 cM genome-wide scan of STR markers was performed
in 585 members of 72 families. The linkage analyses included pre-
and post-bronchodilator values for FEV_1, FEV_1/FVC, FEF_{25-75}, and
FEF_{25-75}/FVC, as well as qualitative phenotypes derived from spirometric
measures and CB. Subgroup analyses in smokers only were performed in
this cohort to identify regions of the genome that may be relevant for
gene-by-smoking interactions.

Qualitative phenotypes in the Boston Early-Onset COPD Study were
investigated using a nonparametric linkage approach (32). In this analysis,
the presence of airflow obstruction was defined by FEV_1/FVC less than
90% predicted. Moderate-to-severe airflow obstruction was defined as
FEV_1 less than 60% predicted, and mild-to-severe airflow obstruction
as FEV_1 less than 80% predicted. LOD scores greater than 1.5 were
observed for moderate-to-severe airflow obstruction on chromosome 12
(LOD 1.70 at 36 cM) and chromosome 19 (LOD 1.54 at 42 cM); the
LOD score for chromosome 19 increased to 1.65 in the smokers-only analysis. LOD scores greater than 1.5 were observed for mild-to-severe airflow
obstruction and CB only in the smokers: LOD > 1.5 for mild-to-severe
airflow obstruction on chromosomes 1, 12, and 19, and for CB on chromosomes 6, 19, and 22. The increase in LOD score with stratification by
smoking may relate to gene-by-smoking interactions in these regions.

Quantitative phenotypes in the Boston Early-Onset COPD Study have
been investigated using a variance component linkage analysis approach.
The initial genome-wide linkage analysis revealed significant linkage to
FEV_1/FVC on chromosome 2q (LOD score = 4.12 at 222 cM). LOD scores
greater than 1.9 (suggestive linkage) were observed on chromosomes 1 and
17 for FEV_1/FVC (14). The inclusion of additional markers on chromosome 12 resulted in a LOD score of 2.43 at 37 cM for linkage to FEV_1.
In a follow-up analysis of postbronchodilator spirometric phenotypes,
the LOD score for FEV_1/FVC on chromosome 2q increased to 4.42 (33).
In general, the use of postbronchodilator FEV_1/FVC in the subsequent
analysis resulted in slight increases in LOD scores. However, comparing
the analyses of pre- and postbronchodilator values of FEV_1, the LOD score

for chromosome 1 increased from 1.24 to 2.24 at 136 cM, and the LOD score for chromosome 8p increased from 1.58 to 3.30 at 2 cM. Of note, linkage analysis results of bronchodilator responsiveness phenotypes did not meet the threshold for suggestive linkage (33).

As described above, the midexpiratory flow phenotypes of FEF_{25-75} and FEF_{25-75}/FVC demonstrated lower values in both smoking and nonsmoking first-degree relatives of probands in the Boston Early-Onset COPD Study versus controls, suggesting that these phenotypes could be useful in genetic studies of COPD susceptibility. LOD scores greater than 1.5 were observed for postbronchodilator FEF_{25-75} on chromosomes 8 and 12, and for postbronchodilator FEF_{25-75}/FVC on chromosome 2 (31).

One relatively unique and important feature of COPD genetic research is that cigarette smoking is known to be the main environmental risk factor for the development of the disease. However, the variable suscept-ibility to develop lung disease in the setting of tobacco smoking suggests the relevance of gene-by-smoking interactions. To further investigate this in the Boston Early-Onset COPD Study, linkage models for quantitative spirometric phenotypes were considered that excluded or included smoking covariates and that stratified by smoking status. For example, the LOD score for FEF_{25-75} on chromosome 12 increased from 3.30 for a model that included pack years as a covariate to a LOD score of 5.03 for the smokers-only analysis. The LOD score in this region of chromosome 12 increased from 2.06 to 3.26 in a similar analysis of FEV_1 (Fig. 1). Despite the loss of power asso-ciated with limiting the cohort to smokers only, LOD scores increased for spirometric phenotypes on chromosomes 2, 12, 16, 19, 20, and 22, suggesting that these genomic regions may contain loci for COPD susceptibility through gene-by-smoking interaction.

The identification of linkage regions of the genome to target for COPD candidate gene investigation and systematic fine mapping represents an important advance in identifying potential genetic determinants of COPD. One important concern in COPD genetic studies is phenotypic heterogeneity, so future research should also focus on more precise pheno-typing of study participants. Replication of the linkage findings from the Boston Early-Onset COPD Study will be essential to confirm the linkage regions of greatest interest.

The linkage peaks for FEV_1/FVC on chromosomes 1, 2, and 19 in the Boston Early-Onset COPD Study approximate regions of the genome where LOD scores greater than 1.0 have been identified in genome scans of lung function: chromosome 1 in Wilk et al. (20), chromosome 2 in Malhotra et al. (16), and chromosome 19 in Joost et al. (15). These overlapping regions likely harbor genes influenced by gene-by-smoking interactions, which may help explain why only some smokers develop COPD. These regions are the focus of ongoing COPD fine mapping and COPD susceptibility gene stu-dies. TGFB1 is a positional candidate gene on chromosome 19; SNPs in TGFB1 have been associated with COPD in two case-control populations,

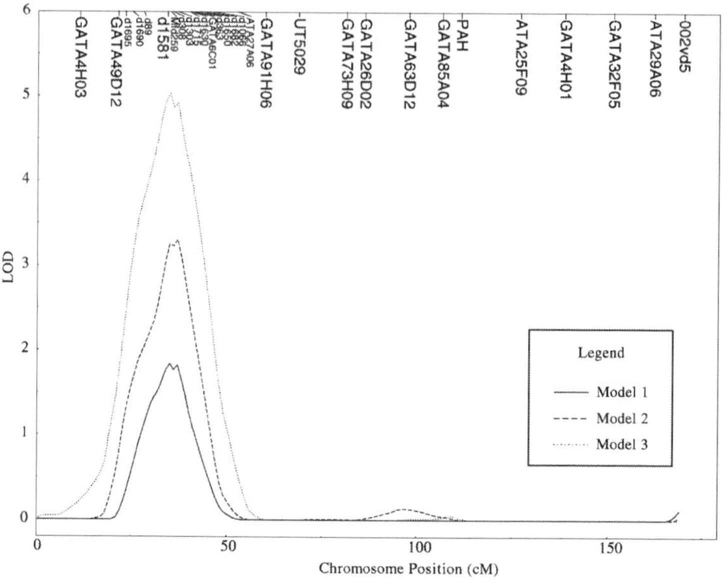

Figure 1 The increase in LOD score for FEV_{25-75} on chromosome 12: Model 1 excluded a covariate for smoking, Model 2 included pack-years of cigarette smoking and Model 3 was a smokers-only analysis. LOD scores increased from 1.83 (no smoking covariate, Model 1) to 3.30 (pack-years of smoking, Model 2) to 5.03 (smokers-only, Model 3).

and one family-based association analysis (34–36). SERPINE2 is a positional candidate gene on chromosome 2q, which has been associated with COPD-related phenotypes in the Boston Early-Onset COPD Study and a case-control study (37). Further study of these genes and other positional candidate genes may lead to confirmed genetic associations and functional genetic determinants of COPD.

Acknowledgment

This work supported by K08 HL 072918 and an ALA Research grant (DLD), K08 HL 080242 and a grant from the Alpha J Foundation (CPH), and R01 HL 68926, 71393 and 075478 (EKS).

References

1. Lander E, Kruglyak L. Genetic dissection of complex traits: guidelines for interpreting and reporting linkage results. Nat Genet 1995; 11(3):241–247.
2. Chen Y. Genetics and pulmonary medicine. 10: genetic epidemiology of pulmonary function. Thorax 1999; 54(9):818–824.
3. Ghio AJ, Crapo RO, Elliott CG. Heritability estimates of pulmonary function. Chest 1989; 96(4):743–746.

4. Hubert HB, Fabsitz RR, Feinleib M, Gwinn C. Genetic and environmental influences on pulmonary function in adult twins. Am Rev Respir Dis 1982; 125(4):409–415.

5. Lewitter FI, Tager IB, McGue M, Tishler PV, Speizer FE. Genetic and environmental determinants of level of pulmonary function. Am J Epidemiol 1984; 120(4):518–530.

6. Devor EJ, Crawford MH. Family resemblance for neuromuscular performance in a Kansas Mennonite community. Am J Phys Anthropol 1984; 64(3):289–296.

7. Astemborski JA, Beaty TH, Cohen BH. Variance components analysis of forced expiration in families. Am J Med Genet 1985; 21(4):741–753.

8. Beaty TH, Liang KY, Seerey S, Cohen BH. Robust inference for variance components models in families ascertained through probands: analysis of spirometric measures. Genet Epidemiol 1987; 4(3):211–221.

9. Cotch MF, Beaty TH, Cohen BH. Path analysis of familial resemblance of pulmonary function and cigarette smoking. Am Rev Respir Dis 1990; 142(6 Pt 1): 1337–1343.

10. Coultas DB, Hanis CL, Howard CA, Skipper BJ, Sarnet JM. Heritability of ventilatory function in smoking and non smoking New Mexico Hispanics. Am Rev Respir Dis 1991; 144(4):770–775.

11. Chen Y, Horne SL, Rennie DC, Dosman JA. Segregation analysis of two lung function indices in a random sample of young families: the Humboldt Family Study. Genet Epidemiol 1996; 13(1):35–47.

12. Wilk JB, Djousse L, Arnett DK, et al. Evidence for major genes influencing pulmonary function in the NHLBI Family Heart Study. Genet Epidemiol 2000; 19(1):81–94.

13. Palmer LJ, Knuiman MW, Divitini ML, et al. Familial aggregation and heritability of adult lung function: results from the Busselton Health Study. Eur Respir J 2001; 17(4):696–702.

14. Silverman EK, Palmer LJ, Mosley JD, et al. Genomewide linkage analysis of quantitative spirometric phenotypes in severe early-onset chronic obstructive pulmonary disease. Am J Hum Genet 2002; 70(5):1229–1239.

15. Joost O, Wilk JB, Cupples LA, et al. Genetic loci influencing lung function: a genome-wide scan in the Framingham Study. Am J Respir Crit Care Med 2002; 165(6):795–799.

16. Malhotra A, Peiffer AP, Ryujin DT, et al. Further evidence for the role of genes on chromosome 2 and chromosome 5 in the inheritance of pulmonary function. Am J Respir Crit Care Med 2003; 168(5):556–561.

17. Kurzius-Spencer M, Sherrill DL, Holberg CJ, Martinez FD, Lebowitz MD. Familial correlation in the decline of forced expi volume in one second. Am J Respir Crit Care Med 2001; 164(7):1261–1265.

18. Gottlieb DJ, Wilk JB, Harmon M, et al. Heritability of longitudinal change in lung function. The Framingham Study. Am J Respir Crit Care Med 2001; 164(9):1655–1659.

19. Wilk JB, DeStefano AL, Joost O, et al. Linkage and association with pulmonary function measures on chromosome 6q27 in the Framingham Heart Study. Hum Mol Genet 2003; 12(21):2745–2751.

20. Wilk JB, DeStefano AL, Amett DK, et al. A genome-wide scan of pulmonary function measures in the National Heart, Lung, and Blood Institute Family Heart Study. Am J Respir Crit Care Med 2003; 167(11):1528–1533.

21. Reinhard C, Meyer B, Fuchs H, et al. Genomewide linkage analysis identifies novel genetic loci for lung function in mice. Am J Respir Crit Care Med 2005; 171(8):880–888.

22. Silverman EK, Province MA, Campbell EJ, Pierce JA, Rao DC. Variability of pulmonary function in alpha-1-antitrypsin deficiency: residual family resemblance beyond the effect of the Pi locus. Hum Hered 1990; 40(6):340–355.

23. Higgins M, Keller J. Familial occurrence of chronic respiratory disease and familial resemblance in ventilatory capacity. J Chronic Dis 1975; 28(4):239–251.

24. Tager IB, Rosner B, Tishler PV, Speizer FE, Kass EH. Household aggregation of pulmonary function and chronic bronchitis. Am Rev Respir Dis 1976; 114(3):485–492.

25. Tager I, Tishler PV, Rosner B, Speizer FE, Litt M. Studies of the familial aggregation of chronic bronchitis and obstructive airways disease. Int J Epidemiol 1978; 7(1):55–62.

26. Khoury MJ, Beaty TH, Tockman MS, Self SG, Cohen BH. Familial aggregation in chronic obstructive pulmonary disease: use of the loglinear model to analyze intermediate environmental and genetic risk factors. Genet Epidemiol 1985; 2(2):155–166.

27. Silverman EK, Chapman HA, Drazen JM, et al. Genetic epidemiology of severe, early-onset chronic obstructive pulmonary disease. Risk to relatives for airflow obstruction and chronic bronchitis. Am J Respir Crit Care Med 1998; 157(6 Pt 1):1770–1778.

28. McCloskey SC, Patel BD, Hinchliffe SJ, Reid ED, Wareham NJ, Lomas DA. Siblings of patients with severe chronic obstructive pulmonary disease have a significant risk of airflow obstruction. Am J Respir Crit Care Med 2001:1419–1424.

29. Celedon JC, Speizer FE, Drazen JM, et al. Bronchodilator responsiveness and serum total IgE levels in families of probands with severe early-onset COPD. Eur Respir J 1999; 14(5):1009–1014.

30. Silverman EK, Weiss ST, Drazen JM, et al. Gender-related differences in severe, early-onset chronic obstructive pulmonary disease. Am J Respir Crit Care Med 2000; 162(6):2152–2158.

31. DeMeo DL, Celedon JC, Lange C, et al. Genomewide linkage of forced midexpiratory flow in chronic obstructive pulmonary disease. Am J Respir Crit Care Med 2004; 170(12): 1294–1301.

32. Silverman EK, Mosley JD, Palmer LJ, et al. Genome-wide linkage analysis of severe, early-onset chronic obstructive pulmonary disease: airflow obstruction and chronic bronchitis phenotypes. Hum Mol Genet 2002; 11(6):623–632.

33. Palmer LJ, Celedon JC, Chapman HA, Speizer FE, Weiss ST, Silverman EK. Genome-wide linkage analysis of bronchodilator responsiveness and postbronchodilator spirometric phenotypes in chronic obstructive pulmonary disease. Hum Mol Genet 2003; 12(10):1199–1210.

34. Celedon JC, Lange C, Raby BA, et al. The transforming growth factor-beta1 (TGFB1) gene is associated with chronic obstructive pulmonary disease (COPD). Hum Mol Genet 2004; 13(15):1649–1656.

35. Su ZG, Wen FQ, Feng YL, Xiao M, Wu XL. Transforming growth factor-beta1 gene polymorphisms associated with chronic obstructive pulmonary disease in Chinese population. Acta Pharmacol Sin 2005; 26(6):714–720.

36. Wu L, Chau J, Young RP. Transforming growth factor beta (1) genotype and susceptibility to chronic obstructive pulmonary disease. Thorax 2004; 59:126–129.

37. DeMeo DL, Mariani TJ, Lange C, et al. The SERPINE2 gene is associated with chronic obstructive pulmonary disease. Am J Hum Genet 2006; 78(2):253–264.

12

Fine Mapping and Whole Genome Association Studies in Asthma and Chronic Obstructive Pulmonary Disease

MIRIAM F. MOFFATT and WILLIAM O. C. COOKSON

The National Heart and Lung Institute, Imperial College,
London, U.K.

I. Introduction

Positional cloning is much more likely to identify novel genetic effects than candidate gene studies. Genetic linkage studies are very powerful for the study of single gene disorders, but have limited power in complex genetic disorders when many genes are likely to be acting and there is no established model for the inheritance of a given disease. Genetic linkage studies in a complex disorder such as asthma typically give an imprecise signal for the localization of the diseased gene that may extend over tens of megabases of DNA. This is because only a proportion of families will actually be linked to the locus, while others will appear randomly linked and nonlinked. In addition, the proportion of individuals with susceptibility alleles who develop the disease will vary between families (i.e., the alleles will have variable penetrance). For this reason, even highly ambitious genetic linkage studies involving several hundreds of families have often failed to deliver conclusive results.

II. Linkage Studies in Asthma and Chronic Obstructive Pulmonary Disease

At least 11 full genome screens have been reported for asthma and its associated phenotypes (1,2). These have identified 10 regions of linkage that were reproducible between screens and four regions that were statistically significant but not replicated by other groups (1). Those regions that were consistently identified are likely to contain the genes with the strongest effect on disease.

A linkage study for chronic obstructive pulmonary disease (COPD) in families with severe early onset COPD identified several regions of weak linkage, but no regions that showed genome-wide significance or unequivocal evidence for a susceptibility gene on a particular chromosomal segment (3). Subsequent recruitment of further families and the study of additional phenotypes such as the forced expiratory volume in one second (FEV_1)/ forced vital capacity (FVC) ratio (4) have increased the evidence for linkage on chromosome 2. An independent genome-wide scan of pulmonary function measures in the National Heart, Lung, and Blood Institute Family Heart Study found that the FEV_1/FVC ratio was significantly linked to the short arm of chromosome 4, with no obvious overlap of linkages with the COPD studies described above (5).

Genome screens have also been carried out for many other immune diseases that have a genetic basis and have identified regions of linkage that are shared (6). Asthma consistently shows linkage to the major histocompatibility complex on the short arm of chromosome 6 (7), and linkage regions for asthma also overlap with loci for ankylosing spondylitis (on chromosomes 1p31–36, 7p13, and 16q23); type 1 diabetes (on chromosomes 1p32–34, 11q13, and 16q22–24); inflammatory bowel disease (IBD) (on chromosomes 7p13 and 12q12–14); and multiple sclerosis and rheumatoid arthritis (on chromosome 17q22–24) (7).

These shared loci are of particular interest, because they may lead to the elucidation of as yet unknown immune processes with important general effects on disease susceptibility.

Although substantial advances have been made in the discovery of the genes underlying asthma, less than 30% of the susceptibility factors have been identified from accepted regions of linkage (8) and there is still an important need for systematic identification of the remaining genes. The study of COPD is less advanced than that of asthma, and novel techniques may greatly speed gene identification for this disorder.

III. Linkage Disequilibrium Mapping

Current technology (as described below) and the completion of the human genome sequence have enormously improved the ability to systematically identify susceptibility genes for common complex diseases. The detection of disease-marker associations and linkage disequilibrium (LD) mapping is much more powerful than traditional linkage studies, and can identify genes of small effect with manageable sample sizes (9). Analytical tools and capabilities for genotyping in common use are now sufficiently powerful for large-scale genome-wide association studies to definitively elucidate complex diseases (10).

LD describes the nonrandom association of DNA variants on contiguous regions of DNA. New polymorphisms first appear on an individual chromosome, and are initially coinherited with every other polymorphism on that chromosome. Polymorphisms may increase in frequency in a population either through selection or through genetic drift. Genetic recombination causes progressive dissociation between the new polymorphism and distant single nucleotide polymorphisms (SNPs), until after many generations only physically close SNPs are coinherited. LD may be detected by population associations between markers or between a disease phenotype and a marker or markers (representing a functional polymorphism).

The detection of disease-marker associations by LD mapping can precisely locate genes of small effect, and could be used to identify common diseased genes in genome-wide scans or to reduce the number of candidate genes in a region where linkage has been established (11–14). In the presence of common disease alleles, or when the frequency of rare alleles is increased through selection, the sample sizes required for LD studies are much smaller than for equivalently powered linkage studies (11).

A. The Nature of Linkage Disequilibrium

Simulations have suggested that LD may extend for less than 5 Kb, even in relatively isolated populations, so that over 1,000,000 equally spaced markers might be required for genome-wide LD scans (15). However, reviews of published data provide examples of LD at distances greater than 100 Kb (16,17), and there is evidence that LD patterns vary between populations (18,19). LD is detectable at 500 Kb in the adenomatous polyposis coli region on chromosome 5 (20), and significant LD between microsatellite loci has been shown to extend to 4.0 cM in some chromosomal regions (17). Other studies have shown that the distribution of LD is irregular in a number of chromosomal regions (21–24).

The D' statistic as a measure of LD, which has a simple interpretation, its scale (between 0 and 1), is independent of allele frequency and it is applicable to both SNP and microsatellite data (9,10).

The fine structure of LD is highly irregular. Forty-five percent of the variation in disequilibrium measures can be explained by physical distance (25). Additional factors such as allele frequency, type of polymorphism, and genomic location explain less than 5% of the variation (25). D' is frequently less than one even for closely linked markers, and SNPs a few base pairs apart on occasion show no LD. Care is therefore required when interpreting allelic association as an evidence of precise localization.

The limit of detection of LD between a disease and a marker is approximately defined by a D' of 0.33 (15,25) and by the size of the sample studied (26). On average, D' declines below 0.33 for distances greater than approximately 35 kb (25). The detection of association between a marker and disease therefore limits the location of the disease gene to within an average of 35 Kb in either direction. Local differences in the extent of LD may modify this figure, which may be approximated to 100 Kb ($\pm$50 Kb).

B. Detection of Association

The key decision in moving from genetic linkage (typically 10–30 Mb) to genetic association (100 Kb) is the number and density of markers to type within the limits for localization of the disease gene. This interval is typically defined by the 1 Lod support unit (the region covered by the linkage curve extending 1 Lod less than the maximum peak), which corresponds approximately to a 90% confidence interval. If LD were to be evenly distributed, then 30 Mb could be covered comprehensively by as few as 300 SNPs (or microsatellites or other polymorphisms). However, the universal observation is that LD is irregular. Much therefore has been made of the presence of "haplotype blocks," which have been defined as "sizeable regions over which there is little evidence for historical recombination and within which only a few common haplotypes are observed" (27,28).

It has been suggested that such blocks may be typified by a limited number of SNPs ("tag SNPs," discussed below in the section on whole-genome association mapping), and that these SNPs may serve to capture all relevant haplotypes and disease associations. However, even within regions of quite high LD, LD still declines with distance, and some markers may be out of LD with their immediate neighbors.

An empirical method of moving from linkage to association may be to type waves of markers of progressive density, until association between disease and a marker is identified. The density of the first wave depends on the resources available for genotyping (budget, subjects, equipment, and workers).

The power of LD mapping depends strongly on matching marker and disease allele frequencies (26,29,30). This means that SNPs with a range of gene frequencies should be tested. Microsatellites reflect LD from multiple alleles simultaneously, and as LD may extend for longer distances around microsatellites (25), they may be more informative than SNPs for low-density scans or when searching for mutations of recent origin. Dense panels of microsatellite markers are already in use for genetic linkage studies (31) and there are 12,000 microsatellites in the public domain, so that these markers also merit consideration in LD mapping.

Association between disease and a marker may be examined in cases and controls, or in families. Cases and controls may be cheaper to collect, but hidden admixture is always a possibility, particularly in countries such as the United States. In the absence of admixture, the power of analysis of association in families may be increased by the inclusion of all family members, correcting for familial correlations in phenotype and genotype. Statistical methods for this type of analysis include regressive models (32) as implemented in Statistical Analysis for Genetic Epidemiology (SAGE) and variance components models as implemented in quantitative transmission disequilibrium test (QTDT) (33) for quantitative traits, and haplotype relative risks (34) for categorical data.

C. Fine Mapping

Assuming that an association has been established between a marker and disease, the next step in localization of an assumed disease gene involves defining the limits of association and the comprehensive identification of polymorphism within those limits. Although the public SNP map is becoming more reliable and comprehensive, it is not so at the time of writing, and the identification of all SNPs in a region will still depend on systematic resequencing.

The nature of the genetic variation underlying complex traits is likely to consist of common alleles that are evolutionarily old (35,36). In addition, rare alleles may require prohibitively large sample sizes to detect associations with complex traits.

Sequencing strategies are therefore typically directed at the identification of alleles with a minimum frequency of 0.15. It has been shown that sequencing 20 haploid genomes gives an approximate 99.9% probability of detecting alleles with a minimal allele frequency of 0.2, and an approximate 99% probability of detecting alleles with a minimum frequency of 0.1 (37). Sequencing of diploid genomes from 10 individuals with and without disease is sufficient to achieve this power.

In general, successful LD mapping will require a systematic understanding of local patterns of LD and haplotype evolution, as exemplified by the mapping of polymorphisms in the ACE gene, which controls circulating ACE levels (38). Haplotype-based tests may be more powerful in the presence of multiple disease alleles (39), but the relationship between haplotype variation and the power of haplotype-based tests has not yet been well described.

IV. Gene Identification

Once an LD and association map has been completed, then the putative gene needs to be identified from the refined genetic region. With luck, only a handful of genes will be implicated by genetic association. Gene identification depends on the examination of sequence for potential genes, the identification of expressed sequences, the pattern of expression of the genes within different tissues, and the inference of gene function from homology searches and examination of domain structure. These steps are considerably facilitated by the completion of the human genetic sequence.

A. Gene Function

Given that positional cloning is capable of finding new and unexpected mechanisms for disease, it is quite possible that at the end of the positional cloning process, there will still be some uncertainty as to the function of the assumed disease gene in the disease process.

The general pattern of expression of the positional candidate genes may be examined by northern blots, such as human Multiple Tissue Northern (MTN) Blots and human immune system MTN blots, which may be obtained commercially. The examination of cDNA panels from multiple tissues by polymerase chain reaction is also very helpful, and allows the examination of splice variants that may not be delineated by Northern blots.

The inclusion of all human genes on commercially available DNA microarrays adds a new dimension to this process. These arrays may be interrogated with a variety of tissues from normal and diseased individuals, and information on the expression levels integrated with positional information from linkage and association studies.

The downstream examination of the function of genes is likely to be highly individual, and difficult to organize with high throughput. The abilities to express proteins in a variety of vectors and systems, to raise antibodies, to localise proteins within cells, to identify ligands, and to knockout in mice or knockdown in cells by RNAi may all be required.

B. The Effects of Polymorphism

The decision, an assumed disease gene has been identified, is easiest if clear mutations are found in the gene, as in the case of the nucleotide oligomerization domain 2 (NOD2) gene and Crohn's disease (40,41). However, it may often be the case that the effects of polymorphism on gene function are more subtle, affecting levels of expression or splice variation. In these circumstances, a definitive understanding of the mechanics of disease may take some time. Systematic examination of polymorphisms for transcription factor binding by electrophoretic mobility shift assay or footprinting experiments may be a helpful first step.

C. Genes Identified by Fine Mapping of Linked Regions

The international effort into the positional cloning of susceptibility genes for asthma has been successful, with the identification of four novel genes: dipeptidyl peptidase 10; chromosome 2q14 (42), G-protein-coupled receptor for asthma susceptibility; chromosome 7p14 (43), plant homeodomain finger protein-11; chromosome 13q14 (44), and a disintegrin and metalloproteinase 33; chromosome 20p (45). In the case of COPD, the results of a very promising study suggest that the *SERPINE2* gene is responsible for COPD susceptibility in the region of established genetic linkage on chromosome 2 (46).

V. Whole Genome Association Mapping

Although the positional cloning of complex disease genes from linked regions has been successful, it has often relied on fortuitous detection of association to microsatellite markers (40,42,44,47,48) as a first step in LD mapping. The low power of linkage studies remains a significant problem for systematic detection of disease genes. Although LD association mapping can by contrast identify genes of small effect with manageable sample sizes (9), detailed LD mapping of established linkage regions is however bioinformatically intensive and inefficient because of limitations on genotype multiplexing.

The International HapMap project has resequenced the human genome to systematically identify all SNPs with a minor allele frequency less than 0.05 (49). Current genotyping technology with whole-genome multiplex arrays, such as the 100 K and 500 K Affymetrix genotyping chips or the Illumina 100 K bead array system, can now deliver costs below $0.01 per genotype. Whole genome association mapping may now be the tool of choice to definitively elucidate complex diseases (50).

The HapMap consortium has provided a public database of SNPs, which is of enormous value to genetic researchers. As it is still impossible to type all 6,000,000 SNPs on cases or families, a key problem remains how to make most efficient use of this data.

Genome-wide studies may concentrate on genes and their regulatory regions (the sequence-based approach), or cover the genome regardless of gene content (the map-based approach) (51,52). Map approaches depend on covering the whole genome evenly with SNPs, with some reduction in the number of genotypes through the identification of tag SNPs that carry most of the relevant genetic information from regions of high LD.

Various scenarios have been explored for the adequate choice of tag SNPs (53), and it is clear that their use may allow some reduction in the need for genotyping in whole genome association studies. Tag SNPs are however being selected on the basis of a very limited number of subjects, and it is unlikely that LD from these individuals can be extrapolated freely. However, there are estimated to be at least 15 million SNPs at frequency 1% or greater in the human genome, 30% of SNPs are not within taggable haplotypic blocks, and 50% of the genome is made up of repeat elements such as short interspersed elements (SINEs) and long interspersed elements (LINEs). This means that definitive map-based whole-genome LD mapping will not be possible in the short term (50).

Our group has made comprehensive high-density SNP maps of seven loci, each of which has been genotyped in more than 1000 subjects (23,25,42,44,54–57). These studies indicate that LD is not simply broken into discrete blocks; that causal SNPs may not be in LD with other SNPs close by; and that the patterns of LD may differ between disease and normal chromosomes. Optimistically, our studies consistently observed that more than one SNP in each gene showed independent association, probably as the result of past positive selection for polymorphism. The common initial localization of positionally cloned genes through association with a microsatellite (40,42,44,47,48) indicates empirically that the detection of association is possible with markers at a moderate density.

A sequence-based strategy has been suggested as an alternative to SNP tagging. The sequence strategy concentrates on genes and their regulatory elements. These sequences are confined to less than 3% of the genome, and may be covered much more easily in a straightforward assay system. Although some fraction of variants responsible for disease may be missed by concentrating on genes, it has been established that examination of association to haplotypes allows efficient detection of untyped disease-causing polymorphisms with a wide range of frequencies in the intervals between SNPs in the genotyping panel (50). The sequence-based approach therefore represents an efficient strategy for disease-gene identification. It does not preclude subsequent map-based LD mapping if non–gene-related sequences are found to be important in complex disease pathogenesis.

A. Genotyping Technology

The choice of technology for whole-genome SNP typing currently rests between the 100 K and 500 K Affymetrix/Perlegen genotyping chips and the Illumina 100 K bead array system. The Affymetrix chip SNPs are randomly spaced and are suitable for map-based LD mapping. The Illumina Sentrix® Human-1 Genotyping BeadChip is sequence based and is designed with approximately 30% of the content directly in genes or within 10 Kb of the coding region. It contains all common coding SNPs. The non–gene-related content targets highly conserved across species noncoding regions and provides uniform spacing across the genome (approximately three SNPs per 200 Kb). Illumina also provide a HapMap chip containing approximately 300 K markers from Phase I of the HapMap project. The optimal strategy for use of these complimentary resources has yet to be resolved.

B. Case–Control and Family Studies

Whole genome association studies may be applied as equally to case–control samples as to families. Large case–control panels are more easily recruited than the families of probands with disease. It is not clear how important hidden population stratification may be in the analysis of cases and controls by whole genome association, or whether this stratification may be managed through the use of genomic controls to identify stratification structure (58). As an alternative, the use of family-based association tests means that the study will be robust to hidden population stratification (59).

Many studies have shown that the risk of transmission of atopic disease from an affected mother is approximately four times higher than from an affected father (60). Similar parent of origin effects have been noted in other immunological diseases, including type-I diabetes (61,62), rheumatoid arthritis (63), psoriasis (64), IBD (65), and selective immunoglobulin A deficiency (66). The use of family-based samples has the additional advantage of allowing the identification of such parent of origin effects in the data.

C. Subject Selection and Power

The cost of whole-genome association can be controlled by strategies to enhance power and reduce the number of subjects in whom genotyping is to be carried out.

Quantitative intermediate phenotypes have more power to detect linkage and association than diagnostic categories, because they do not present difficulties with marginal cases and they may be more heritable than categories. The power to detect association is considerably augmented by selection of probands with extreme phenotypes (typically within the top 10% of the population distribution of trait) (67), together with siblings that are either highly concordant or discordant for the trait (68). Simulations show that an efficient strategy for association studies is to recruit probands with severe disease and to include their siblings (and parents) in the study regardless of affection status (68).

Whatever study design is used, whole-genome association studies will only be effective when large numbers of subjects are included (typically 1000–3000 and an equal number of controls) and where still larger numbers of cases and controls are available for replication studies.

D. Statistical Analyses

The comparison of 100,000 to 500,000 markers with multiple phenotypes requires some method to define significance levels of statistical tests of association. In general, this may be dealt with by the use of modern statistical techniques that assume a dataset will derive multiple true positives, and that accept some level of false positives among results that identify the true positives. The control of the false discovery rate offers more than 100% increase in statistical power over simple control of the "experiment-wise" type-I error (69,70). Typically, a 5% rate of false positives may be accepted in highly dimensional datasets. Replication may then be used to determine true genetic effects in independent family, case–control samples, and population samples.

Rare variants that will not have been identified by the HapMap may have very significant effects on disease [as exemplified by *NOD2* mutations and IBD (40)]. These may be detected by the systematic "exhaustive" examination of haplotypes across the genome (50).

The use of whole genome data will allow the systematic testing for epistasis (gene–gene interactions) between markers. However, this type of testing is very demanding because of the small numbers of subjects who may have the interacting genotypes (two SNPs of 10% frequency will interact in 1% of the population), and the very large numbers of comparisons that will be possible between 500,000 genotypes. Definitive results may therefore depend on datasets of 10,000 subjects.

VI. Expression Quantitative Trait Loci

Transcript abundances of disease susceptibility genes in cells and tissues are significantly correlated with disease traits in families (71,72). These gene expression levels can be used as a surrogate for classical quantitative traits, and have been named expression quantitative trait loci (eQTLs). As gene expression is directly modified by polymorphism in regulatory elements, eQTLs can exhibit remarkable power to identify disease-associated genes and genetic variants.

Comprehensive genetic screens of eQTLs have been successfully carried out with mouse, plant, and human transcriptomes (72). In one study, the authors examined 111 F2 mice for expression eQTLs of 21,320 genes. They identified Lod scores greater than 4.3 with 2123 genes (compared to 400 expected), and observed a maximum Lod score of 80. A study of Epstein-Barr Virus transformed (EBV) cell lines from extended Center d'Etude Du Polymorphisme Humain (CEPH) families containing approximately 100 siblings identified 142 expression phenotypes with a Lod score for linkage greater than 5.3 ($p < 4.3 \times 10^{-7}$), and a minimum $p < 10^{-11}$ (73). These results indicate the detection of linkage to eQTLs to be a very powerful tool for dissecting the genetics of complex traits. The use of a single cell type harvested in controlled conditions is desirable for the detection of subtle differences in expression levels between individuals. In human studies, it has been shown that EBV-transformed lymphoblastoid cell lines provide general information about gene expression, even for genes whose primary function is not in such cells (47,72,74,75). Thirty percent of gene expression levels in EBV lines show significant heritability and may be mapped as eQTLs (72,76). These genes are very significantly enriched in gene ontology categories of "immune response" and "defense/immunity protein activity" (76), and so are excellent targets for investigation in asthma and COPD.

VII. Conclusions

Genetic studies of asthma and COPD are making remarkable advances. The successful positional cloning of several susceptibility genes for these diseases indicates that systematic gene identification is not only possible but also likely. In addition to fine mapping studies of regions of accepted genetic linkage, the next generation of genetic studies will rely on whole-genome association and eQTL mapping to bring about definitive identification of all of the major genetic effects on airway disease.

References

1. Cookson W. A new gene for asthma: would you ADAM and Eve it? Trends Genet 2003; 19(4):169–172.
2. Wills-Karp M, Ewart SL. Time to draw breath: asthma-susceptibility genes are identified. Nat Rev Genet 2004; 5(5):376–387.
3. Silverman EK, Mosley JD, Palmer LJ, et al. Genome-wide linkage analysis of severe, early-onset chronic obstructive pulmonary disease: airflow obstruction and chronic bronchitis phenotypes. Hum Mol Genet 2002; 11(6):623–632.
4. Silverman EK, Palmer LJ, Mosley JD, et al. Genomewide linkage analysis of quantitative spirometric phenotypes in severe early-onset chronic obstructive pulmonary disease. Am J Hum Genet 2002; 70(5):1229–1239.
5. Wilk JB, DeStefano AL, Arnett DK, et al. A genome-wide scan of pulmonary function measures in the National Heart, Lung, and Blood Institute Family Heart Study. Am J Respir Crit Care Med 2003; 167(11):1528–1533.
6. Becker K, Simon R, Bailey-Wilson J, et al. Clustering of non-major histocompatibility complex susceptibility candidate loci in human autoimmune diseases. Proc Natl Acad Sci USA 1998; 95(17):9979–9984.
7. Cookson W. Genetics and genomics of asthma and allergic diseases. Immunol Rev 2002; 190:195–206.
8. Cookson W, Moffatt M. Making sense of asthma genes. N Engl J Med 2004; 351(17):1794–1796.
9. Hedrick PW. Gametic disequilibrium measures: proceed with caution. Genetics 1987; 117(2):331–341.
10. Devlin B, Risch N. A comparison of linkage disequilibrium measures for fine-scale mapping. Genomics 1995; 29(2):311–322.
11. Risch N, Merikangas K. The future of genetic studies of complex human diseases. Science 1996; 273(5281):1516–1517.
12. Lander ES. The new genomics: global views of biology [see comments]. Science 1996; 274(5287):536–539.
13. Collins FS, Guyer MS, Charkravarti A. Variations on a theme: cataloging human DNA sequence variation. Science 1997; 278(5343):1580–1581.
14. Lai E, Riley J, Purvis I, Roses A. A 4-Mb high-density single nucleotide polymorphism-based map around human APOE. Genomics 1998; 54(1):31–38.
15. Kruglyak L. Prospects for whole-genome linkage disequilibrium mapping of common disease genes. Nat Genet 1999; 22(2):139–144.

16. Collins A, Lonjou C, Morton NE. Genetic epidemiology of single-nucleotide polymorphisms. Proc Natl Acad Sci USA 1999; 96(26):15173–15177.

17. Huttley GA, Smith MW, Carrington M, O'Brien SJ. A scan for linkage disequilibrium across the human genome. Genetics 1999; 152(4):1711–1722.

18. Kidd JR, Pakstis AJ, Zhao H, et al. Haplotypes and linkage disequilibrium at the phenylalanine hydroxylase locus, PAH, in a global representation of populations. Am J Hum Genet 2000; 66(6):1882–1899.

19. Goddard KA, Hopkins PJ, Hall JM, Witte JS. Linkage disequilibrium and allele-frequency distributions for 114 single-nucleotide polymorphisms in five populations. Am J Hum Genet 2000; 66(1):216–234.

20. Jorde LB, Watkins WS, Carlson M, et al. Linkage disequilibrium predicts physical distance in the adenomatous polyposis coli region [see comments]. Am J Hum Genet 1994; 54(5):884–898.

21. Clark AG, Weiss KM, Nickerson DA, et al. Haplotype structure and population genetic inferences from nucleotide-sequence variation in human lipoprotein lipase. Am J Hum Genet 1998; 63(2):595–612.

22. Rieder MJ, Taylor SL, Clark AG, Nickerson DA. Sequence variation in the human angiotensin converting enzyme. Nat Genet 1999; 22(1):59–62.

23. Moffatt MF, Traherne JA, Abecasis GR, Cookson WO. Single nucleotide polymorphism and linkage disequilibrium within the TCR alpha/delta locus. Hum Mol Genet 2000; 9(7):1011–1019.

24. Templeton AR, Clark AG, Weiss KM, Nickerson DA, Boerwinkle E, Sing CF. Recombinational and mutational hotspots within the human lipoprotein lipase gene. Am J Hum Genet 2000; 66(1):69–83.

25. Abecasis GR, Noguchi E, Heinzmann A, et al. Extent and distribution of linkage disequilibrium in three genomic regions. Am J Hum Genet 2001; 68(1): 191–197.

26. Abecasis GR, Cookson WO, Cardon LR. The power to detect linkage disequilibrium with quantitative traits in selected samples. Am J Hum Genet 2001; 68(6):1463–1474.

27. Daly MJ, Rioux JD, Schaffner SF, Hudson TJ, Lander ES. High-resolution haplotype structure in the human genome. Nat Genet 2001; 29(2):229–232.

28. Gabriel SB, Schaffner SF, Nguyen H, et al. The structure of haplotype blocks in the human genome. Science 2002; 296(5576):2225–2229.

29. Muller-Myhsok B, Abel L. Genetic analysis of complex diseases [letter; comment]. Science 1997; 275(5304):1328–1329; discussion 1329–1330.

30. Tu IP, Whittemore AS. Power of association and linkage tests when the disease alleles are unobserved. Am J Hum Genet 1999; 64(2):641–649.

31. Weissenbach J, Gypay G, Dib C, et al. A second generation linkage map of the human genome. Nature 1992; 359:794–801.

32. George VT, Elston RC. Testing the association between polymorphic markers and quantitative traits in pedigrees. Genet Epidemiol 1987; 4(3):193–201.

33. Abecasis GR, Cardon LR, Cookson WO. A general test of association for quantitative traits in nuclear families. Am J Hum Genet 2000; 66(1):279–292.

34. Terwilliger JD, Ott J. A haplotype-based "haplotype relative risk" approach to detecting allelic associations. Hum Hered 1992; 42(6):337–346.

35. Chakravarti A. Population genetics—making sense out of sequence. Nat Genet 1999; 21(suppl 1):56–60.
36. Reich DE, Lander ES. On the allelic spectrum of human disease. Trends Genet 2001; 17(9):502–510.
37. Kruglyak L, Nickerson DA. Variation is the spice of life. Nat Genet 2001; 27(3):234–236.
38. Farrall M, Keavney B, McKenzie C, Delepine M, Matsuda F, Lathrop GM. Fine-mapping of an ancestral recombination breakpoint in DCP1 [letter]. Nat Genet 1999; 23(3):270–271.
39. Morris RW, Kaplan NL. On the advantage of haplotype analysis in the presence of multiple disease susceptibility alleles. Genet Epidemiol 2002; 23(3):221–233.
40. Hugot JP, Chamaillard M, Zouali H, et al. Association of NOD2 leucine-rich repeat variants with susceptibility to Crohn's disease. Nature 2001; 411(6837): 599–603.
41. Ogura Y, Bonen DK, Inohara N, et al. A frameshift mutation in NOD2 associated with susceptibility to Crohn's disease. Nature 2001; 411(6837):603–606.
42. Allen M, Heinzmann A, Noguchi E, et al. Positional cloning of a novel gene influencing asthma from Chromosome 2q14. Nat Genet 2003; 35(3):258–263.
43. Laitinen T, Polvi A, Rydman P, et al. Characterization of a common susceptibility locus for asthma-related traits. Science 2004; 304(5668):300–304.
44. Zhang Y, Leaves NI, Anderson GG, et al. Positional cloning of a quantitative trait locus on chromosome 13q14 that influences immunoglobulin E levels and asthma. Nat Genet 2003; 34(2):181–186.
45. Van Eerdewegh P, Little RD, Dupuis J, et al. Association of the ADAM33 gene with asthma and bronchial hyperresponsiveness. Nature 2002; 418(6896):426–430.
46. Demeo DL, Mariani TJ, Lange C, et al. The SERPINE2 Gene Is Associated with chronic obstructive pulmonary disease. Am J Hum Genet 2006; 78(2): 253–264.
47. Gretarsdottir S, Thorleifsson G, Reynisdottir ST, et al. The gene encoding phosphodiesterase 4D confers risk of ischemic stroke. Nat Genet 2003; 35(2): 131–138.
48. Helms C, Cao L, Krueger JG, et al. A putative RUNX1 binding site variant between SLC9A3R1 and NAT9 is associated with susceptibility to psoriasis. Nat Genet 2003; 35(4):349–356.
49. Altshuler D, Brooks LD, Chakravarti A, Collins FS, Daly MJ, Donnelly P. A haplotype map of the human genome. Nature 2005; 437(7063):1299–1320.
50. Lin S, Chakravarti A, Cutler DJ. Exhaustive allelic transmission disequilibrium tests as a new approach to genome-wide association studies. Nat Genet 2004; 36(11):1181–1188.
51. Peltonen L, McKusick VA. Genomics and medicine. Dissecting human disease in the postgenomic era. Science 2001; 291(5507):1224–1229.
52. Botstein D, Risch N. Discovering genotypes underlying human phenotypes: past successes for mendelian disease, future approaches for complex disease. Nat Genet 2003; 33(suppl):228–237.
53. de Bakker PI, Yelensky R, Pe'er I, Gabriel SB, Daly MJ, Altshuler D. Efficiency and power in genetic association studies. Nat Genet 2005; 37(11):1217–1223.

54. James ES, Harney S, Wordsworth BP, Cookson WO, Davis SJ, Moffatt MF. PDCD1: a tissue-specific susceptibility locus for inherited inflammatory disorders. Genes Immun 2005; 6(5):430–437.

55. Traherne JA, Hill MR, Hysi P, et al. LD mapping of maternally and nonmaternally derived alleles and atopy in FcepsilonRI-beta. Hum Mol Genet 2003; 12(20):2577–2585.

56. Walley AJ, Chavanas S, Moffatt MF, et al. Gene polymorphism in Netherton and common atopic disease. Nat Genet 2001; 29(2):175–178.

57. Hysi P, Kabesch M, Moffatt MF, et al. NOD1 variation, immunoglobulin E and asthma. Hum Mol Genet 2005; 14(7):935–941.

58. Devlin B, Roeder K, Wasserman L. Genomic control, a new approach to genetic-based association studies. Theor Popul Biol 2001; 60(3):155–166.

59. Spielman RS, Ewens WJ. The TDT and other family-based tests for linkage disequilibrium and association. Am J Hum Genet 1996; 59(5):983–989.

60. Moffatt M, Cookson W. The genetics of asthma. Maternal effects in atopic disease. Clin Exp Allergy 1998; 28(Suppl 1):56–61.

61. Bennett S, Todd J. Human type 1 diabetes and the insulin gene: principles of mapping polygenes. Annu Rev Genet 1996; 30:343–370.

62. Warram JH, Krolewski AS, Gottlieb MS, Kahn CR. Differences in risk of insulin-dependent diabetes in offspring of diabetic mothers and diabetic fathers. N Engl J Med 1984; 311(3):149–152.

63. Koumantaki Y, Giziaki E, Linos A, et al. Family history as a risk factor for rheumatoid arthritis: a case-control study. J Rheumatol 1997; 24(8):1522–1526.

64. Burden A, Javed S, Bailey M, Hodgins M, Connor M, Tillman D. Genetics of psoriasis: paternal inheritance and a locus on chromosome 6p [see comments]. J Invest Dermatol 1998; 110(6):958–960.

65. Akolkar PN, Gulwani-Akolkar B, Heresbach D, et al. Differences in risk of Crohn's disease in offspring of mothers and fathers with inflammatory bowel disease. Am J Gastroenterol 1997; 92(12):2241–2244.

66. Vorechovsky I, Webster AD, Plebani A, Hammarstrom L. Genetic linkage of IgA deficiency to the major histocompatibility complex: evidence for allele segregation distortion, parent-of-origin penetrance differences, and the role of anti-IgA antibodies in disease predisposition. Am J Hum Genet 1999; 64(4):1096–1109.

67. Zhang H, Risch N. Mapping quantitative-trait loci in humans by use of extreme concordant sib pairs: selected sampling by parental phenotypes. Am J Hum Genet 1996; 59(4):951–957.

68. Abecasis G, Cardon. L, Cookson W. Selection strategies for disequilibrium mapping of quantitative traits in nuclear families. Am J Hum Genet 1999; 65: A245.

69. Sabatti C, Service S, Freimer N. False discovery rate in linkage and association genome screens for complex disorders. Genetics 2003; 164(2):829–833.

70. Weller JI, Song JZ, Heyen DW, Lewin HA, Ron M. A new approach to the problem of multiple comparisons in the genetic dissection of complex traits. Genetics 1998; 150(4):1699–1706.

71. Eaves IA, Wicker LS, Ghandour G, et al. Combining mouse congenic strains and microarray gene expression analyses to study a complex trait: the NOD model of type 1 diabetes. Genome Res 2002; 12(2):232–243.

72. Schadt EE, Monks SA, Drake TA, et al. Genetics of gene expression surveyed in maize, mouse and man. Nature 2003; 422(6929):297–302.
73. Morley M, Molony CM, Weber TM, et al. Genetic analysis of genome-wide variation in human gene expression. Nature 2004; 430(7001):743–747.
74. Yan H, Yuan W, Velculescu VE, Vogelstein B, Kinzler KW. Allelic variation in human gene expression. Science 2002; 297(5584):1143.
75. Cheung VG, Conlin LK, Weber TM, et al. Natural variation in human gene expression assessed in lymphoblastoid cells. Nat Genet 2003; 33(3):422–425.
76. Monks SA, Leonardson A, Zhu H, et al. Genetic inheritance of gene expression in human cell lines. Am J Hum Genet 2004; 75(6):1094–1105.

13

Association Studies in Asthma

INGRID A. LAING

Telethon Institute for Child Health Research,
Centre for Child Health Research, and
School of Paediatrics and Child Health,
University of Western Australia,
Perth, Western Australia, and
Australian Respiratory Council,
Sydney, South Wales, Australia

PETER N. LE SOUËF

School of Paediatrics and Child Health,
University of Western Australia,
Perth, Western Australia, Australia

I. Introduction

Association studies may be defined as population-based genetic studies that examine whether a particular allele or a series of alleles in one or more genes occur at a significantly higher rate with a disease phenotype than would otherwise be expected. This method yields statistical estimates of whether a polymorphism is a marker, or contributor, to disease susceptibility. A positive association may occur because: (i) the polymorphism is a true causal variant, (ii) of a type I error (an association was detected that occurred by chance), (iii) of inherent study biases, or (iv) of linkage with a causal variant. The inability to detect an association may be because of: (i) the polymorphism is not causal, (ii) type II error (not detecting an association when one exists) usually because of a lack of statistical power, or (iii) lack or weakness of a necessary environmental stimulus (1). Despite the high potential for erroneously identifying a polymorphism as a causal variant, association studies to date have been highly successful in identifying genes involved in the development of asthma. This is likely to be because of the large number of association studies completed due to their relatively low cost and the process by which a candidate gene is selected.

Unselected cohorts and populations of asthmatics that have been genotyped for asthma candidate genes were mostly already recruited, often for another purpose. The time and cost of obtaining consent and DNA for such association studies has been relatively small compared with other methods of identifying susceptibility genes, although this approach may necessitate collecting a suitable control sample with which to compare the asthmatic cases. However, as a consequence, this field has suffered from the copious publication of results of poorly designed and inadequately powered studies, where readily available populations have been used to study the genetic epidemiology of asthma rather than populations specifically recruited to test candidate genes.

Despite these potential limitations, the very large number of association studies has enabled the repeated assessment of some candidates in many different populations with a wide variety of environmental exposures and ethnic backgrounds engendering rapid development of the field. This is particularly true for some of the candidate genes that were among the first to be described and have therefore provided sufficient time for many different studies to be performed. For example, IL4 C-589T was first reported in 1995 and over 10 publications have reported positive associations between this polymorphism and asthma-related phenotypes in cohorts from at least seven different countries (2,3). IL13 polymorphisms were first described in 1999 and more than 10 publications from at least eight different countries have reported positive associations with these genetic variations (2,3). CD14 C-159T was also first reported in 1999, and similar numbers of studies as for IL13 have found positive associations (2,3).

Interestingly, there does appear to be an association between year of first report of a candidate gene and the number of positive associations reported, particularly for those with over 10 positive reports (3). Whether this is because the earliest candidate genes reported were both the most obvious and the most important, or that there has simply been more time for studies to have been completed and reported is unclear. If the latter is true, a very large number of genetic variations that are causally related to the development of asthma may eventually be confirmed.

Alternatively, given that there is no way of knowing how many negative studies go unreported, the possibility also exists that an earlier discovery date could allow more time for chance associations to be reported. Hence, although some authorities have stated that replication of association findings in six or more separate studies would allow a gene to be considered as a "true susceptibility gene" (3), we would suggest a somewhat more cautious approach and the inclusion of the stringent criteria as outlined below, related to establishment of an asthma gene, before considering such a conclusion.

II. Selection of an Asthma Candidate Gene

The process of selecting a candidate also facilitates the chances of identifying an asthma gene. All available data on the potential of that gene/protein to be involved in the pathogenesis of asthma is utilized. Preference is given to those with a high likelihood of being involved in the development of asthma, increasing the probability of identifying positive associations. Candidate genes are most often selected using a number of criteria (4,5) including:

1. The gene structure, sequence, and its product have been at least partially characterized.
2. The gene is located in a chromosomal region previously linked to asthma/related phenotype or identified by positional cloning.
3. The function of the gene product has a biologically plausible role in the pathogenesis of asthma.
4. Differences in levels of gene product (mRNA or protein) have been found in the circulation, bronchoalveolar lavage fluid (BALF), or tissues/cells of asthmatic compared with healthy subjects.
5. The tissue-specific expression profile of the gene is consistent with it being involved in the pathogenesis of asthma.

Once a candidate gene is selected, the polymorphisms investigated in an association study may be (i) those identified by screening a candidate gene for novel mutations or (ii) those previously identified.

III. Identification of Polymorphisms

Candidate gene screening aims to identify novel sequence variants that functionally or quantitatively alter the gene product and thus contribute to the development of asthma. Several methodologies have been used to detect polymorphisms in genes of interest, including DNA sequencing, DNA mis-match and enzyme cleavage, denaturing high performance liquid chromatography, single stranded conformational polymorphism analysis, and heteroduplex analysis. The need for candidate gene screening has diminished since the completion of the human genome project and the establishment of public access databases of polymorphisms. The National Centre for Biotechnology Information has established the single nucleotide polymorphism database (dbSNP) database for both single base nucleotide substitutions and short deletion and insertion polymorphisms (6). The human data in dbSNP comprises records from the single nucleotide polymorphism (SNP) Consortium, variations mined from genome sequence as part of the human genome project and individual laboratory contributions of variations in specific genes, mRNAs, ESTs, or genomic regions. The unique reference number for each polymorphism on this database also provides an invaluable method for cross-referencing genes and/or polymorphisms that have been assigned multiple names or loci in the literature. Unfortunately, because of the sheer volume of recorded polymorphisms, many of the polymorphisms described on the database have not been verified in an independent sample and the database is likely to contain many mistakes. Furthermore, little information is available on variations unique to, or the polymorphism frequencies within different ethnic groups. These limitations are at least partly addressed by data available on other public access databases such as the Innate Immunity Program for Genomic Applications website (7) and published articles. Nevertheless, it is still common practice to DNA sequence the regions of interest in each association study candidate gene to determine or verify genotypes and also identify any sequence variations other than the polymorphisms being studied.

IV. Selection of Polymorphisms for Association Studies

In an association study of a novel asthma candidate gene, all of the poly-morphisms identified may be genotyped in a population to establish their frequency, haplotype arrangement, and association with disease. However, in an association study of a known candidate gene, the polymorphisms selected for genotyping should have the potential to, or have been shown to, alter the gene or protein function and thereby alter protein expression levels or structure. Promoter- and gene-coding regions, exon–intron bound-aries, and sequences conserved between species are those regions most likely to contain polymorphisms that affect gene or protein function. The polymorphisms characterising a haplotype that has previously been associated with disease should also be assessed. Furthermore, the poly-morphisms should ideally be sufficiently prevalent to: (i) detect statistically significant differences in affected and unaffected subjects; (ii) be biologi-cally relevant and important in the general disease process; and (iii) be of general relevance to diagnosed cases of asthma (4,5).

V. Population Selection/Study Design

Several association study designs have been used to identify genes that pre-dispose subjects to developing asthma. Case control, family/triplet, selected or unselected prospective cohorts and cross sectional and longitudinal populations have been recruited for study. Each has their advantages and limitations. Case control studies assume that there is no bias in the enrol-ment and assessment of asthmatic subjects compared with the control subjects. In analyses of affected families or triplets (both parents and a child), it was assumed that the subjects are all genetically related, the asthma is caused by inheritance of the same set of alleles, and that the phenotype assessments are not influenced by the age of each subject. In such studies, nonpaternity, which is common in some communities, needs to be detected to avoid loss of power. Both selected and unselected prospective cohorts require a constant, unbiased level of participation from subjects. The results of association studies of unselected cohorts should reflect those in the wider community from which they are drawn. Cross-sectional studies assess subjects at a single time point and lose a great deal of power because of the very high degree of within subject variability over time. Populations followed longitudinally usually suffer from a loss of subjects with increasing numbers of follow-up visits and are likely to retain a disproportionate number of affected subjects over time (8).

A. Population Bias

Recruiting a population without introducing bias is extremely difficult, and even a small degree of population stratification has been shown to significantly skew the results found in case control populations (9). Many factors involved in the recruitment, enrolment, and assessment of subjects in a population may affect the results of association studies. These can include the age of the population, definitions of outcome measures, study design, and uniformity of the environmental exposures (10).

Participation of subjects in research studies is voluntary and thus, subject self selection can result in an unselected population with a disproportionate number of affected participants entering the study (11) and, as noted above, an even greater number of affected subjects may remain in the study. Selection of cases and controls must be done with care to minimise population stratification introduced by the use of different recruitment and phenotype assessment methods (12,13).

Phenotype assessment may also introduce bias or errors. Asthmatics and their parents are more likely to recognise and report symptoms, once diagnosed with asthma (14). Reporting of qualitative phenotypes relies on the recall of parents and/or subjects, as well as equivalent diagnosis of different physicians (15). Furthermore, bias in the estimated influence of maternal/paternal effects can be introduced if only one parent provides responses to respiratory and environmental history questionnaires on behalf of both parents. The interviewed parent's knowledge of their own current status and life-long history of respiratory problems will inevitably be much more accurate than their knowledge or recollection of this information for their absent partner. This may be the reason for results showing that maternal inheritance is more important than paternal inheritance for susceptibility to disease (16). Alternatively, there may indeed be a greater maternal influence, as the in utero environment may have a role in determining the outcome of the offspring. Data collection can also become distorted if the phenotype assessments are not made contemporaneously by the same investigators. Associations may be identified in isolated or founder populations that may be related to the altered allele frequencies caused by founder effect and random drift (13) rather than associations reflecting a potentially causative relationship.

The introduction of biases can be minimized with careful attention to study design, planning of the recruitment/assessment methods, and appropriate analysis of the results (17). Identifying whether the genotype of interest is in Hardy–Weinberg equilibrium for the population being studied provides a further method of detecting population bias (18). Hardy–Weinberg equilibrium states that population genotype frequencies remain constant from generation to generation where mating is random and mutation, selection, immigration, and emigration do not occur. Thus, the genotype distribution for a particular polymorphism in a population occurs in a mathematically predictable proportion. A population with genotype frequencies that differ from those expected may be biased or affected by one of the factors described, such as natural selection.

VI. Methods Used to Identify New Asthma Candidate Genes

Association studies may be done on newly characterized genes and/or proteins, which have been identified using several methods. Serial analysis of gene expression, high-density oligonucleotide microarrays, and cDNA microarrays are the three methods of mass detection of gene expression that have been utilized for the identification of candidate genes in human disease (19). Differential gene mRNA expression studies employing either DNA microarray technology or polymerase chain reaction (PCR)-based cDNA subtraction (20) have been used. Differential protein studies employ proteomic technology to discover new genes (21). Differential expression methods compare expression levels from either human or animal samples that were affected/unaffected or pre/post-challenge.

New candidate genes may be identified through genome linkage analysis and positional cloning. Linkage analysis of asthma in many populations, using both qualitative and quantitative traits as outcome measures, has identified a large number of regions of the human chromosome linked to disease. Positional cloning or fine mapping techniques have been used to refine these results so that both candidate and novel genes located within the chromosomal region may be targeted for association analysis (21).

VII. Environmental Exposures

The interaction of environmental factors with genetic predisposition confers susceptibility to asthma. Appropriate assessment of breast feeding in infancy, diet, timing and load of allergen exposure, pollutants, and infections is required in the populations to adequately determine their involvement. Investigation of the quantity and timing of environmental exposures may be able to delineate the interaction of these factors with the polymorphisms. Adjustment for environmental influences can reveal a genetic predisposition, as seen in the recent genome screen study of a Dutch cohort in which linkage between a region on chromosome 5q was only revealed when the population consisting of the offspring of smokers was segregated and examined separately (22). The level of exposure to an environmental factor may also affect outcome, with opposite results being found for high versus low exposure. For example, IgE levels were associated with one homozygous CD14 genotype in children with high levels of endotoxin exposure or exposure to stable animals, but an association with the other homozygous genotype was found in children with exposure to pets and therefore, presumably, low levels of endotoxin exposure (23). On the contrary, theoretically, if a potent environmental exposure is in a very high dose, all individuals could be affected regardless of their level of genetic susceptibility to that exposure. Thus, those who have a low genetic susceptibility to the exposure would produce the same phenotype and be indistinguishable from those with a high genetic susceptibility to that exposure.

VIII. Association Study Limitations

There are several limitations that should be carefully considered of association studies. The polymorphism analyzed may be falsely associated with the disease because of introduced bias, random error, and confounders (13).

A. Linkage Disequilibrium

Linkage disequilibrium is the nonrandom distribution of alleles at different loci in haplotypes. With respect to disease, linkage disequilibrium is considered to be present when a marker allele is co-inherited with a disease more often than would usually occur randomly with recombination. As such, multiple markers may be inherited together and may co-segregate with disease, although only one may alter gene function and contribute to disease. An association of one polymorphism with asthma does not preclude the possibility that another linked polymorphism is the causative locus.

B. Multiple Testing/Sample Size

The power to detect an association in a population is limited by the number of subjects assessed, polymorphisms analyzed, and the statistical tests completed.

The size of populations in asthma genetic epidemiology studies is a key factor in establishing a particular variant as contributing to the asthma diathesis. Smaller populations increase type II errors (not identifying a significant difference between groups when one exists) and result in wider confidence intervals. The number of subjects available for analysis in each population may also be limited by missing phenotype or genotype data. Experts in the field have suggested that the minimum number of subjects needed for recessive models, in asthma association studies of single polymorphisms, should be at least 1000 subjects, unless the polymorphism is very common (24,25). Studies that used meta analysis of pooled data were done to investigate effects in a larger number of subjects: "these problems of replication are unlikely to be resolved until results are pooled and the true significance of a positive linkage result can be evaluated in a larger data set" (26). This approach has been endorsed by more recent comment (27). However, there is a problem with the concept that if an effect is not seen in a small population, then a larger population should be used. This assumes that the environmental effect and ethnicity mix in a larger population or pooled data will be reasonably uniform. Yet, the larger the population, the greater the likelihood that it will be recruited from a wider range of environments, some of which may lack critical environmental factors. Furthermore, this method may pool data from smaller populations selected using self-identified ethnicity, but may inadvertently bias the results because these populations have very different proportions of genetic admixture.

To assist in evaluating these issues, each population should also be analyzed separately before meta analysis, although results may not be helpful because of the limited numbers of subjects. For these reasons, meta analyses in asthma genetics need very careful interpretation. Recruiting large numbers of subjects is expensive, and if the subjects are drawn from one particular local environment, the results may still be of limited value, as the findings may only be relevant for that population group and that location and may not be generalisable. Therefore, replicating association results in numerous smaller studies may be more cost effective than using a limited number of very large studies.

C. Confounders

Age, gender, and ethnicity are potential confounders of asthma studies. Several studies have reported on asthma phenotypes in early life and have identified differences in the nature and causes of asthma that begin in early childhood compared with early- to mid-adult onset (28,29). In the subset of infants with lower lung function, those with a parental history of atopy have the greatest likelihood of having a persistent reduction in lung function and of developing asthma by the age of six years (30). The risk of asthma in early life is thought to be influenced by environmental factors such as tobacco smoke exposure, duration of breastfeeding (31–33), timing, number and type of respiratory infections (34–36), and allergen exposure. Risk factors for persistent asthma and late onset asthma in adulthood include atopy (37), airway responsiveness, personal tobacco smoking, occupational exposure to specific irritants or allergens (solvents, latex, and bakers flour), and environmental pollutants (diesel, wood smoke, gas fuels, and smog) (38–40). Epidemiological studies suggest that 10% to 25% of adult asthma is work related and is because of mixed exposures to low molecular weight chemicals and high molecular weight antigens (41). An age-specific association between the CD14 C-159T polymorphism and atopy in mid-childhood, but not in early adulthood, has been found in an Australian unselected longitudinal population (42).

Gender differences in the prevalence of asthma have been previously reported (43,44). From birth to age six, more boys than girls develop asthma (45). During adolescence, the gender prevalence of asthma equalizes (46,47) and becomes more predominant in women in early adulthood (48). These differences may be partly physiological as male infants have smaller, size-corrected airways (49) and a higher decrement to forced expiratory flows as a result of passive tobacco smoke exposure (50). Alterations to the gender-specific pattern of asthma prevalence may be because of hormonal changes in adolescence influencing airway inflammation (51). Furthermore, an increase in interleukin 10 (IL10) and a reduction in interferon gamma (IFNγ) during the peri-menstrual cycle of women not taking an oral contraceptive (52) may contribute to an atopic profile. There has been some suggestion that in later life, there may be gender differences in physician diagnosis and treatment for a similar profile of symptoms (53).

Relatedness of study subjects is a particular issue when a study population is recruited from a small and/or isolated community. Adjustments for genetic admixture or familial relationships are possible but rely on adequate recall of the participants or quantitative molecular techniques. Often it is not appropriate to attempt such a statistical adjustment because of the complexities and inherent errors involved. Furthermore, correction for familial relationships may be inappropriate if the members of a small population are all related within three generations. A further consideration that will always be of concern is that genetic association studies may identify associations that are only relevant to that ethnic group.

D. Methodological Limitations

Errors may be introduced through the molecular techniques utilized. Suboptimal DNA extraction could result in inadequate PCR amplification of samples, leading to missing data. Amplification by PCR may introduce changes to the sequence studied, and inaccuracies in the methodology used to genotype populations and observer error may also lead to missing data or mis-identification of genotypes.

Inclusion of controls in each experiment, repeat experiments, and DNA sequencing a random sample of subjects for each gene region screened or for each genotype can be used to confirm the results obtained and to minimize the occurrence of errors. DNA sequencing is the "gold standard" for detecting SNPs, but relies on adequate amplification of template DNA by PCR.

IX. Association Study Interpretation

In the early years of the study of asthma genetics, it was suggested that failure to replicate results of associations previously identified was because of type I statistical errors made in the initial study (26,54). However, a true association may also be missed because of lack of the appropriate environmental factor or interactions with other genotypes not found in other populations. An important point is that the presence of an association between a polymorphism and an asthma-related phenotype in one population and the absence of that relationship in another population do not necessarily mean that either finding is incorrect. There are many possible reasons that such a discrepancy could be found including:

- Absence of, or less of, a critical environmental influence in one of the populations.
- Presence of an additional environmental factor in one of the populations that counteracts the effect of an environmental factor present in both populations.
- A powerful environmental influence in one of the populations that leads to the presentation of a phenotype in all subjects, irrespective of their genetic susceptibility.
- Presence of modifier genes that negate the effect of the polymorphism in one of the populations.
- Presence of an as yet unidentified polymorphism in the same gene that counteracts the effect of the polymorphism being examined.

These possibilities are mostly theoretical and would be very difficult to study, as the critical environmental factors that contribute to asthma are still largely unknown.

X. How to Establish an Asthma Gene

Association studies have been extremely successful in identifying genes that are potentially involved in the development of asthma. There are now over 100 genes that have been associated with the asthma diathesis. However, relatively few genes have demonstrated the level of evidence required to define them as established asthma genes. For reasonable substantiation, an asthma gene should fulfill the following criteria. A particular allele or haplotype should have been associated with (i) asthma phenotypic outcomes in

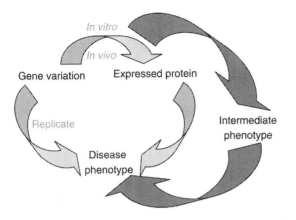

Figure 1 Substantiating an asthma gene.

more than one population of similar age, regardless of polymorphism frequency, (ii) altered protein levels or shown to alter protein function in vivo and (iii) in vitro, (iv) an intermediate phenotype, such as cellular cytokine responses, and (iv) the alteration to protein level or function is associated with susceptibility to the asthma phenotype (Fig. 1).

Several strategies may be used to minimize the number of statistical tests used and thus, type I errors (detecting an association that occurred by chance). One strategy, is to use one population for initial genotype/phenotype association studies testing multiple outcomes, and use a second population with a specific set of hypotheses based on the results of the first association study. However, the difficulty and expense of adopting this strategy often precludes its use. Recruiting two contemporaneous populations or dividing one population into two also limits the power to detect associations (10). Another strategy is to correct for multiple testing by using a more conservative p value such as using the Bonferroni method. Yet, asthma is a disease with multigenic components that are likely to have low penetrance, and reducing the level of significance increases the rate of type II errors (failing to detect an association). Asthma genotype/phenotype association studies most often use "constructive" replication (13) by evaluating similar hypotheses in populations independently recruited worldwide. Although for genes of small or moderate effect, geographically dispersed populations may not replicate the findings because of differences in ethnicity and environmental exposures. In all studies, all statistical tests completed should be reported regardless of significance to account for type I errors by allowing appropriate interpretation of results (55). A hypothesis can also be addressed a priori, so that there is no need for multiple statistical testing.

XI. Asthma Associations Reported

Over the last few years, several comprehensive reviews of the literature on asthma association studies have been published. The number of genes reported to be related to asthma continues to increase, now over 100 (3); there are now many hundreds of associations study references in asthma genetics. Of the genes reported, fewer have had positive associations reported in more than one study (3). Table 1 lists those genes with sequence variations that have been associated with asthma or asthma quantitative traits in more than one study (Table 1). The proportion of studies that detected an association compared with the total number reported and the variety of populations examined was included to provide some indication of the extent to which a gene had been investigated. However, the total number of studies reported is not likely to represent the total number completed, as many studies that did not detect an association may not have been published. Furthermore, no judgment was made regarding the study design or the power to detect association.

The exponential increase in information on asthma genetics (3,67,68) creates difficulties in providing an overview or summary of the topic. Hence, in the following summary, only selected genes have been mentioned to demonstrate examples of important genes and to highlight areas of potential future interest. Emphasis has been given to genes that are either well established as asthma candidate genes or are of particular interest because of their position on an inflammatory or immunological pathway or their role in mechanisms related to asthma.

A. Genes Involved in Th1/Th2 Responses and Innate Immunity

The most important group of genes involved in the mechanisms of airway inflammation in asthma are those that contribute to Th1 and Th2 lymphocyte responses and innate immunity. This group contains several of the genes that have the highest number of reported replication studies as well as the strongest supporting data that fulfill the candidate selection criteria noted above.

CD14

There is more evidence for CD14 having a role in asthma genetics than for almost any other gene. CD14 plays a critical role by being both a major receptor for lipopolysaccharide (LPS) and for determining Th1/Th2 differentiation (69). The most important SNP is the promoter polymorphism C-159T (69). This has been associated with total IgE levels in subjects with a positive skin prick test (SPT) (69,70) or specific IgE levels (71), circulating CD14 levels (69,71,72), total IgE levels in nonatopic subjects (73),

(Text continues on page 256.)

Table 1 Genes with Sequence Variations Associated with Asthma-Related Phenotype in More Than One Study

Gene[a]	Chromosomal position	Individual sequence variants analyzed	Haplotypes analyzed	Positive/total number of association studies	Populations studied[b]
GSTM1	1p13	✓		6/10	E, R, EA, I, B, T, Tw, G
IL10	1q32	✓	✓	8/12	EA, J, C, Ic, Hutt, Ind, Tw, K, G, F
ACP1	2p25	✓		4/4	It, B, Ch
IL1A	2q13	✓	✓	4/5	F, K
IL1B	2q13	✓	✓	3/8	F, Tw, G, K, B
IL1RN	2q13	✓	✓	5/7	J, Tw, F, G
DPP10	2q14	✓	✓	3/3	A, B, G
CTLA4	2q33	✓		7/9	G, J, K, Hutt, Tw, D, E
IL5RA	3p26	✓		2/3	Hutt, K
CCR5	3p21	✓		4/9	B, A, H, Can, En, G, Ind
TLR10	4p14	✓		2/2	EA
TLR6	4p13	✓		2/2	AA, G
TLR2	4q31	✓		2/3	Au/G, G, J
CSF2	5q23	✓		4/5	S, Ic, Can, Hutt, B
IL5	5q23	✓		2/2	J, K
IL13	5q23	✓		18/21	D, Ic, J, Sc, AA, G, EA, B, Hutt, Ch, CR, C
IL4	5q23	✓	✓	19/34	EA, A, B, J, C, Hutt, Can, Kuw, Ic, G, Ch, Tw, Ind, P, K, AA, His, Tun, Sp
CD14	5q31	✓		16/24	EA, A, B, J, Hutt, D, Ic, SG, G, C Cz, Ch, A, F, Ind, Bb, M, PR, EA, Tw
SPINK5	5q32	✓		5/7	B, J, G, D

(Continued)

Table 1 Genes with Sequence Variations Associated with Asthma-Related Phenotype in More Than One Study (*Continued*)

Gene[a]	Chromosomal position	Individual sequence variants analyzed	Haplotypes analyzed	Positive/total number of association studies	Populations studied[b]
ADRB2	5q32–34	✓	✓	33/44	EA, B, G, J, NZ, Hutt, K, Ic, Ch (56,57), PR, M, Can, A, Is, Ind, It, C
IL12B	5q31–33	✓	✓	5/6	A, EA, J (58)
HAVCR1 (TIM1)	5q33	✓	✓	4/5	K, USm, AA, J
HAVCR2 (TIM3)	5q33	✓	✓	3/3	K, EA, AA
LTC4S	5q35	✓	✓	7/16	J, P, EA (59), Ic, C, Hutt, B, A, Sp, K (59,60), AA
EDN1	6p24	✓		2/4	C, Cz, B, J
HLAG	6p22	✓		3/3	C, Hutt, D
LTA	6p21	✓		9/19	A, B, It, Mal, Ch, Sp, Cz, SG, C, USm, EA, J, Tw
TNFA	6p21	✓	✓	17/30	A, It, C, B, Mal, Ch, Can, Sp, SA, USm, Tw, Cz, EA, G, K, Hutt, J, Ind (61)
HLA-DRB1	6p21	✓		34/40	C, Au, Sp, B, J, It, Is, Fr, G, Hutt, AA, K, Tw, SG, P, T, AbA, Gr
HLA-DQA1	6p21	✓		4/6	B, Fr, G, Hutt, AA, Ch
HLA-DQB1	6p21	✓		12/18	J, Sp, Fr, B, G, C, Hutt, AA, Tw, T, EA, Ch, Au, Gr
TAP1	6p21	✓		2/4	Tun, Cz, J, Tw
HLA-DPB1	6p21	✓		5/9	G, B, Fr, C, Tw, K
HLA	6p21		✓	7/7	A, V, SG, P, Tw, F, K

Gene	Location			Ratio	Populations
PAFAH	6p12		✓	4/5	J, G, B
IFNGR1	6q23		✓	2/4	B, J
NOD1 (CARD4)	7p15	✓	✓	4/4	G, A, B
GPRA	7p14	✓	✓	5/8	F, Can, G, E, Sw, K, C
CCL26 (Eotaxin 3)	7q11	✓	✓	2/3	K
CCL24 (Eotaxin 2)	7q11	✓	✓	3/3	K
CFTR	7q31	✓	✓	4/9	EA, B, Da, It, F, Ic, Sp, Gr
NOS3	7q36		✓	4/8	K, Cz, C, AA, T, B, Hutt, Ch
DEFB1	8p23	✓	✓	2/2	EA
NAT2	8p22		✓	5/6	P, T, R, F, Fr
TLR4	9q33	✓	✓	2/4	EA, Can, C, G, F
C5	9q33	✓	✓	2/2	Hutt, J
ALOX5	10q11	✓	✓	4/6	EA (59), B, C, K
FCER1B	11q12	✓	✓	18/30	B, WSA, BSA, FC, Ic, A, KA, J, S, Can, Ch, Mal, Ind, P, Sp, Sw, SG
CRTH2	11q12		✓	2/2	AA, Ch
CCI6	11q12		✓	7/12	A, B, J, D, Ic, C, G, I, Da, Ind
GSTP1	11q13	✓	✓	9/13	E, Ic, It, EA, R, T, B, Tw, G, K (62)
ILI8	11q23	✓	✓	5/7	G, J, K, S (63), Sing Ch, Mal, Ind (63,64)
AICDA	12p13	✓	✓	2/4	J, Ch, Sp
VDR	12q13	✓	✓	4/5	Can, EA, G
STAT6	12q13	✓	✓	10/13	J, B, G, Ind, C, F
IFNG	12q15	✓	✓	3/4	Hutt, J, Ind
NOS1	12q24	✓	✓	7/8	C, B, J, Hutt, A, Cz, Ch
CYSLTR2	13q14	✓	✓	4/6	TdC, C, AA, Da/EA, Int, J

(Continued)

Table 1 Genes with Sequence Variations Associated with Asthma-Related Phenotype in More Than One Study (*Continued*)

Gene[a]	Chromosomal position	Individual sequence variants analyzed	Haplotypes analyzed	Positive/total number of association studies	Populations studied[b]
PHF11	13q14	✓	✓	4/4	A, B, E
TCRA/D	14q11	✓		2/2	A, SG
CMA1	14q11	✓	✓	6/8	J, It, B, G, Ind
PTGDR	14q22	✓	✓	2/3	J, EA, AA
IL4RA	16p12	✓	✓	24/38	J, Sing, Da, M, It, K, G, D, Haw, EA, Mal, Can, B, Ch, Sp, F, Hutt, Sw
CARD15	16q12	✓	✓	4/4	G
NOS2A	17q11	✓		2/3	J, B, Hutt
CCL11 (*Eotaxin*)	17q12	✓		4/7	EA, J, Ic, K, Hutt
CCL5 (*RANTES*)	17q12	✓	✓	7/10	G, C, H, J, Ch, B, AA, K
CRHR1	17q21	✓	✓	3/3	C
ITGB3	17q21	✓	✓	3/3	Hutt, C, AA
TBX21 (*T-bet*)	17q21	✓	✓	4/6	EA, K, J, F, C
ACE	17q23	✓		4/13	Fr, Cz, J, B, K, C, SA, T
TBXA2R	19p13	✓	✓	6/6	J, K
C3	19p13	✓	✓	3/3	Hutt, J, AC (65)
TGFB1	19q13	✓	✓	8/11	EA, B, Cz, Ic, G, Ind, Ch (66)
ADAM33	20p13	✓	✓	11/13	C, EA, AA, His, D, M, PR, G, J, K, B

MIF	22q11		✓		2/2	J
GSTT1	22q11	✓	✓		4/6	E, R, I, T, G

[a] GSTM1, glutathione S-transferase M1; IL10, interleukin 10; ACP1, acid phosphatase 1; IL1A/B, interleukin 1 A/B; IL1RN, interleukin 1 receptor antagonist; DPP10, dipeptidyl peptidase; CTLA4, cytotoxic T lymphocyte-antigen 4; IL5RA, interleukin 5 receptor alpha; CCR5, chemokine receptor 5; TLR10/6/2, toll-like receptor 10/6/2; CSF2, colony stimulating factor 2; IL5/13/4, interleukin 5/13/4; CD14, monocyte differentiation antigen 14; SPINK5, serine protease inhibitor, Kazal-type, 5; ADRB2, beta 2 adrenergic receptor; IL12B, interleukin 12B; HAVCR1/2, hepatitis A virus cellular receptor 1/2; TIM1/3, T cell immunoglobulin and mucin 1/3; LTC4S, leukotriene C4 synthase; EDN1, endothelin 1; HLA, human leukocyte antigen; LTA, lymphotoxin-alpha; TNFA, tumour necrosis factor alpha; TAP1, transporter, ATP-binding cassette 1; PAFAH, platelet activating factor acetylhydrolase; IFNGR1, interferon gamma receptor 1; NOD1/CARD4, caspase recruitment domain-containing protein 4; GPRA, G protein-coupled receptor 154; CCL26/Eotaxin 3, chemokine, CC motive, ligand 26; CCL24/Eotaxin 2, chemokine, CC motive, ligand 24; CFTR, cystic fibrosis transmembrane conductance regulator; NOS3, nitric oxide synthase 3; DEFB1, defensin beta 1; NAT2, N-acetyl transferase 2; TLR4, toll-like receptor 4; C5, complement factor 5; ALOX5, arachidonate 5-lipoxygenase; FCER1B, high affinity IgE receptor beta chain; CRTH2, G protein-coupled receptor 44; CC16, vita-Clara cell specific 16kD protein; GSTP1, glutathione S-transferase P1; IL18, interleukin 18; AICDA, activation-induced cytidine deaminase; VDR, vitamin D receptor; STAT6, signal transducer and activator of transcription 6; IFNG, interferon gamma; NOS1, nitric oxide synthase; CYSLTR2, cysteinyl leukotriene receptor 2; PHF11, PHD finger protein 11; TCRA/D, T cell antigen receptor alpha/delta; CMA1, mast cell chymase 1; PTGDR, prostaglandin D2 receptor; IL4RA, interleukin 4 receptor alpha chain; CARD15, caspase recruitment domain-containing protein 15; NOS2A, nitric oxide synthase 2A; CCL11/Eotaxin, chemokine, CC motif, ligand 11; CCL5/RANTES, chemokine, CC motif, ligand 5; ITGB3, integrin beta 3; TBX21/T-bet, T-box 21; ACE, angiotensin 1-converting enzyme; TBXA2R, thromboxane A2 receptor; C3, complement factor 3; TGFB1, transforming growth factor beta 1; ADAM33, a disintegrin and metalloproteinase domain 33; MIF, macrophage migration inhibitory factor 1; GSTT1, glutathione S-transferase T1.

[b] A—Australian, AA—African American, AbA—Aboriginal Australian, AC—African Caribbean, Au—Austrian, B—British, Bb—Barbados, BSA—Black South African, C—Caucasian, Can—Canadian, Ch—Chinese, CR—Costa Rican, Cz—Czech, D—Dutch, Da—Danish, E—European (includes Northern European, Western European), EA—European American (includes American, United States of America, US white, Northern American), En—English, F—Finnish, FC—French Canadian, Fr—French, G—German, Gr—Greek, H—Hawaiian, Haw—Hawaiian, His—Hispanic, Hutt—Hutterites, I—Iranian, Ic—Icelandic, Ind—Indian (includes Northern Indians), Int—International, Is—Israelian, It—Italian, J—Japanese, K—Korean, KA—Kuwaiti Arabs, Kuw—Kuwaiti, M—Mexican, Mal—Malays, NZ—New Zealand, P—Polish, PR—Puerto Rican, R—Russian, S—Swiss, SA—South Asian, Sc—Scandinavian, SG—Spanish Gypsies, Sing—Singapore, Sp—Spanish, Sw—Swedish, T—Turkish, TdC—Tristan de Cuhna, Tun—Tunisian, Tw—Taiwanese, USm—US mixed, V—Venezuelan, WSA—White South African.

Source: Adapted and updated with permission from Ober and Hoffjan, 2006 (Ref. 3).

severity of atopy, allergic symptoms (70), positive SPT to moulds, particularly in atopic subjects with asthma or rhinitis (74), and atopic asthma (75) in ethnically diverse populations. The gene for CD14 is also located in the chromosomal region 5q31 to 33. Functional studies have confirmed that the T allele enhances transcription compared with the C allele (76). Four other promoter SNPs have been reported and these are in tight linkage disequilibrium (77). Haplotypes of these polymorphisms show even more significant associations with total IgE compared with the individual genotypes (77). In a recent study, serum CD14 levels have been shown to have allele-specific increases in levels during viral-related acute asthma attacks in children (78) with corresponding associations in asthma severity.

Interleukin 4

The gene for IL4 was one of the first genes being investigated in asthma genetics and reported in 1995 (79), and there is evidence to support its being a true asthma susceptibility gene. IL4 is a key Th2 cytokine, and it has a central role in the production of IgE (80). A promoter polymorphism (C-589T) was the first polymorphism that was reported and there have been over 10 publications since then that have also described positive associations with asthma phenotypic features (3). These associations have included clinical evidence of asthma and asthma severity (81–83), lung function (84), atopy (85), and airway responsiveness in asthmatics (86). The gene also fulfills all of the asthma candidate gene selection criteria outlined above. For example, the gene is located in the 5q31 to 33 chromosomal region that has been linked in several populations to atopy and asthma and functional studies have shown altered transcription with the -589 allele (79).

Interleukin 4 Receptor

The gene for IL4R has strong supporting evidence for a causal role in asthma. The IL4 receptor has an alpha and a gamma chain (87). The close relationship between IL4 and IL13 is demonstrated by the observation that the alpha chain binds both IL4 and IL13 (87). Eight of the 13 polymorphisms in IL4R change the amino acid produced, and three of those eight have also been shown to affect gene function (88). Of these, Ile50Val has been most studied, and it has been associated with various asthma phenotypes including IgE levels and clinical evidence of asthma (86,89).

Interleukin 13

IL13 is another important Th2 cytokine and has a role in IgE isotype switching (90). The gene has also been investigated for a number of years, and its most studied SNP is the promoter polymorphism C-1111T, but 10 other SNPs have been identified and three of these have been examined for asthma phenotype associations (91). The T allele of C-1111T has been associated with asthma and related phenotypes (91–93). Arg130Gln and a 3'UTR polymorphism have also been associated with asthma and IgE related phenotypes (91,94–97). Given that the alpha chain of IL4R binds both IL4 and IL13, the observed interactions between genotypes for IL4R, IL4, and IL13 are not unexpected. Haplotypes that include variations in two of these three genes produced stronger associations between genotype and atopic outcomes than were obtained by any of the component genotypes on their own (98).

Interleukin 10

Interleukin 10 is considered a regulatory cytokine due to its role in limiting or terminating inflammatory responses (99). The gene for IL10 contains several polymorphisms, three of which are in the promoter and these form various haplotypes that are associated with serum IL10 levels (100). Haplotypes associated with low IL10 levels are also associated with severe asthma (101). IL10 secretion may have a particularly important role in viral-induced asthma, as its secretion has been shown to be increased in subjects with acute asthma associated with rhinovirus infection (102).

Interleukin 12B

The gene for interleukin 12B (IL12B) is a good example of a gene that is likely to be an excellent candidate gene for asthma by virtue of its known role in the immune system, but for which there are limited data. The reason why data are limited is most probably because of the relatively recent publication date of papers describing polymorphisms in IL12. IL12 has an important role in enhancing Th1 immune responses and suppressing Th2 deviation (103). The IL12B gene encodes the p40 subunit of IL12 (104) and a promoter polymorphism has been associated with asthma severity (105) and total IgE levels (106).

Interferon Gamma

IFNγ is one of the most important Th1 cytokines, as it enhances Th1 cell differentiation and suppresses Th2 deviation, as well as directly suppressing IgE synthesis (107). IFNγ itself has no important polymorphisms in either its promoter or its exons, but intronic variations have been noted and these have been associated with various asthma-related phenotypes and with altered function in vitro and possibly an increase in susceptibility to tuberculosis (108–110).

Interferon Gamma Receptor 1

The gene for Interferon gamma receptor (IFNγR1) has several polymorphisms of which several have been reported as showing associations with asthma. A promoter polymorphism has been shown to affect gene function (111) and an intronic polymorphism has been associated with altered total serum IgE levels (112).

Toll-Like Receptor Genes

Genes for the Toll-like receptor (TLRs) are likely to be important in asthma genetics by virtue of the critical role played by TLRs in immune responses. TLRs are part of the innate immune system's defence against infective pathogens that includes pattern recognition receptors. The number of TLRs continues to increase, but those likely to be important for asthma are TLR2, TLR3, and TLR4. TLR2 recognizes a wide variety of cell membrane components (113), TLR3 is involved in viral recognition (114), and TLR4 is specific for bacterial LPS (115,116). The TLR2 gene has four SNPs that are reasonably common (117). Association data for the -16934 SNP are most interesting, as the T allele was associated with a reduction in the incidence and severity of asthma in the children of farmers (117). Functional studies on another SNP, Arg753Gln, showed differences in responsive to bacterial peptides in vivo (118). The gene for TLR3 contains polymorphisms, but these have not been linked to asthma as yet. However, a potential role for TLR3 is likely because it is a recognition receptor for rhinovirus (114), which is the most common virus associated with acute asthma at all ages (119).

The gene for TLR4 gene have been extensively studied for SNPs (117,120,121). Associations have been reported between Asp299Gly and Thr399Ile and hypo-responsiveness to LPS (115,122), but none of the SNPs have been associated with asthma to date (121).

Transforming Growth Factor Beta 1

Transforming growth factor beta (TGFB1) is a cytokine with several roles, and its levels have been shown to be increased in the bronchoalveolar lavage of asthmatics compared to control subjects (123). C-509T has been shown to be associated with asthma (124,125), asthma severity (124) and elevated total serum IgE levels (126). The -509T allele has been associated with increased TGFB1 levels (127) and with increased activity in functional studies (125).

Interleukin 1 Beta

Interleukin 1 beta (IL1B) is a proinflammatory cytokine and a promoter polymorphism C-511T has been associated with level of lung function in asthmatics (128) and with asthma susceptibility (129). A haplotype containing the C3953T exon 5 polymorphism was associated with atopy (130).

Interleukin 6

Interleukin 6 (IL6) is a pro-inflammatory Th1 cytokine and has an important role in the acute phase response (131). Haplotypes of the IL6 SNPs have been shown to influence IL6 transcription in vitro (132).

B. Genes Involved in the Leukotriene Pathway

The leukotriene pathway is of interest as it is known to be important in asthma and there are several genes that may be important in asthma genetics. However, there are as yet limited studies to substantiate the importance of the genetic influence of this pathway. Genes of interest include the genes for 5-LO, 5 lipoxygenase activating protein (FLAP), LTC_4 synthase, phospholipid hydroperoxide glutathione peroxidase (GPX_4), CysLTR1, and CysLTR2 receptors and polymorphisms in these genes have been reported (133–157). Many of these polymorphisms occur in the 5' flanking regions of the genes where regulatory elements may be located and could therefore affect gene transcription and levels of the encoded protein. Others are located in coding regions and alter the amino acid sequence of the protein whereas one is in a functionally important part of the 3'UTR. Leukotriene pathway variations could influence leukotriene levels, the severity of asthma and/or response to anti-leukotriene treatment.

C. Other Genes

Beta 2 Adrenoreceptor

This is one of the most important genes in asthma genetics, and polymorphisms in it were first described in 1993; nine polymorphisms were initially identified of which four conferred alteration to amino acids at positions (149,158–161). The two most common amino acid polymorphisms were arginine 16 glycine (Arg16Gly) and glutamine 27 glutamic acid (Gln27Glu) and have been extensively studied. In a number of ethnically diverse populations, the Arg16Gly polymorphism has been associated with severity of asthma (160,162) nocturnal asthma (163,164), desensitization to bronchodilator that persisted for six hours (165), atopy (166), % predicted forced expiratory volume in one second (FEV_1) (167–169), % predicted forced vital capacity (FVC) (167,168), acute exacerbations when regularly treated with β_2 agonists (170), airway responsiveness to methacholine, but not adenosine monophosphate (171), altered protection following β_2 agonist treatment (172), infant lung function (173), airway responsiveness to histamine in infancy (169) and bronchodilator response, particularly in those with FEV_1 less than 80% (174). This polymorphism was also associated with egg count,

SPT wheal size, and specific IgE levels to the Helminth *Ascaris lumbricoides* (175). The Gln27Glu polymorphism was associated with airway responsiveness to methacholine (176), total IgE levels (177,178), desensitization to bronchodilator that persisted for six hours (165), asthma in children attending a hospital emergency department (179), % predicted FEV_1 (167), asthma (163), and infant lung function (173). Haplotype analyses of the 13 SNPs in the beta 2 adrenoreceptor gene identified three common haplotypes and these were associated with differences in response to beta agonists (167,180) and affected gene expression and protein levels (180). Preliminary results from our study of children presenting with acute asthma show that Gln homozygotes had a delayed response to beta agonist treatment compared to the other variant 27 genotypes.

Clara Cell Secretory Protein 16

Clara cell secretory protein (CC16) is an anti-inflammatory protein and the most abundant protein in the airways accounting for 7% of total protein in the BALF of healthy nonsmokers (181). The A38G polymorphism in the noncoding region of exon 1 was reported, and homozygotes for the AA genotype were associated with a 6.9-fold increased risk of asthma (182) and decreased levels of plasma CC16 (183). Recently, serum CC16 levels have also been shown to have allele specific increases in levels during viral related acute asthma attacks in children (78) with corresponding associations in asthma severity.

A Disintigrin and Metalloproteinase

A disintigrin and metalloproteinase (ADAM33) is one of the few genes related to asthma that have been found through positional cloning. ADAM proteins have a role in cell fusion, adhesion, signaling and proteolysis (184). The gene for ADAM33 is highly polymorphic containing over 55 SNPs but in association studies only six were significantly associated with asthma in a U.K. population (185). When analyzed as haplotypes, the significance was greatly increased (185). These initial associations with asthma have been replicated in some (186,187) but not all studies (188) and an association with accelerated lung function decline in asthma has also been reported (189). Over 10 studies have now been reported showing positive associations between ADAM33 genotypes and asthma-related phenontypes (3).

XII. Conclusions

Association studies have been used for many years to investigate candidate genes for asthma. These studies have yielded some of the most important information about the genetic susceptibility to asthma. They have also undoubtedly produced a great deal results of dubious reliability. These reliability issues have led to a call for larger, more comprehensive and much more expensive studies. However, since there is such great variability in results derived from different locations and different populations, larger studies that draw subjects from a wider area may not produce positive findings and miss true relationships existing within them. The results of larger studies performed in single locations may also continue to be dominated by local environmental conditions and not be relevant to other locations or populations. This dilemma may only be solved if there is a much better understanding of the environmental risk factors that produce asthma and these remain very poorly understood. This chapter has attempted to summaries the approaches that have been used to design association studies and generate and interpret their results. In the future, these approaches will need to be further refined and they may also benefit from being broadened to include more novel approaches including assessments using data obtained during perturbations and exacerbations of asthma.

References

1. Palmer LJ. Linkages and associations to intermediate phenotypes underlying asthma and allergic disease. Curr Opin Allergy Clin Immunol 2001; 1:393–398.
2. Hoffjan S, Nicolae D, Ober C. Association studies for asthma and atopic diseases: a comprehensive review of the literature. Respir Res 2003; 4:14.
3. Ober C, Hoffjan S. Asthma genetics 2006: the long and winding road to gene discovery. Genes Immun 2006.
4. Hall IP. Genetics and pulmonary medicine: asthma. Thorax 1999; 54:65–69.
5. Le Souef PN. Genetics. In: Silverman M, ed. Childhood Asthma and Other Wheezing Disorders. 2nd ed. London: Arnold, 2002:85–92.
6. http://www.ncbi.nlm.nih.gov/SNP/index.html
7. http://innateimmunity.net//
8. Turner SW, Le Souef PN. Is patient dropout from a longitudinal study of lung function predictable and reversible? Pediatr Pulmonol 2003; 35:29–33.
9. Cardon LR, Palmer LJ. Population stratification and spurious allelic association. Lancet 2003; 361:598–604.
10. Palmer LJ, Cookson WO. Using single nucleotide polymorphisms as a means to understanding the pathophysiology of asthma. Respir Res 2001; 2:102–112.
11. Ronckers C, Land C, Hayes R, et al. Factors impacting questionnaire response in a Dutch retrospective cohort study. Ann Epidemiol 2004; 14:66–72.
12. Little J, Bradley L, Bray MS, et al. Reporting, appraising, and integrating data on genotype prevalence and gene-disease associations. Am J Epidemiol 2002; 156:300–310.
13. Page GP, George V, Go RC, et al. "Are we there yet?" Deciding when one has demonstrated specific genetic causation in complex diseases and quantitative traits. Am J Hum Genet 2003; 73:711–719.

14. Renzoni E, Forastiere F, Biggeri A, et al. Differences in parental- and self-report of asthma, rhinitis and eczema among Italian adolescents. SIDRIA collaborative group. Eur Respir J 1999; 14:597–604.

15. Toren K, Brisman J, Jarvholm B. Asthma and asthma-like symptoms in adults assessed by questionnaires. A literature review. Chest 1993; 104:600–608.

16. Barnes KC. Gene-environment and gene-gene interaction studies in the molecular genetic analysis of asthma and atopy. Clin Exp Allergy 1999; 29 (Suppl 4):47–51.

17. Aitken L, Gallagher R, Madronio C. Principles of recruitment and retention in clinical trials. Int J Nurs Pract 2003; 9:338–346.

18. Wittke-Thompson JK, Pluzhnikov A, Cox NJ. Rational inferences about departures from Hardy-Weinberg equilibrium. Am J Hum Genet 2005; 76: 967–986.

19. Venter JC, Levy S, Stockwell T, et al. Massive parallelism, randomness and genomic advances. Nat Genet 2003; 33(suppl):219–227.

20. Amatschek S, Koenig U, Auer H, et al. Tissue-wide expression profiling using cDNA subtraction and microarrays to identify tumor-specific genes. Cancer Res 2004; 64:844–856.

21. Brutsche MH, Joos L, Carlen Brutsche IE, et al. Array-based diagnostic gene-expression score for atopy and asthma. J Allergy Clin Immunol 2002; 109:271–273.

22. Meyers DA, Postma DS, Stine OC, et al. Genome screen for asthma and bronchial hyperresponsiveness: interactions with passive smoke exposure. J Allergy Clin Immunol 2005; 115:1169–1175.

23. Eder W, Klimecki W, Yu L, et al. Opposite effects of CD 14/-260 on serum IgE levels in children raised in different environments. J Allergy Clin Immunol 2005; 116:601–607.

24. Hall IP, Blakey JD. Genetic association studies in Thorax. Thorax 2005; 60:357–359.

25. Palmer LJ, Silverman ES, Weiss ST, et al. Pharmacogenetics of asthma. Am J Respir Crit Care Med 2002; 165:861–866.

26. Simon Thomas N, Wilkinson J, Lonjou C, et al. Linkage analysis of markers on chromosome 11q13 with asthma and atopy in a United Kingdom population. Am J Respir Crit Care Med 2000; 162:1268–1272.

27. Blakey J, Halapi E, Bjornsdottir US, et al. Contribution of ADAM33 polymorphisms to the population risk of asthma. Thorax 2005; 60:274–276.

28. De Marco R, Locatelli F, Cerveri I, et al. Incidence and remission of asthma: a retrospective study on the natural history of asthma in Italy. J Allergy Clin Immunol 2002; 110:228–235.

29. Silvestri M, Sabatini F, Defilippi AC, et al. The wheezy infant — immunological and molecular considerations. Paediatr Respir Rev 2004; 5(suppl A):S81–S87.

30. Martinez FD, Wright AL, Taussig LM, et al. Asthma and wheezing in the first six years of life. The Group Health Medical Associates. N Engl J Med 1995; 332:133–138.

31. Oddy WH, Holt PG, Sly PD, et al. Association between breast feeding and asthma in 6 year old children: findings of a prospective birth cohort study. Br Med J 1999; 319:815–819.

32. Oddy WH, Peat JK, de Klerk NH. Maternal asthma, infant feeding, and the risk of asthma in childhood. J Allergy Clin Immunol 2002; 110:65–67.
33. Wright AL, Holberg CJ, Taussig LM, et al. Factors influencing the relation of infant feeding to asthma and recurrent wheeze in childhood. Thorax 2001; 56:192–197.
34. Holt PG, Sly PD. Interactions between RSV infection, asthma, and atopy: unraveling the complexities. J Exp Med 2002; 196:1271–1275.
35. Holt PG, Sly PD. Interactions between respiratory tract infections and atopy in the aetiology of asthma. Eur Respir J 2002; 19:538–545.
36. Message SD, Johnston SL. Viruses in asthma. Br Med Bull 2002; 61:29–43.
37. Toren K, Olin AC, Hellgren J, et al. Rhinitis increase the risk for adult-onset asthma—a Swedish population-based case-control study (MAP-study). Respir Med 2002; 96:635–641.
38. Gautrin D, Newman-Taylor AJ, Nordman H, et al. Controversies in epidemiology of occupational asthma. Eur Respir J 2003; 22:551–559.
39. Sears MR. Consequences of long-term inflammation. The natural history of asthma. Clin Chest Med 2000; 21:315–329.
40. Thorn J, Brisman J, Toren K. Adult-onset asthma is associated with self-reported mold or environmental tobacco smoke exposures in the home. Allergy 2001; 56:287–292.
41. Petsonk EL. Work-related asthma and implications for the general public. Environ Health Perspect 2002; 110(suppl 4):569–572.
42. O'Donnell AR, Toelle BG, Marks GB, et al. Age-specific relationship between CD14 and atopy in a cohort assessed from age 8 to 25 years. Am J Respir Crit Care Med 2004; 169:615–622.
43. Kjellman B, Gustafsson PM. Asthma from childhood to adulthood: asthma severity, allergies, sensitization, living conditions, gender influence and social consequences. Respir Med 2000; 94:454–465.
44. Strachan DP, Butland BK, Anderson HR. Incidence and prognosis of asthma and wheezing illness from early childhood to age 33 in a national British cohort. Br Med J 1996; 312:1195–1199.
45. Horwood LJ, Fergusson DM, Shannon FT. Social and familial factors in the development of early childhood asthma. Pediatrics 1985; 75:859–868.
46. Abramson M, Kutin JJ, Raven J, et al. Risk factors for asthma among young adults in Melbourne, Australia. Respirology 1996; 1:291–297.
47. Martin AJ, McLennan LA, Landau LI, et al. The natural history of childhood asthma to adult life. Br Med J 1980; 280:1397–1400.
48. Sunyer J, Anto JM, Kogevinas M, et al. Risk factors for asthma in young adults. Spanish Group of the European Community Respiratory Health Survey. Eur Respir J 1997; 10:2490–2494.
49. Tepper RS, Morgan WJ, Cota K, et al. Physiologic growth and development of the lung during the first year of life. Am Rev Respir Dis 1986; 134:513–519.
50. Tepper RS, Reister T. Forced expiratory flows and lung volumes in normal infants. Pediatr Pulmonol 1993; 15:357–361.
51. von Mutius E. Progression of allergy and asthma through childhood to adolescence. Thorax 1996; 51(suppl 1):S3–S6.

52. Agarwal SK, Marshall GD Jr. Perimenstrual alterations in type-1/type-2 cytokine balance of normal women. Ann Allergy Asthma Immunol 1999; 83: 222–228.
53. Dodge R, Cline MG, Burrows B. Comparisons of asthma, emphysema, and chronic bronchitis diagnoses in a general population sample. Am Rev Respir Dis 1986; 133:981–986.
54. Amelung PJ, Postma DS, Xu J, et al. Exclusion of chromosome 11q and the FcepsilonRI-beta gene as aetiological factors in allergy and asthma in a population of Dutch asthmatic families. Clin Exp Allergy 1998; 28:397–403.
55. Rothman KJ. Modern Epidemiology. Boston: Little Brown, 1986:358.
56. Yin K, Zhang X, Qiu Y. Association between beta(2)-adrenergic receptor genetic polymorphisms and nocturnal asthmatic patients of Chinese Han Nationality. Respiration 2006; 73:464–467.
57. Qiu YY, Zhang XL, Yin KS. Association between beta(2)-adrenergic receptor genetic polymorphisms and total serum IgE in asthmatic patients of Chinese Han Nationality. Respiration 2006; 73:180–184.
58. Hirota T, Suzuki Y, Hasegawa K, et al. Functional haplotypes of IL-12B are associated with childhood atopic asthma. J Allergy Clin Immunol 2005; 116:789–795.
59. Lima JJ, Zhang S, Grant A, et al. Influence of leukotriene pathway polymorphisms on response to Montelukast in asthma. Am J Respir Crit Care Med 2005.
60. Choi JH, Kim SH, Bae JS, et al. Lack of an association between a newly identified promoter polymorphism (-1702G > A) of the leukotriene C4 synthase gene and aspirin-intolerant asthma in a Korean population. Tohoku J Exp Med 2006; 208:49–56.
61. Gupta V, Sarin BC, Changotra H, et al. Association of G-308A TNF-alpha polymorphism with bronchial asthma in a North Indian population. J Asthma 2005; 42:839–841.
62. Oh JM, Kim SH, Suh CH, et al. Lack of association of glutathione S-transferase P1 Ile105Val polymorphism with aspirin-intolerant asthma. Korean J Intern Med 2005; 20:232–236.
63. Imboden M, Nicod L, Nieters A, et al. The common G-allele of interleukin-18 single-nucleotide polymorphism is a genetic risk factor for atopic asthma. The SAPALDIA Cohort Study. Clin Exp Allergy 2006; 36:211–218.
64. Liang XH, Cheung W, Heng CK, et al. Reduced transcriptional activity in individuals with IL-18 gene variants detected from functional but not association study. Biochem Biophys Res Commun 2005; 338:736–741.
65. Barnes KC, Grant AV, Baltadzhieva D, et al. Variants in the gene encoding C3 are associated with asthma and related phenotypes among African Caribbean families. Genes Immun 2006; 7:27–35.
66. Mak JC, Leung HC, Ho SP, et al. Analysis of TGF-beta(1) gene polymorphisms in Hong Kong Chinese patients with asthma. J Allergy Clin Immunol 2006; 117:92–96.
67. Cookson W, Moffatt M. Making sense of asthma genes. N Engl J Med 2004; 351:1794–1796.
68. Cookson WO. Asthma genetics. Chest 2002; 121:7S–13S.

69. Baldini M, Lohman IC, Halonen M, et al. A Polymorphism* in the 5' flanking region of the CD14 gene is associated with circulating soluble CD14 levels and with total serum immunoglobulin E. Am J Respir Cell Mol Biol 1999; 20:976–983.

70. Koppelman GH, Reijmerink NE, Colin Stine O, et al. Association of a promoter polymorphism of the CD14 gene and atopy. Am J Respir Crit Care Med 2001; 163:965–969.

71. Leung TF, Tang NL, Sung YM, et al. The C-159T polymorphism in the CD14 promoter is associated with serum total IgE concentration in atopic Chinese children. Pediatr Allergy Immunol 2003; 14:255–260.

72. Kabesch M, Hasemann K, Schickinger V, et al. A promoter polymorphism in the CD14 gene is associated with elevated levels of soluble CD14 but not with IgE or atopic diseases. Allergy 2004; 59:520–525.

73. Gao PS, Mao XQ, Baldini M, et al. Serum total IgE levels and CD14 on chromosome 5q31. Clin Genet 1999; 56:164–165.

74. Buckova D, Holla LI, Schuller M, et al. Two CD14 promoter polymorphisms and atopic phenotypes in Czech patients with IgE-mediated allergy. Allergy 2003; 58:1023–1026.

75. Sharma M, Batra J, Mabalirajan U, et al. Suggestive evidence of association of C-159T functional polymorphism of the CD14 gene with atopic asthma in northern and northwestern Indian populations. Immunogenetics 2004; 56: 544–547.

76. LeVan TD, Bloom JW, Bailey TJ, et al. A common single nucleotide polymorphism in the CD14 promoter decreases the affinity of Sp protein binding and enhances transcriptional activity. J Immunol 2001; 167:5838–5844.

77. Vercelli D, Baldini M, Martinez F. The monocyte/IgE connection: may polymorphisms in the CD14 gene teach us about IgE regulation? Int Arch Allergy Immunol 2001; 124:20–24.

78. Martin AC, Laing IA, Khoo SK, et al. Acute asthma in children: relationship between CD14 and CC16 genotype, plasma levels and severity. Am J Respir Crit Care Med 2005.

79. Rosenwasser LJ, Klemm DJ, Dresback JK, et al. Promoter polymorphisms in the chromosome 5 gene cluster in asthma and atopy. Clin Exp Allergy 1995; 25(suppl 2):74–78; discussion 95–96.

80. Paul WE. Interleukin-4: a prototypic immunoregulatory lymphokine. Blood 1991; 77:1859–1870.

81. Kabesch M, Tzotcheva I, Carr D, et al. A complete screening of the IL4 gene: novel polymorphisms and their association with asthma and IgE in childhood. J Allergy Clin Immunol 2003; 112:893–898.

82. Noguchi E, Shibasaki M, Arinami T, et al. Association of asthma and the interleukin-4 promoter gene in Japanese. Clin Exp Allergy 1998; 28:449–453.

83. Sandford AJ, Chagani T, Zhu S, et al. Polymorphisms in the IL4, IL4RA, and FCERIB genes and asthma severity. J Allergy Clin Immunol 2000; 106: 135–140.

84. Burchard EG, Silverman EK, Rosenwasser LJ, et al. Association between a sequence variant in the IL-4 gene promoter and FEV(1) in asthma. Am J Respir Crit Care Med 1999; 160:919–922.

85. Zhu S, Chan-Yeung M, Becker AB, et al. Polymorphisms of the IL-4, TNF-alpha, and Fcepsilon RIbeta genes and the risk of allergic disorders in at-risk infants. Am J Respir Crit Care Med 2000; 161:1655–1659.

86. Beghe B, Barton S, Rorke S, et al. Polymorphisms in the interleukin-4 and interleukin-4 receptor alpha chain genes confer susceptibility to asthma and atopy in a Caucasian population. Clin Exp Allergy 2003; 33:1111–1117.

87. Kammer W, Lischke A, Moriggl R, et al. Homodimerization of interleukin-4 receptor alpha chain can induce intracellular signaling. J Biol Chem 1996; 271:23634–23637.

88. Wjst M, Kruse S, Illig T, et al. Asthma and IL-4 receptor alpha gene variants. Eur J Immunogenet 2002; 29:263–268.

89. Ober C, Leavitt SA, Tsalenko A, et al. Variation in the interleukin 4-receptor alpha gene confers susceptibility to asthma and atopy in ethnically diverse populations. Am J Hum Genet 2000; 66:517–526.

90. Wills-Karp M, Chiaramonte M. Interleukin-13 in asthma. Curr Opin Pulm Med 2003; 9:21–27.

91. Howard TD, Whittaker PA, Zaiman AL, et al. Identification and association of polymorphisms in the interleukin-13 gene with asthma and atopy in a Dutch population. Am J Respir Cell Mol Biol 2001; 25:377–384.

92. Hummelshoj T, Bodtger U, Datta P, et al. Association between an interleukin-13 promoter polymorphism and atopy. Eur J Immunogenet 2003; 30:355–359.

93. van der Pouw Kraan TC, van Veen A, Boeije LC, et al. An IL-13 promoter polymorphism associated with increased risk of allergic asthma. Genes Immun 1999; 1:61–65.

94. Graves PE, Kabesch M, Halonen M, et al. A cluster of seven tightly linked polymorphisms in the IL-13 gene is associated with total serum IgE levels in three populations of white children. J Allergy Clin Immunol 2000; 105: 506–513.

95. Heinzmann A, Jerkic SP, Ganter K, et al. Association study of the IL13 variant Arg110Gln in atopic diseases and juvenile idiopathic arthritis. J Allergy Clin Immunol 2003; 112:735–739.

96. Liu X, Nickel R, Beyer K, et al. An IL13 coding region variant is associated with a high total serum IgE level and atopic dermatitis in the German multi-center atopy study. J Allergy Clin Immunol 2000; 106:167–170.

97. Wang M, Xing ZM, Lu C, et al. A common IL-13 Arg130Gln single nucleotide polymorphism among Chinese atopy patients with allergic rhinitis. Hum Genet 2003; 113:387–390.

98. He JQ, Chan-Yeung M, Becker AB, et al. Genetic variants of the IL13 and IL4 genes and atopic diseases in at-risk children. Genes Immun 2003; 4:385–389.

99. Moore KW, de Waal Malefyt R, Coffman RL, et al. Interleukin-10 and the interleukin-10 receptor. Annu Rev Immunol 2001; 19:683–765.

100. Turner DM, Williams DM, Sankaran D, et al. An investigation of polymorphism in the interleukin-10 gene promoter. Eur J Immunogenet 1997; 24:1–8.

101. Lim S, Crawley E, Woo P, et al. Haplotype associated with low interleukin-10 production in patients with severe asthma. Lancet 1998; 352:113.

102. Papadopoulos NG, Stanciu LA, Papi A, et al. A defective type 1 response to rhinovirus in atopic asthma. Thorax 2002; 57:328–332.

103. Wills-Karp M. IL-12/IL-13 axis in allergic asthma. J Allergy Clin Immunol 2001; 107:9–18.
104. Sieburth D, Jabs EW, Warrington JA, et al. Assignment of genes encoding a unique cytokine (IL12) composed of two unrelated subunits to chromosomes 3 and 5. Genomics 1992; 14:59–62.
105. Morahan G, Huang D, Wu M, et al. Association of IL12B promoter polymorphism with severity of atopic and non-atopic asthma in children. Lancet 2002; 360:455–459.
106. Khoo SK, Hayden CM, Roberts M, et al. Associations of the IL12B promoter polymorphism in longitudinal data from asthmatic patients 7 to 42 years of age. J Allergy Clin Immunol 2004; 113:475–481.
107. Pene J, Chretien I, Rousset F, et al. Modulation of IL-4-induced human IgE production in vitro by IFN-gamma and IL-5: the role of soluble CD23 (s-CD23). J Cell Biochem 1989; 39:253–264.
108. Lopez-Maderuelo D, Arnalich F, Serantes R, et al. Interferon-gamma and interleukin-10 gene polymorphisms in pulmonary tuberculosis. Am J Respir Crit Care Med 2003; 167:970–975.
109. Pravica V, Perrey C, Stevens A, et al. A single nucleotide polymorphism in the first intron of the human IFN-gamma gene: absolute correlation with a polymorphic CA microsatellite marker of high IFN-gamma production. Hum Immunol 2000; 61:863–866.
110. Rossouw M, Nel HJ, Cooke GS, et al. Association between tuberculosis and a polymorphic NFkappaB binding site in the interferon gamma gene. Lancet 2003; 361:1871–1872.
111. Juliger S, Bongartz M, Luty AJ, et al. Functional analysis of a promoter variant of the gene encoding the interferon-gamma receptor chain I. Immunogenetics 2003; 54:675–680.
112. Gao PS, Mao XQ, Jouanguy E, et al. Nonpathogenic common variants of IFNGR1 and IFNGR2 in association with total serum IgE levels. Biochem Biophys Res Commun 1999; 263:425–429.
113. Lien E, Sellati TJ, Yoshimura A, et al. Toll-like receptor 2 functions as a pattern recognition receptor for diverse bacterial products. J Biol Chem 1999; 274:33,419–33,425.
114. Takeda K, Kaisho T, Akira S. Toll-like receptors. Annu Rev Immunol 2003; 21:335–376.
115. Michel O, LeVan TD, Stern D, et al. Systemic responsiveness to lipopolysaccharide and polymorphisms in the toll-like receptor 4 gene in human beings. J Allergy Clin Immunol 2003; 112:923–929.
116. Hirschfeld M, Ma Y, Weis JH, et al. Cutting edge: repurification of lipopolysaccharide eliminates signaling through both human and murine toll-like receptor 2. J Immunol 2000; 165:618–622.
117. Eder W, Klimecki W, Yu L, et al. Toll-like receptor 2 as a major gene for asthma in children of European farmers. J Allergy Clin Immunol 2004; 113:482–488.
118. Lorenz E, Mira JP, Cornish KL, et al. A novel polymorphism in the toll-like receptor 2 gene and its potential association with staphylococcal infection. Infect Immun 2000; 68:6398–6401.

119. Papadopoulos NG, Papi A, Psarras S, et al. Mechanisms of rhinovirus-induced asthma. Paediatr Respir Rev 2004; 5:255–260.

120. Noguchi E, Nishimura F, Fukai H, et al. An association study of asthma and total serum immunoglobin E levels for Toll-like receptor polymorphisms in a Japanese population. Clin Exp Allergy 2004; 34:177–183.

121. Raby BA, Klimecki WT, Laprise C, et al. Polymorphisms in toll-like receptor 4 are not associated with asthma or atopy-related phenotypes. Am J Respir Crit Care Med 2002; 166:1449–1456.

122. Arbour NC, Lorenz E, Schutte BC, et al. TLR4 mutations are associated with endotoxin hyporesponsiveness in humans. Nat Genet 2000; 25:187–191.

123. Redington AE, Madden J, Frew AJ, et al. Transforming growth factor-beta 1 in asthma. Measurement in bronchoalveolar lavage fluid. Am J Respir Crit Care Med 1997; 156:642–647.

124. Pulleyn LJ, Newton R, Adcock IM, et al. TGFbeta1 allele association with asthma severity. Hum Genet 2001; 109:623–627.

125. Silverman ES, Palmer LJ, Subramaniam V, et al. Transforming growth factor-beta1 promoter polymorphism C-509T is associated with asthma. Am J Respir Crit Care Med 2004; 169:214–219.

126. Hobbs K, Negri J, Klinnert M, et al. Interleukin-10 and transforming growth factor-beta promoter polymorphisms in allergies and asthma. Am J Respir Crit Care Med 1998; 158:1958–1962.

127. Grainger DJ, Heathcote K, Chiano M, et al. Genetic control of the circulating concentration of transforming growth factor type beta1. Hum Mol Genet 1999; 8:93–97.

128. Karjalainen J, Hulkkonen J, Hurme M. IL-1 haplotypes and lung function decline. Thorax 2002; 57:561–562; author reply 562.

129. Karjalainen J, Nieminen MM, Aromaa A, et al. The IL-1beta genotype carries asthma susceptibility only in men. J Allergy Clin Immunol 2002; 109:514–516.

130. Pessi T, Karjalainen J, Hulkkonen J, et al. A common IL-1 complex haplotype is associated with an increased risk of atopy. J Med Genet 2003; 40:e66.

131. Jansky L, Vybiral S, Pospisilova D, et al. Production of systemic and hypotha-lamic cytokines during the early phase of endotoxin fever. Neuroendocrinology 1995; 62:55–61.

132. Terry CF, Loukaci V, Green FR. Cooperative influence of genetic polymor-phisms on interleukin 6 transcriptional regulation. J Biol Chem 2000; 275: 18,138–18,144.

133. Choi JH, Park HS, Oh HB, et al. Leukotriene-related gene polymorphisms in ASA-intolerant asthma: an association with a haplotype of 5-lipoxygenase. Hum Genet 2004; 114:337–344.

134. Drazen JM, Yandava CN, Dube L, et al. Pharmacogenetic association between ALOX5 promoter genotype and the response to anti-asthma treatment. Nat Genet 1999; 22:168–170.

135. In KH, Asano K, Beier D, et al. Naturally occurring mutations in the human 5-lipoxygenase gene promoter that modify transcription factor binding and reporter gene transcription. J Clin Invest 1997; 99:1130–1137.

136. Sayers I, Barton S, Rorke S, et al. Promoter polymorphism in the 5-lipoxygenase (ALOX5) and 5-lipoxygenase-activating protein (ALOX5AP) genes and

asthma susceptibility in a Caucasian population. Clin Exp Allergy 2003; 33: 1103–1110.

137. Silverman ES, Du J, De Sanctis GT, et al. Egr-1 and Sp1 interact functionally with the 5-lipoxygenase promoter and its naturally occurring mutants. Am J Respir Cell Mol Biol 1998; 19:316–323.

138. Hatzelmann A, Schatz M, Ullrich V. Involvement of glutathione peroxidase activity in the stimulation of 5-lipoxygenase activity by glutathione-depleting agents in human polymorphonuclear leukocytes. Eur J Biochem 1989; 180:527–533.

139. Hatzelmann A, Ullrich V. Regulation of 5-lipoxygenase activity by the glutathione status in human polymorphonuclear leukocytes. Eur J Biochem 1987; 169:175–184.

140. Imai H, Narashima K, Arai M, et al. Suppression of leukotriene formation in RBL-2H3 cells that overexpressed phospholipid hydroperoxide glutathione peroxidase. J Biol Chem 1998; 273:1990–1997.

141. Koshino T, Takano S, Houjo T, et al. Expression of 5-lipoxygenase and 5-lipoxygenase-activating protein mRNAs in the peripheral blood leukocytes of asthmatics. Biochem Biophys Res Commun 1998; 247:510–513.

142. Koshino T, Takano S, Kitani S, et al. Novel polymorphism of the 5-lipoxygenase activating protein (FLAP) promoter gene associated with asthma. Mol Cell Biol Res Comm 1999; 2:32–35.

143. Maiorino M, Bosello V, Ursini F, et al. Genetic variations of gpx-4 and male infertility in humans. Biol Reprod 2003; 68:1134–1141.

144. Sayers I, Barton S, Rorke S, et al. Allelic association and functional studies of promoter polymorphism in the leukotriene C4 synthase gene (LTC4S) in asthma. Thorax 2003; 58:417–424.

145. Kawagishi Y, Mita H, Taniguchi M, et al. Leukotriene C4 synthase promoter polymorphism in Japanese patients with aspirin-induced asthma. J Allergy Clin Immunol 2002; 109:936–942.

146. Sampson AP, Siddiqui S, Buchanan D, et al. Variant LTC(4) synthase allele modifies cysteinyl leukotriene synthesis in eosinophils and predicts clinical response to zafirlukast. Thorax 2000; 55(suppl 2):S28–S31.

147. Sanak M, Pierzchalska M, Bazan-Socha S, et al. Enhanced expression of the leukotriene C(4) synthase due to overactive transcription of an allelic variant associated with aspirin-intolerant asthma. Am J Respir Cell Mol Biol 2000; 23:290–296.

148. Sanak M, Simon HU, Szczeklik A. Leukotriene C4 synthase promoter polymorphism and risk of aspirin-induced asthma. Lancet 1997; 350:1599–1600.

149. Van Sambeek R, Stevenson DD, Baldasaro M, et al. 5′ flanking region polymorphism of the gene encoding leukotriene C4 synthase does not correlate with the aspirin-intolerant asthma phenotype in the United States. J Allergy Clin Immunol 2000; 106:72–76.

150. Villette S, Kyle JA, Brown KM, et al. A novel single nucleotide polymorphism in the 3′ untranslated region of human glutathione peroxidase 4 influences lipoxygenase metabolism. Blood Cells Mol Dis 2002; 29:174–178.

151. Whelan GJ, Blake K, Kissoon N, et al. Effect of montelukast on time-course of exhaled nitric oxide in asthma: influence of LTC4 synthase A(-444)C polymorphism. Pediatr Pulmonol 2003; 36:413–420.

152. Asano K, Shiomi T, Hasegawa N, et al. Leukotriene C4 synthase gene A(-444)C polymorphism and clinical response to a CYS-LT(1) antagonist, pranlukast, in Japanese patients with moderate asthma. Pharmacogenetics 2002; 12:565–570.

153. Currie GP, Lima JJ, Sylvester JE, et al. Leukotriene C4 synthase polymorphisms and responsiveness to leukotriene antagonists in asthma. Br J Clin Pharmacol 2003; 56:422–426.

154. Hui Y, Funk CD. Cysteinyl leukotriene receptors. Biochem Pharmacol 2002; 64:1549–1557.

155. Hui Y, Yang G, Galczenski H, et al. The murine cysteinyl leukotriene 2 (CysLT2) receptor. cDNA and genomic cloning, alternative splicing, and in vitro characterization. J Biol Chem 2001; 276:47489–47495.

156. Mastalerz L, Nizankowska E, Sanak M, et al. Clinical and genetic features underlying the response of patients with bronchial asthma to treatment with a leukotriene receptor antagonist. Eur J Clin Invest 2002; 32:949–955.

157. Thompson MD, van's Gravesande KS, Galczenski H, et al. A cysteinyl leukotriene 2 receptor variant is associated with atopy in the population of Tristan da Cunha. Pharmacogenetics 2003; 13:641–649.

158. Huh JC, Strickland DH, Jahnsen FL, et al. Bidirectional interactions between antigen-bearing respiratory tract dendritic cells (DCs) and T cells precede the late phase reaction in experimental asthma: DC activation occurs in the airway mucosa but not in the lung parenchyma. J Exp Med 2003; 198:19–30.

159. Knorr B, Franchi LM, Bisgaard H, et al. Montelukast, a leukotriene receptor antagonist, for the treatment of persistent asthma in children aged 2 to 5 years. Pediatrics 2001; 108:E48.

160. Reihsaus E, Innis M, MacIntyre N, et al. Mutations in the gene encoding for the beta 2-adrenergic receptor in normal and asthmatic subjects. Am J Respir Cell Mol Biol 1993; 8:334–339.

161. Samuelsson B, Dahlen SE, Lindgren JA, et al. Leukotrienes and lipoxins: structures, biosynthesis, and biological effects. Science 1987; 237:1171–1176.

162. Holloway JW, Dunbar PR, Riley GA, et al. Association of beta2-adrenergic receptor polymorphisms with severe asthma. Clin Exp Allergy 2000; 30:1097–1103.

163. Santillan AA, Camargo CA Jr., Ramirez-Rivera A, et al. Association between beta2-adrenoceptor polymorphisms and asthma diagnosis among Mexican adults. J Allergy Clin Immunol 2003; 112:1095–1100.

164. Turki J, Pak J, Green SA, et al. Genetic polymorphisms of the beta 2-adrenergic receptor in nocturnal and nonnocturnal asthma. Evidence that Gly16 correlates with the nocturnal phenotype. J Clin Invest 1995; 95:1635–1641.

165. Tan S, Hall IP, Dewar J, et al. Association between beta 2-adrenoceptor polymorphism and susceptibility to bronchodilator desensitisation in moderately severe stable asthmatics. Lancet 1997; 350:995–999.

166. Dewar JC, Wheatley AP, Venn A, et al. Beta2-adrenoceptor polymorphisms are in linkage disequilibrium, but are not associated with asthma in an adult population. Clin Exp Allergy 1998; 28:442–448.

167. Silverman EK, Kwiatkowski DJ, Sylvia JS, et al. Family-based association analysis of beta2-adrenergic receptor polymorphisms in the childhood asthma management program. J Allergy Clin Immunol 2003; 112:870–876.

168. Summerhill E, Leavitt SA, Gidley H, et al. beta(2)-adrenergic receptor Arg16/Arg16 genotype is associated with reduced lung function, but not with asthma, in the Hutterites. Am J Respir Crit Care Med 2000; 162:599–602.

169. Turner SW, Khoo SK, Laing IA, et al. beta2 adrenoceptor Arg16Gly polymorphism, airway responsiveness, lung function and asthma in infants and children. Clin Exp Allergy 2004; 34:1043–1048.

170. Taylor DR, Drazen JM, Herbison GP, et al. Asthma exacerbations during long term beta agonist use: influence of beta(2) adrenoceptor polymorphism. Thorax 2000; 55:762–767.

171. Fowler SJ, Dempsey OJ, Sims EJ, et al. Screening for bronchial hyperresponsiveness using methacholine and adenosine monophosphate. Relationship to asthma severity and beta(2)-receptor genotype. Am J Respir Crit Care Med 2000; 162:1318–1322.

172. Lee DK, Currie GP, Hall IP, et al. The arginine-16 beta2-adrenoceptor polymorphism predisposes to bronchoprotective subsensitivity in patients treated with formoterol and salmeterol. Br J Clin Pharmacol 2004; 57:68–75.

173. Wilson NM, Lamprill JR, Mak JC, et al. Symptoms, lung function, and beta2-adrenoceptor polymorphisms in a birth cohort followed for 10 years. Pediatr Pulmonol 2004; 38:75–81.

174. Choudhry S, Ung N, Avila PC, et al. Pharmacogenetic differences in response to Albuterol between Puerto Rican and Mexican asthmatics. Am J Respir Crit Care Med 2005; 171:563–570.

175. Ramsay CE, Hayden CM, Tiller KJ, et al. Association of polymorphisms in the beta2-adrenoreceptor gene with higher levels of parasitic infection. Hum Genet 1999; 104:269–274.

176. Hall IP, Wheatley A, Wilding P, et al. Association of Glu 27 beta 2-adrenoceptor polymorphism with lower airway reactivity in asthmatic subjects. Lancet 1995; 345:1213–1214.

177. Dewar J, Wheatley A, Wilkinson J, et al. Association of the Gln 27 beta 2-adrenoceptor polymorphism and IgE variability in asthmatic families. Chest 1997; 111:78S–79S.

178. Dewar JC, Wilkinson J, Wheatley A, et al. The glutamine 27 beta2-adrenoceptor polymorphism is associated with elevated IgE levels in asthmatic families. J Allergy Clin Immunol 1997; 100:261–265.

179. Hopes E, McDougall C, Christie G, et al. Association of glutamine 27 polymorphism of beta 2 adrenoceptor with reported childhood asthma: population based study. Br Med J 1998; 316:664.

180. Drysdale CM, McGraw DW, Stack CB, et al. Complex promoter and coding region beta 2-adrenergic receptor haplotypes alter receptor expression and predict in vivo responsiveness. Proc Natl Acad Sci USA 2000; 97:10,483–10,488.

181. Van Vyve T, Chanez P, Bernard A, et al. Protein content in bronchoalveolar lavage fluid of patients with asthma and control subjects. J Allergy Clin Immunol 1995; 95:60–68.

182. Laing IA, Goldblatt J, Eber E, et al. A polymorphism of the CC16 gene is associated with an increased risk of asthma. J Med Genet 1998; 35:463–467.

183. Laing IA, Hermans C, Bernard A, et al. Association between plasma CC16 levels, the A38G polymorphism, and asthma. Am J Respir Crit Care Med 2000; 161:124–127.

184. Primakoff P, Myles DG. The ADAM gene family: surface proteins with adhesion and protease activity. Trends Genet 2000; 16:83–87.

185. Van Eerdewegh P, Little RD, Dupuis J, et al. Association of the ADAM33 gene with asthma and bronchial hyperresponsiveness. Nature 2002; 418:426–430.

186. Howard TD, Postma DS, Jongepier H, et al. Association of a disintegrin and metalloprotease 33 (ADAM33) gene with asthma in ethnically diverse populations. J Allergy Clin Immunol 2003; 112:717–722.

187. Werner M, Herbon N, Gohlke H, et al. Asthma is associated with single-nucleotide polymorphisms in ADAM33. Clin Exp Allergy 2004; 34:26–31.

188. Lind DL, Choudhry S, Ung N, et al. ADAM33 is not associated with asthma in Puerto Rican or Mexican populations. Am J Respir Crit Care Med 2003; 168: 1312–1316.

189. Jongepier H, Boezen HM, Dijkstra A, et al. Polymorphisms of the ADAM33 gene are associated with accelerated lung function decline in asthma. Clin Exp Allergy 2004; 34:757–760.

14

Association Studies in Chronic Obstructive Pulmonary Disease

TAKEO ISHII and ANDREW J. SANDFORD

The James Hogg iCAPTURE Centre for Cardiovascular and Pulmonary Disease,
University of British Columbia,
Vancouver, British Columbia, Canada

I. Introduction

As written in the previous chapters, it is clear that exposure to cigarette smoke, by itself, is not sufficient to explain the development of chronic obstructive pulmonary disease (COPD), and other factors including genetic and environmental risk factors must contribute to its pathogenesis. Epidemiological studies (family studies, twin studies, and segregation analyses) demonstrate that COPD is a complex genetic disease, i.e., there is a genetic component to COPD, but it is unlikely that there is a major susceptibility gene in the majority of families.

Two major strategies have been used to identify genes containing mutations or polymorphisms (common sequence variants), which contribute to the development of COPD. The first strategy is linkage analysis (as shown in Chapter 1), and the second strategy is the association study in which individual genes are directly tested for their involvement in a disease process.

In this chapter, we review the genes that have been investigated as potential susceptibility factors for COPD. COPD is characterized by a slowly progressive irreversible airflow limitation that is primarily due to two pathophysiological changes in the lung: peripheral airway inflammation and a loss of lung elastic recoil resulting from parenchymal destruction (Fig. 1). Many inflammatory cells, mediators, and enzymes have been implicated, and these offer potential targets for genetic investigations. It seems certain that there will be a complex interaction between several different genetic and environmental factors. To date, the genes that have been implicated in the pathogenesis of airflow limitation are involved in the protease/antiprotease balance, the metabolism of toxic substances in cigarette smoke, the oxidant/antioxidant balance, the inflammatory response to cigarette smoke, and mucociliary clearance. The genes involved or potentially involved in the pathogenesis of COPD are summarized in Table 1 .

Recently, Sandford and Silverman (1) and Molfino (2) presented comprehensive reviews of the literature regarding candidate genes for COPD. In this chapter, we will concentrate on recent developments and selected genes for which there is strong evidence that they are susceptibility loci for COPD.

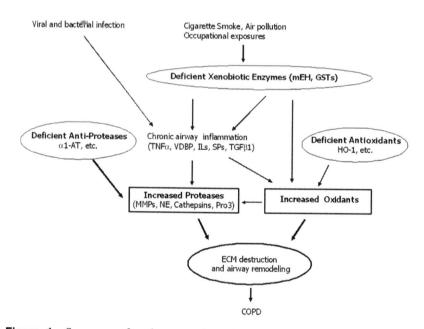

Figure 1 Summary of pathways and possible candidate genes involved in the pathogenesis of chronic obstructive pulmonary disease. *Abbreviations:* COPD, chronic obstructive pulmonary disease; TNFα, tumor necrosis factor α; VDBP, vitamin D binding protein; IL, interleukin; SP, surfactant protein; TGFβ1, transforming growth factor-β1; α1-AT, α1-antitrypsin; MMPs, matrix metalloproteinases; NE, neutrophil elastase; Pro3, proteinase 3; mEH, microsomal epoxide hydrolase; GST, glutathione S-transferase; HO-1, heme oxygenase-1; ECM, extracellular matrix.

Table 1 Genes Involved or Potentially Involved in the Pathogenesis of COPD Grouped by Gene Function

Category	Genes
Protease/antiprotease balance	α_1-Antitrypsin
	MMPs
	MMP1
	MMP9
	MMP12
	α_1-Antichymotrypsin
Xenobiotic metabolizing enzymes	Microsomal epoxide hydrolase
	Glutathione S-transferases
Antioxidants	Heme oxygenase
Inflammatory mediators	Vitamin D binding protein
	Tumor necrosis factor α
	IL-1
	IL-1α
	IL-1β
	IL-1 receptor antagonist
	IL-10
	IL-13
	IL-13
	IL-13 receptor
	SP
	SP-A
	SP-B
	Transforming growth factor-β1
Mucociliary clearance	Cystic fibrosis transmembrane conductance regulator
Others	β-Defensin-1
	β2-Adrenoceptor

Abbreviations: MMP, matrix metalloproteinase; IL, interleukin; SP, surfactant proteins.

II. Association Studies of Candidate Genes

A. Protease/Antiprotease Balance

α_1-Antitrypsin Deficiency

α_1-antitrypsin (α_1-AT) is an acute phase protein synthesized in the liver and to a lesser extent by alveolar macrophages. This antiprotease provides the major defense against proteolytic digestion of the lung by neutrophil elastase, cathepsin G, and proteinase 3 (3). It has been known since the early 1960s that individuals who have extremely low levels of α_1-AT have an increased prevalence of emphysema, which partly introduced the protease versus antiprotease hypothesis into our understanding of the pathogenesis of COPD.

Severe α_1-Antitrypsin Deficiency

A genetic basis for α_1-AT deficiency was demonstrated by the observation that the deficiency followed a simple Mendelian pattern of inheritance and was usually associated with the Z isoform of α_1-AT (4). The two most common deficiency variants of α_1-AT, S and Z, result from point mutations in the α_1-AT gene and are named on the basis of their altered electrophoretic mobility on isoelectric focusing gels compared with the normal M allele (5).

In contrast to the fact that α_1-AT deficiency is one of the most common hereditary disorders of Caucasians, deficient variants among Asians have been recognized to be extremely rare (6). Thus, in the following, we discuss α_1-AT deficiency mainly in Caucasian populations.

Homozygosity of the Z variant (which contains lysine rather than glutamic acid at amino acid position 342) results in a severe deficiency that is characterized by plasma α_1-AT levels approximately 15% of the normal M allele. Individuals with the ZZ genotype have a clearly accelerated rate of decline in lung function (7), sometimes even in the absence of smoking. However, the homozygous state is rare in the population ($<1\%$ of Caucasians) and thus can explain only a small percentage of the genetic susceptibility to cigarette smoke.

Despite the strong association of the ZZ genotype with early-onset COPD, the clinical course of the disease is highly variable (8) as is common with other genetic disorders. Exposure to cigarette smoke plays an important role in determining this variability. However, the rate of decline of lung function in ZZ subjects who are lifelong nonsmokers is also highly variable. In studies in which index and nonindex cases have been compared, many nonindex ZZ subjects show normal lung function and a survival similar to the normal population (8) if they are nonsmokers. It is possible that other genetic factors influence the clinical course in ZZ homozygotes. Polymorphisms in the endothelial nitric oxide synthase gene and glutathione S-transferase P1 (GSTP1) gene were shown to contribute to the development of COPD in ZZ individuals (9,10).

Intermediate α_1-AT Deficiency Alleles

With the clear association of severe α_1-AT deficiency with COPD, it was natural to ask whether individuals with intermediate deficiency were also at risk for airflow limitation. The results of many case–control studies have shown an increased prevalence of MZ heterozygotes in COPD patients compared with controls (1,2).

Investigators have also assessed the risk of the MZ genotype by studying lung function in the general population (1,2). In these studies, a population sample is phenotyped for α_1-AT variants, and the prevalence of COPD in those with the MZ phenotype is compared with the prevalence in those with the MM phenotype. In a recent large cohort study from Denmark, Seersholm et al. compared the prevalence of obstructive pulmonary disease in 1551 MZ individuals versus 14,484 controls from the general population of unknown α_1-AT genotype (11). The risk for obstructive pulmonary disease was significantly increased in the MZ individuals compared to the controls (relative risk $= 2.2$). However, only first-degree relatives of ZZ COPD patients had a significantly increased risk, suggesting that other genetic or environmental factors were contributing to the increased risk in these patients. Dahl et al. performed a large cross-sectional study of 9187 individuals from the general population of Copenhagen in Denmark (12). Only the SZ and ZZ individuals in this population showed an increased prevalence of airflow limitation [forced expiratory volume in one second (FEV_1) $< 80\%$ predicted]. There was no association of either the MS or MZ genotype with lower level of lung function in individuals without clinically established COPD. However, among the COPD patients FEV_1 was 655 mL less in MZ individuals compared with MM individuals ($p < 0.05$), after adjustment for confounding variables. The observation that the MZ genotype was associated with airflow limitation only in those with COPD suggests that other predisposing factors exist, consistent with the results of Seersholm et al. (11).

In addition to this cross-sectional study, Dahl et al. performed a longitudinal study to test whether MZ genotype affects lung function decrease and other clinical outcomes of COPD on the same study cohort (13). Three lung function measurements obtained during 1976–1978, 1981–1983, and 1991–1994 were used to calculate annual change in FEV_1. The results showed that the MZ genotype was more prevalent in subjects with airway obstruction and COPD, and was associated with more rapid decline rate in FEV_1 than did the MM genotype. The authors also concluded that the MZ genotype accounts for almost the same proportion of COPD cases as do the ZZ genotype. However, Silva et al. could not duplicate the association between MZ genotype and FEV_1 decline rate in their study with 2016 adult subjects in a community population in Tucson, Arizona (14).

Because the risk of COPD in MZ or MS heterozygous individuals is controversial as shown above, two meta-analyses were reported to evaluate the association between COPD and these genotypes (15,16). In these studies, it was shown that the SZ genotype was a significant risk factor for COPD and that the risk of COPD due to the MS or MZ genotype was not substantially elevated. As the authors of these meta-analyses suggest, future studies that adjust for smoking and include other COPD-related phenotypes are required to conclusively determine the risk of COPD in MS or MZ heterozygotes.

The Other α_1-AT Mutations

There are several polymorphisms of the α_1-AT gene that are not associated with α_1-AT deficiency, e.g., a polymorphism in the $3'$ untranslated region of the α_1-AT gene was associated with COPD in some populations but not others (1,2).

In a recent study, a single nucleotide polymorphism (SNP) in intron 1 of the α_1-AT gene was found to have a functional effect on transcriptional regulation observed by luciferase assay (17). Thus, in future studies, it will be necessary to investigate the association between α_1-AT haplotypes including this functional SNP and COPD phenotypes.

Matrix Metalloproteinases and Their Inhibitors

Matrix metalloproteinases (MMPs) are a structurally and functionally related family of proteolytic enzymes that play an essential role in tissue remodeling and repair associated with development and inflammation. Several studies in animals and humans have provided evidence that MMP1 (interstitial collagenase), MMP12 (human macrophage elastase), and MMP9 (gelatinase B) are important in airway inflammation and in the development of emphysema. Transgenic mice overexpressing human *MMP1* in their lungs developed morphologic changes similar to human pulmonary emphysema (18). *MMP12* knockout mice did not develop emphysema following exposure to cigarette smoke (19), suggesting that the presence of MMP12 is critical in smoke-induced lung injury. Smokers with airway obstruction show increased expression of MMP1 and MMP9 compared with smokers without COPD and nonsmokers (20).

There are several reports on the association between polymorphisms in MMP1, -9, and -12 genes and COPD or related phenotypes, which are shown in Table 2 (21–25). Most recently, it was reported that a genetic polymorphism in the promoter of the MMP9 gene was associated with susceptibility to COPD in the Han population of South China (23).

Tissue inhibitors of metalloproteinases (TIMPs) are inhibitors of MMPs, and they regulate extracellular matrix degradation. The allele frequency of the +853 G/A SNP in TIMP2 was associated with COPD in a Japanese population (26), and its genotype frequency was associated with COPD in Egyptians (27). It will be important to investigate association between TIMPs and COPD, including other TIMPs (TIMP1, -3, and -4) and other populations (Caucasian and African American), utilizing larger study groups.

Other Genes Related to Protease–Antiprotease Balance

The association of airflow limitation with genetic defects in the α_1-AT gene also led to a search for genetic variants of other antiproteases that may be involved in protection against lung destruction. For example, a polymorphism in the signal peptide of α_1-antichymotrypsin (Ala-15) was shown to be associated with susceptibility to the development of COPD in a Japanese population (28). However, this association was not observed in a Caucasian population.

Cathepsins, cysteine proteinases that are capable of degrading elastin, and their inhibitor cystatin C are also thought to be related to the

Table 2 Summary of Association Studies of Matrix Metalloproteinases

Cases	Controls	Population	Polymorphism	Minor allele frequency: cases vs. controls	Result	References
45 COPD patients with emphysema on CT-scan	65 subjects without emphysema on CT-scan	Japanese	MMP-9 C-1562T	0.244 vs. 0.123	T allele frequency was higher in subjects with emphysema on chest CT-scans than in those without emphysema. DL$_{CO}$/VA was lower and emphysematous changes were more conspicuous in subjects with C/T or T/T than in those with C/C	21
284 smokers with rapid decline of lung function	306 smokers with no decline in lung function	Caucasian (North America)	MMP1 G-1607GG	0.59 vs. 0.49	Of the five polymorphisms, only the -1607GG allele was associated with a fast rate of decline of lung function Haplotypes consisting of alleles from the MMP1 G-1607GG and MMP12 Asn357Ser polymorphisms were associated with rate of decline of lung function	22
			MMP9 CA repeat	[a]		
			MMP9 C-1562T	0.16 vs. 0.14		
			MMP12 A-82G	0.12 vs. 0.11		
			MMP12 Asn357Ser	0.04 vs. 0.05		
100 COPD patients	98 healthy smokers	Chinese (South China)	MMP9 C-1562T	0.07 vs. 0.01	The frequencies of C/T heterozygotes and that of the T allele were significantly higher in COPD patients	23

(Continued)

Table 2 Summary of Association Studies of Matrix Metalloproteinases (*Continued*)

Cases	Controls	Population	Polymorphism	Minor allele frequency: cases vs. controls	Result	References
304 COPD patients	441 non-COPD smokers	Caucasian U.S.A.	MMP1 G-1607GG	0.49 vs. 0.48	No association with COPD	24
			MMP9 CA repeat	[a]		
Family-based association study of 127 early-onset COPD pedigrees				NA		
84 COPD patients	85 healthy smokers	Japanese	MMP-9 C-1562T	0.14 vs. 0.15	There was no difference in genotype frequency between COPD patients and controls In the HRCT study, COPD patients with a T-allele (C/T or T/T) showed larger LAA%, and smaller mean-CTv in the upper lung compared to patients without T-alleles (C/C)	25

Note: Allele frequencies refer to MMP9-1562T, MMP1-1607GG, MMP12-82G, and MMP12 357Ser.
[a]The MMP9 CA repeat contains a large number of alleles, and there were no associations either considering the complete allelic distribution or collapsing the distribution into small, $(CA)_{\geq16}$, or large, $(CA)_{\leq17}$, repeats.
Abbreviations: MMP, matrix metalloproteinase; COPD, chronic obstructive pulmonary disease; NA, not applicable; DL, diffusing capacity of the lung; VA, alveolar volume; HRCT, high-resolution computed tomography; LAA, law attenuation area.

susceptibility to COPD, and it was reported that the concentration of cathepsin L and cystatin C in bronchoalveolar lavage was elevated in subclinical emphysema (29). However, there are no reports on the association between polymorphisms in these genes and COPD.

It was recently reported that the Gly773Asp variant of the elastin gene confers structural and functional consequences relevant to the pathogenesis of COPD (30). Although this variant was not associated with COPD in this study, it remains an important candidate for COPD that should be definitively tested in a much larger population (due to the rarity of the variant).

B. Xenobiotic Metabolizing Enzymes

Xenobiotic metabolizing enzymes are a class of molecules that play an important role in detoxifying potentially damaging organic compounds found in cigarette smoke. There is considerable interindividual variation in the catalytic efficiencies of these enzymes in many, if not all, human populations. Therefore, these molecules have been studied to determine whether genetically determined deficiencies in xenobiotic metabolism predispose an individual to the development of COPD (1,2).

Microsomal Epoxide Hydrolase

Microsomal epoxide hydrolase (mEH) is an enzyme that plays a critical role in the lung's ability to metabolize highly reactive epoxide intermediates found in cigarette smoke. mEH is expressed in a variety of different cell types including hepatocytes and bronchial epithelial cells.

Two relatively common genetic polymorphisms have been identified in the coding region of the mEH gene (31). Overall, the published data suggest that genetic variation in the mEH gene does modify an individual's risk of COPD in Caucasian populations (1,2). In contrast, mEH genotype was not associated with COPD in a Japanese population (32) or in a Korean population (33). Because it has been shown that the slow metabolizing form of mEH was associated with more severe COPD (32) and was associated with COPD when combined with the GSTM1 null and homozygous GSTP1 isoleucine 105 genotypes (34), it is possible that mEH variants are related to susceptibility to COPD in Asian populations, although to a lesser degree than in Caucasians.

Glutathione S-Transferases

Glutathione (GSH) S-transferases are members of a family of enzymes that play an important role in detoxifying various aromatic hydrocarbons found in cigarette smoke, and can be divided into four main classes, α (A), μ (M), π (P), and θ (T). GSTM1 is expressed in the liver and the lung. Homozygous deletion of the GSTM1 gene occurs in approximately 50% of Caucasians and therefore results in complete absence of this enzyme in these individuals. Homozygous deficiency for GSTM1 was associated with emphysema in Caucasian patients who had lung cancer (35) and severe chronic bronchitis in heavy smokers (36).

GSTP1 is an enzyme expressed in the same cell types as GSTM1, although at a higher level. There is a polymorphism at position 105 ($Ile^{105} \rightarrow$ Val), leading to an increased catalytic activity of the enzyme in vitro. Homozygotes for the isoleucine allele were significantly increased in Japanese patients with COPD compared with the controls [odds ratio (OR)= 3.5] (37), and there was a trend toward association between GSTP1 haplotypes and COPD in a recent Caucasian case–control study (24).

He et al. investigated the association between the polymorphisms of the GSTM1, GSTT1, and GSTP1 gene and accelerated decline rate in FEV_1 in a Caucasian population (38). None of the polymorphisms individually had a significant effect on the decline of lung function. However, a significant association was observed for concurrent deletion of the GSTM1 and GSTT1 genes, and presence of homozygous GSTP1 Ile allele (OR = 2.83, $p = 0.03$). Similarly, the combination of genetic variants including at least one mutant mEH exon-3 allele, GSTM1 null, and homozygosity for the GSTP1 Ile allele was a risk factor for COPD in the Taiwanese population (34). These data suggest that individuals who had a defective genotype for more than one of these genes were at greater risk for susceptibility to COPD than those who had only one defective genotype.

The association between polymorphisms of GSTP1, M1, or T1 was not replicated in a Korean COPD population (33,39). However, these studies may not have had sufficient samples sizes to confirm the association, and it is important to perform other replication studies with larger Asian populations, in a similar manner to the replication study in the Caucasian population (24).

C. Antioxidants

Heme Oxygenase-1

Heme oxygenase (HO) degrades heme to biliverdin and has been demonstrated to provide cellular protection against heme and nonheme-mediated oxidant injury. There is a polymorphism consisting of variable numbers of guanine-thymine (GT) nucleotides within the HO-1 gene promoter. The distribution of the number of (GT) n repeats was trimodal: short alleles (S: < 27 GT), medium alleles (M: 27–32 GT), and long alleles (L: ≥ 33 GT) (40).

An association study in a Japanese population found that the L allele was associated with pulmonary emphysema in smokers, yielding an OR of 2.4 (40). The authors showed that high numbers of GT repeats resulted in decreased in vitro gene expression in response to hydrogen peroxide.

In a recent study, Hirai et al. (41) reported different HO-1 mRNA expression level and HO-1 activity between the S/S genotype and the L/L genotype, and cell lines with the S/S genotype were more resistant to oxidant-induced apoptosis than those with the L/L genotype. These data provide another possible mechanism for association with susceptibility to oxidative stress–mediated diseases.

There was no association found between HO (GT) n alleles and the rate of decline in lung function in smokers in a subsequent study of Caucasian individuals (38). However, Hersh et al. reported recently that the 30 GT allele was significantly associated with COPD in a case–control analysis using an additive genetic model, whereas the 31 GT allele was significantly associated with early-onset COPD in a family-based study in a Caucasian population (24).

Other Antioxidants

GSH is an important protective antioxidant in lung epithelial cells and epithelial lining fluid, and the rate-limiting enzyme for de novo GSH synthesis is gamma-glutamylcysteine synthetase (gamma-GCS). However, there have been no genetic investigations of the association between the pathway including gamma-GCS and COPD.

Nuclear factor, erythroid-derived 2, like 2 (Nrf2) is a redox-sensitive basic leucine zipper protein transcription factor that is involved in the regulation of many detoxification and antioxidant genes. It was recently reported that disruption of the Nrf2 gene in mice led to earlier-onset and more extensive cigarette smoke–induced emphysema than that was found in wild-type littermates (42). This study indicates that Nrf2 is a strong candidate susceptibility gene for COPD.

D. Inflammatory Mediators

Vitamin D Binding Protein

Vitamin D binding protein (VDBP) is a protein secreted by the liver, which is able to bind vitamin D, extracellular actin, and endotoxin. VDBP enhances the chemotactic activity of two complement factors (C5a and C5a des-Arg) for neutrophils by one to two orders of magnitude (43). In addition, VDBP can be converted to a potent macrophage-activating factor (44). Thus, besides its vitamin D binding function, VDBP could have important influences on the intensity of the inflammatory reaction in the lung in response to cigarette smoke.

There are three major isoforms of this protein termed 1S, 1F, and 2, and these isoforms are due to two common substitutions in exon 11 of the VDBP gene. It was shown that individuals who had one or two copies of allele 2 were shown to be protected against COPD and that 1F homozygous Caucasian individuals had an increased risk of developing COPD (1,2).

However, no association of this genotype with accelerated decline of lung function was found in a more recent study with another Caucasian population (1,2). This association was also reported in a Japanese population (45), and was replicated in a study with another Japanese population (46). It was also reported that the 1F and 2 alleles are associated with sputum hypersecretion (47), which might also increase the risk of developing COPD (48).

Tumor Necrosis Factor

Tumor necrosis factor α (TNFα) and TNFβ (lymphotoxin) are proinflammatory cytokines that have many effects of relevance to the pathogenesis of COPD, e.g., neutrophil release from the bone marrow and neutrophil activation.

Fujita et al. reported that mice overexpressing TNFα in alveolar type II cells showed an increase in lung volumes and a decrease in elastic recoil characteristic of emphysema (49). Churg et al. also reported that control mice demonstrated increases in gene expression of TNFα, macrophage inflammatory protein-1 and -2 two hours after smoke exposure, and also demonstrated increases in lavage neutrophils, macrophages, desmosine (a measure of elastin breakdown), and hydroxyproline (a measure of collagen breakdown) at 24 hours, whereas TNFα-receptor knockout (RKO) mice did not. They concluded that TNFα is central to acute smoke-induced inflammation and resulting connective tissue breakdown, the precursor of emphysema (50).

Elevated TNFα was found in bronchoalveolar lavage (BAL) fluid, bronchial biopsy specimens, and induced sputum of patients with COPD (51). It was also observed that TNFα (52) and soluble TNFα receptors (53) were increased in the peripheral blood of COPD patients, which implies an association with systemic inflammation in COPD. A recent in vitro study suggested that metalloproteases mediate cigarette smoke–induced inflammation via the release of TNFα from macrophages (54).

The TNFα and TNFβ genes contain several polymorphisms including a G → A transition in the TNFα gene promoter (TNFα G-308A) and an A → G transition in the first intron of the TNFβ gene (TNFβ A252G). These polymorphisms have been shown to be associated with the level of TNFα and TNFβ production in vitro.

An association of the TNFα-308A allele with COPD was found in a Taiwanese population (55). The prevalence of the TNFα-308A allele was considerably increased in the patients compared with the controls, yielding an OR of 11.1 for chronic bronchitis. Sakao et al. reported in 2001 that TNFα-308∗1/2 alleles are significantly associated with the presence of smoking-related COPD in a Japanese population (56). Sakao et al. also reported in 2002 that the TNFα-308∗1/2 allele frequency tended to be associated with severity of emphysema evaluated with CT-scan; however, this was not statistically significant (57).

In contrast, Ishii et al. reported that no association of the -308A allele with COPD was found in a study of 53 physician diagnosed COPD patients and 65 controls from the Japanese population (58), and Hegab et al. also reported that no association was observed between -308A allele and COPD in another Japanese population (59).

Studies of Caucasian populations have found no association of TNFα-308A with COPD or rate of decline of lung function (1,2). A study of a Caucasian population from the Netherlands also reported that no associa-tion was found between TNFα-308A with COPD (60), although these authors did find an association of COPD with the presence of the A allele of another TNFα polymorphism (TNFα G489A). However, Hersh et al. reported recently that significant associations with quantitative and qualitative COPD-related phenotypes were found for the TNFα-308G >A polymorphism in the Boston Early-Onset COPD Study families; but no association was found in their case–control population (24).

Therefore, we believe that there is a need to investigate the association between the -308A allele and the other SNPs of TNF and COPD in a much larger populations of both Caucasians and Asians. We have summarized the previous reports on the association between polymorphisms in TNF genes and COPD or related phenotypes in Table 3 (24,55–58,60–65).

Interleukin-1 Complex

The interleukin (IL)-1 family consists of two proinflammatory cytokines, IL-1α and IL-1β, and a naturally occurring anti-inflammatory agent, the IL-1 receptor antagonist (IL1RN). IL1RN is a protein that binds to the IL-1 receptor with the same affinity as IL-1 but does not possess agonist activity and therefore acts as a competitive inhibitor of IL-1. It was recently reported that chronic production of IL-1β in respiratory epithelial cells of adult transgenic mice causes lung inflammation, enlargement of distal air-spaces, mucus metaplasia, and airway fibrosis in the adult mouse (66).

The IL-1β gene (IL1B) has an SNP in the promoter region (C-511T), and the IL1RN gene has a polymorphic site in intron 2 containing two to six repeats of an 86 base pair sequence. The *IL1B* C-511T polymorphism has been associated with plasma levels of IL1B and IL1RN (67).

Individual IL-1 genotypes were not associated with rate of decline of lung function in Caucasian smokers. However, there was a significant influ-ence of combinations of IL1RN/IL1B alleles in these individuals (68). A smaller study in a Japanese population found no association with indivi-dual IL1B and IL1RN genotypes and COPD (58), and this result was replicated with another Japanese population (59). In the same study, Hegab et al. also showed that the distributions of the IL1B haplotype (-31 T/C:+3954 C/T) were significantly different between the COPD patients and the controls in the Egyptian population.

Table 3 Summary of Association Studies of TNFα and TNFβ Polymorphisms

Cases	Controls	Population	Polymorphism	Allele frequency: cases vs. controls	Result	References
42 chronic bronchitis patients	42 matched controls	Taiwanese	TNFα G-308A	0.19 vs. 0.02	Frequency of A allele increased in patients. OR for AA+AG vs. GG = 11.1	55
86 COPD patients	63 non-COPD smokers and 199 blood donors	Caucasian (U.K.)	TNFα G-308A	0.15 vs. 0.15	No association with COPD, FEV$_1$, FEV$_1$/VC, K$_{CO}$, DL$_{CO}$	61
106 COPD patients	99 non-COPD smokers	Caucasian (Ireland)	TNFα G-308A	0.24 vs. 0.22	No association with COPD or FEV$_1$. AA homozygotes had ↓ bronchodilator response and ↑ mortality due to respiratory failure	62
53 COPD patients	65 non-COPD smokers	Japanese	TNFα G-308A	0.01 vs. 0.01	No association with COPD	58
66 COPD patients	45 nonobstructive pulmonary disease patients	Caucasian (Italy)	TNFα G-308A TNFβ A252G	0.11 vs. 0.18 0.28 vs. 0.29	No association of either polymorphism with COPD	63
106 COPD patients	110 non-COPD smokers	Japanese	TNFα G-308A	0.16 vs. 0.08	A allele increased in patients. OR for AA+AG vs. GG = 2.6	56

Cases	Controls	Population	Polymorphism	Allele frequencies	Results	Ref.
283 smokers with rapid decline of lung function	308 smokers with no decline in lung function	Caucasian (North America)	TNFα G-308A TNFβ A252G	0.19 vs. 0.18 0.33 vs. 0.36	No association of either polymorphism with rapid decline of lung function	64
169 COPD patients	358 healthy blood donors	Caucasian (Holland)	TNFα G-376A TNFα G-308A TNFα G-238A TNFα G489A	0.01 vs. 0.01 0.16 vs. 0.16 0.04 vs. 0.03 0.13 vs. 0.09	For G489A and COPD, OR for AG vs. GG = 1.9. For G489A and COPD without emphysema, OR for AG vs. GG = 1.9.	60
44 patients with severe emphysema	40 patients with mild/moderate emphysema	Japanese	TNFα G-308A	0.19 vs. 0.10	No association with emphysema assessed by CT-scan	57
63 COPD patients	86 non-COPD smokers	Caucasian (Italy)	TNFα G-308A TNFβ A252G	0.07 vs. 0.08 0.17 vs. 0.25	No association with COPD	65
Family-based association study of 127 early-onset COPD pedigrees		Caucasian (U.S.A.)	TNFα G-308A	NA	Association with FEV$_1$ ($p = 0.002$) and FEV$_1$/FVC ($p = 0.002$)	24

Note: Allele frequencies refer to TNFα-308A, TNFβ+252G, TNF376A, TNFα-238A, and TNFα+489A.

Abbreviations: TNF, tumor necrosis factor; OR, odds ratio; NA, not applicable; COPD, chronic obstructive pulmonary disease; FEV, forced expiratory volume at one second.

Interleukin-13 and Its Receptor

Targeted expression of IL-13 in the adult murine lung has been shown to cause emphysema, elevated mucus production, and inflammation reminiscent of human COPD (69). IL-13 operates through the IL-13 receptor, which is composed of one IL-4 receptor α (IL4RA) subunit and either a low-affinity IL13RA1 or a high-affinity IL13RA2 subunit.

A study found an association of a promoter polymorphism (C-1055T) of IL-13 with COPD in a Caucasian population (70). Another recent study suggested the IL4RA 551ArgArg genotype was associated with rapid decline of lung function (OR = 2.24) (71). There was no association between SNPs in IL-13 and COPD in a Japanese population and an Egyptian population (72).

Lanone et al. compared the remodeling and inflammatory effects of an IL-13 transgene in lungs of wild-type, MMP9-deficient, or MMP12-deficient mice and showed that IL-13 acts via MMP9 and MMP12 to induce alveolar enlargement, respiratory failure, and death (73). Therefore, not only SNPs in one gene (e.g., IL-13) but also gene–gene interaction studies (e.g., interaction between IL-13 and MMPs) might also be important avenues of research in the future.

Interleukin-10

IL-10 is an immunoregulatory cytokine produced by many cell types, and its main biological function is to inhibit the production of a variety of proinflammatory mediators. In addition, IL-10 may regulate the balance between proteases and antiproteases produced by airway macrophages. Studies have found that airway IL-10 level was significantly lower in asthma and COPD patients and healthy smokers compared with healthy nonsmokers (74).

Polymorphisms in the IL-10 promoter could affect the level of IL-10 expression (75). Seifart et al. reported that in comparison with an age-, sex-, and smoking-matched control group, COPD patients had a significant increase in genotypes carrying the G allele of the IL-10–1082 A/G polymorphism (76). Burgess et al. also reported that a statistically significant difference in decline in lung function was related to IL-10 SNP at position 1668 in 1204 firefighters (77).

Surfactant Proteins

Surfactant proteins contribute to immune and inflammatory regulation within the lung. It was reported that increased metalloproteinase activity, oxidant production, and emphysema were observed in surfactant protein D gene–inactivated mice (78). Another group reported that sequential targeted deficiency of SP-A and -D leads to progressive alveolar lipoproteinosis and emphysema (79). Glasser et al. reported that SP-C-deficient

(SP-C -/-) mice developed a severe pulmonary disorder associated with emphysema and pneumonitis (80).

Guo et al. have shown that variants in the surfactant protein genes A and B were associated with COPD in a Mexican population (81). One of these variants (B1580) changes the encoded amino acid from a threonine to a serine and results in the elimination of a potential N-linked glycosylation site. One of the same genetic variants in the surfactant B gene (D2S388_5) was also associated with COPD in a case–control study by Hersh et al. (24).

Transforming Growth Factor-β1

Transforming growth factor-β1 (TGFβ1) has anti-inflammatory properties and prorepair properties, i.e., it increases elastin and collagen synthesis after inflammation (82).

It was reported that loss of activation of latent TGFβ1 causes pulmonary emphysema in mice (83). De Boer et al. reported that twofold higher levels of TGFβ1 mRNA and protein were observed in bronchiolar and alveolar epithelium as compared with subjects without COPD and the epithelial expression of TGFβ1 mRNA and protein correlated with the number of intraepithelial macrophages, and suggested a role for TGFβ1 1 in recruiting macrophages into the airway epithelium in COPD (84).

Three association studies show that the Leu10 or -509C variants of TGFβ1 were associated with COPD in the United States (85), New Zealand (86), and China (87). Because genetic linkage analysis also showed that genetic variants in or near the TGFβ1 gene influence the pathogenesis of COPD among cigarette smokers (85), TGFβ1 is a strong candidate susceptibility gene for COPD.

E. Mucociliary Clearance

The rate at which particulate matter is cleared from the lungs is highly variable between individuals (88). The tracheobronchial clearance rate of 6 to 7 μm particles was studied in nine pairs of MZ and nine pairs of DZ twins (89). The intrapair correlation in clearance rates was significantly higher in the MZ twins versus the DZ twins, suggesting that genetic factors may affect an individual's mucociliary clearance rate. This may have important implications for an individual's cumulative exposure to the compounds found in cigarette smoke.

Cystic Fibrosis Transmembrane Regulator

The cystic fibrosis transmembrane conductance regulator (CFTR) forms a chloride channel at the apical surface of airway epithelial cells and is involved in the control of airway secretions. Mutations in the *CFTR* gene were identified as the cause of cystic fibrosis (CF) in 1989. The most frequent CF-causing variant is ΔF508, and heterozygosity for this mutation was increased in patients who had disseminated bronchiectasis (90,91), and in patients who had "bronchial hypersecretion." The prevalence of the most frequent CF-causing variant (ΔF508) was not increased in patients who had chronic bronchitis (91). Other *CFTR* mutations were increased in patients who had disseminated bronchiectasis and normal sweat chloride levels. A variable length thymine repeat in intron 8 of the *CFTR* gene (IVS8) has an allele (IVS8-5T) that results in reduced *CFTR* gene expression. Studies of IVS8-5T as a risk factor for COPD have yielded conflicting results (92,93).

Tzetis et al. screened patients with obstructive lung diseases for variants in the whole *CFTR*-coding region (94). The study compared 12 COPD patients with 52 controls, both groups from the Greek population. There was no significant increase in CF-causing mutations in the patients versus the controls. However, the frequency of the methionine allele of the Met470Val polymorphism was increased in the patients (71%) compared with the controls (36%). Divac et al. reported that the Arg75Gln polymorphism in the *CFTR* gene was significantly overrepresented in COPD patients, and all patients carrying 75Gln were homozygous for the Val470 allele (95). The Met470 variant is associated with increased CFTR chloride channel activity compared with the Val variant.

Other Genes

Matsushita et al. showed in a Japanese population that genetic variations in β-defensin-1, an endogenous antimicrobial peptide in the airway, may define a high-risk subgroup of COPD patients, where the component of chronic bronchitis is predominant (96).

Hegab et al. reported that the +79 C/G polymorphism of the β2-adrenoceptor and its haplotypes may be involved in the pathogenesis of COPD in Egyptians (72).

III. Future Directions of Association Studies in COPD

Although there is clear evidence of a genetic contribution to the pathogenesis of COPD, few specific genes have been convincingly implicated to date. Candidate genes can be selected based on previous genetic linkage analysis results, e.g., the TGFβ1 gene (85). However, the reported studies have been mostly limited to known biologically plausible candidates. To select appropriate candidate genes, it is necessary to search the entire human genome for disease-causing genes with linkage analysis for late-onset general COPD with populations of various races. In fact, as we have shown in this chapter, ethnic group–specific genetic risk factors possibly exist in some genes, e.g., TNFα and VDBP.

Most association studies were too small in size to be powerful enough to detect genes of modest effect, and these studies have been also criticized because of a lack of replication (97). Meta-analyses and replication studies should be performed to check the results of the previous association studies.

Now the Human Genome Project accomplished its goal of sequencing one human genome, and population-specific genetic variation is being investigated by the International HapMap Project (98); genome-wide association studies should be performed by genotyping SNPs across the whole genome, not only for a Caucasian population but also for Asian and African populations. Because so many noncoding RNA transcripts have been found recently to be functional in, e.g., transcriptional regulation (99), it becomes more important to genotype SNPs covering not only the protein-coding region but also intergenic regions. In this way, we believe that the role of genetic risk factors in the development of COPD will be elucidated.

References

1. Sandford AJ, Silverman EK. Chronic obstructive pulmonary disease. 1: Susceptibility factors for COPD the genotype-environment interaction. Thorax 2002; 57(8):736–741.
2. Molfino NA. Genetics of COPD. Chest 2004; 125(5):1929–1940.
3. Pierce JA. Antitrypsin and emphysema. Perspective and prospects. JAMA 1988; 259(19):2890–2895.
4. Kueppers F, Briscoe WA, Bearn AG. Hereditary deficiency of α_1-antitrypsin. Science 1964; 146:1678–1679.
5. Brantly M, Nukiwa T, Crystal RG. Molecular basis of α_1-antitrypsin deficiency. Am J Med 1988; 84(6A):13–31.
6. Seyama K, Nukiwa T, Souma S, et al. Alpha 1-antitrypsin-deficient variant Siiyama [Ser53(TCC) to Phe53(TTC)] is prevalent in Japan. Status of alpha 1-antitrypsin deficiency in Japan. Am J Respir Crit Care Med 1995; 152(6 Pt 1): 2119–2126.
7. Brantly ML, Paul LD, Miller BH, et al. Clinical features and history of the destructive lung disease associated with α_1-antitrypsin deficiency of adults with pulmonary symptoms. Am Rev Respir Dis 1988; 138(2):327–336.
8. Seersholm N, Kok-Jensen A, Dirksen A. Survival of patients with severe α_1-antitrypsin deficiency with special reference to non-index cases. Thorax 1994; 49(7):695–698.
9. Novoradovsky A, Brantly ML, Waclawiw MA, et al. Endothelial nitric oxide synthase as a potential susceptibility gene in the pathogenesis of emphysema in alpha 1-antitrypsin deficiency. Am J Respir Cell Mol Biol 1999; 20(3):441–447.
10. Rodriguez F, de la Roza C, Jardi R, et al. Glutathione S-transferase P1 and lung function in patients with alpha1-antitrypsin deficiency and COPD. Chest 2005; 127(5):1537–1543.

11. Seersholm N, Wilcke JT, Kok-Jensen A, et al. Risk of hospital admission for obstructive pulmonary disease in alpha(1)-antitrypsin heterozygotes of phenotype PiMZ. Am J Respir Crit Care Med 2000; 161(1):81–84.

12. Dahl M, Nordestgaard BG, Lange P, et al. Molecular diagnosis of intermediate and severe alpha(1)-antitrypsin deficiency: MZ individuals with chronic obstructive pulmonary disease may have lower lung function than MM individuals. Clin Chem 2001; 47(1):56–62.

13. Dahl M, Tybjaerg-Hansen A, Lange P, et al. Change in lung function and morbidity from chronic obstructive pulmonary disease in alpha1-antitrypsin MZ heterozygotes: a longitudinal study of the general population. Ann Intern Med 2002; 136(4):270–279.

14. Silva GE, Sherrill DL, Guerra S, et al. A longitudinal study of alpha1-antitrypsin phenotypes and decline in FEV_1 in a community population. Chest 2003; 123(5):1435–1440.

15. Hersh CP, Dahl M, Ly NP, et al. Chronic obstructive pulmonary disease in alpha1-antitrypsin PI MZ heterozygotes: a meta-analysis. Thorax 2004; 59(10):843–849.

16. Dahl M, Hersh CP, Ly NP, et al. The protease inhibitor PI*S allele and COPD: a meta-analysis. Eur Respir J 2005; 26(1):67–76.

17. Chappell S, Guetta-Baranes T, Batowski K, et al. Haplotypes of the alpha-1 antitrypsin gene in healthy controls and Z deficiency patients. Hum Mutat 2004; 24(6):535–536.

18. D'Armiento J, Dalal SS, Okada Y, et al. Collagenase expression in the lungs of transgenic mice causes pulmonary emphysema. Cell 1992; 71(6):955–961.

19. Hautamaki RD, Kobayashi DK, Senior RM, et al. Requirement for macrophage elastase for cigarette smoke-induced emphysema in mice. Science 1997; 277(5334):2002–2004.

20. Segura-Valdez L, Pardo A, Gaxiola M, et al. Upregulation of gelatinases A and B, collagenases 1 and 2, and increased parenchymal cell death in COPD. Chest 2000; 117(3):684–694.

21. Minematsu N, Nakamura H, Tateno H, et al. Genetic polymorphism in matrix metalloproteinase-9 and pulmonary emphysema. Biochem Biophys Res Commun 2001; 289(1):116–119.

22. Joos L, He JQ, Shepherdson MB, et al. The role of matrix metalloproteinase polymorphisms in the rate of decline in lung function. Hum Mol Genet 2002; 11(5):569–576.

23. Zhou M, Huang SG, Wan HY, et al. Genetic polymorphism in matrix metalloproteinase-9 and the susceptibility to chronic obstructive pulmonary disease in Han population of south China. Chin Med J (Engl) 2004; 117(10):1481–1484.

24. Hersh CP, Demeo DL, Lange C, et al. Attempted replication of reported chronic obstructive pulmonary disease candidate gene associations. Am J Respir Cell Mol Biol 2005; 33(1):71–78. Epub 2005, Apr 2007.

25. Ito I, Nagai S, Handa T, et al. Matrix metalloproteinase-9 promoter polymorphism associated with upper lung dominant emphysema. Am J Respir Crit Care Med 2005; 172(11):1378–1382.

26. Hirano K, Sakamoto T, Uchida Y, et al. Tissue inhibitor of metalloproteinases-2 gene polymorphisms in chronic obstructive pulmonary disease. Eur Respir J 2001; 18(5):748–752.

27. Hegab AE, Sakamoto T, Uchida Y, et al. Association analysis of tissue inhibitor of metalloproteinase2 gene polymorphisms with COPD in Egyptians. Respir Med 2005; 99(1):107–110.

28. Ishii T, Matsuse T, Teramoto S, et al. Association between alpha-1-antichymotrypsin polymorphism and susceptibility to chronic obstructive pulmonary disease. Eur J Clin Invest 2000; 30(6):543–548.

29. Takeyabu K, Betsuyaku T, Nishimura M, et al. Cysteine proteinases and cystatin C in bronchoalveolar lavage fluid from subjects with subclinical emphysema. Eur Respir J 1998; 12(5):1033–1039.

30. Kelleher CM, Silverman EK, Broekelmann T, et al. A functional mutation in the terminal exon of elastin in severe, early-onset chronic obstructive pulmonary disease. Am J Respir Cell Mol Biol 2005; 33(4):355–362. Epub 2005, Aug 2004.

31. Hassett C, Aicher L, Sidhu JS, et al. Human microsomal epoxide hydrolase: genetic polymorphism and functional expression in vitro of amino acid variants. Hum Mol Genet 1994; 3(3):421–428.

32. Yoshikawa M, Hiyama K, Ishioka S, et al. Microsomal epoxide hydrolase genotypes and chronic obstructive pulmonary disease in Japanese. Int J Mol Med 2000; 5(1):49–53.

33. Yim JJ, Park GY, Lee CT, et al. Genetic susceptibility to chronic obstructive pulmonary disease in Koreans: combined analysis of polymorphic genotypes for microsomal epoxide hydrolase and glutathione S-transferase M1 and T1. Thorax 2000; 55(2):121–125.

34. Cheng SL, Yu CJ, Chen CJ, et al. Genetic polymorphism of epoxide hydrolase and glutathione S-transferase in COPD. Eur Respir J 2004; 23(6):818–824.

35. Harrison DJ, Cantlay AM, Rae F, et al. Frequency of glutathione S-transferase M1 deletion in smokers with emphysema and lung cancer. Hum Exp Toxicol 1997; 16(7):356–360.

36. Baranova H, Perriot J, Albuisson E, et al. Peculiarities of the GSTM1 0/0 genotype in French heavy smokers with various types of chronic bronchitis. Hum Genet 1997; 99(6):822–826.

37. Ishii T, Matsuse T, Teramoto S, et al. Glutathione S-transferase P1 (GSTP1) polymorphism in patients with chronic obstructive pulmonary disease. Thorax 1999; 54(8):693–696.

38. He JQ, Ruan J, Connett JE, et al. Antioxidant gene polymorphisms and susceptibility to a rapid decline in lung function in smokers. Am J Respir Crit Care Med 2002; 166(3):323–328.

39. Yim JJ, Yoo CG, Lee CT, et al. Lack of association between glutathione S-transferase P1 polymorphism and COPD in Koreans. Lung 2002; 180(2):119–125.

40. Yamada N, Yamaya M, Okinaga S, et al. Microsatellite polymorphism in the heme oxygenase-1 gene promoter is associated with susceptibility to emphysema. Am J Hum Genet 2000; 66(1):187–195.

41. Hirai H, Kubo H, Yamaya M, et al. Microsatellite polymorphism in heme oxygenase-1 gene promoter is associated with susceptibility to oxidant-induced apoptosis in lymphoblastoid cell lines. Blood 2003; 102(5):1619–1621. Epub 2003, May 1611.

42. Rangasamy T, Cho CY, Thimmulappa RK, et al. Genetic ablation of Nrf2 enhances susceptibility to cigarette smoke-induced emphysema in mice. J Clin Invest 2004; 114(9):1248–1259.

43. Kew RR, Webster RO. Gc-globulin (vitamin D-binding protein) enhances the neutrophil chemotactic activity of C5a and C5a des Arg. J Clin Invest 1988; 82(1):364–369.
44. Yamamoto N, Homma S. Vitamin D-binding protein (group-specific component) is a precursor for the macrophage-activating signal factor from lysophosphatidylcholine-treated lymphocytes. Proc Natl Acad Sci USA 1991; 88(19):8539–8543.
45. Ishii T, Keicho N, Teramoto S, et al. Association of Gc-globulin variation with susceptibility to COPD and diffuse panbronchiolitis. Eur Respir J 2001; 18(5): 753–757.
46. Ito I, Nagai S, Hoshino Y, et al. Risk and severity of COPD is associated with the group-specific component of serum globulin 1F allele. Chest 2004; 125(1):63–70.
47. Laufs J, Andrason H, Sigvaldason A, et al. Association of vitamin D binding protein variants with chronic mucus hypersecretion in Iceland. Am J Pharmacogenomics 2004; 4(1):63–68.
48. Vestbo J, Prescott E, Lange P. Association of chronic mucus hypersecretion with FEV$_1$ decline and chronic obstructive pulmonary disease morbidity. Copenhagen City Heart Study Group. Am J Respir Crit Care Med 1996; 153(5): 1530–1535.
49. Fujita M, Shannon JM, Irvin CG, et al. Overexpression of tumor necrosis factor-alpha produces an increase in lung volumes and pulmonary hypertension. Am J Physiol Lung Cell Mol Physiol 2001; 280(1):L39–L49.
50. Churg A, Dai J, Tai H, et al. Tumor necrosis factor-alpha is central to acute cigarette smoke-induced inflammation and connective tissue breakdown. Am J Respir Crit Care Med 2002; 166(6):849–854.
51. Keatings VM, Collins PD, Scott DM, et al. Differences in interleukin-8 and tumor necrosis factor-alpha in induced sputum from patients with chronic obstructive pulmonary disease or asthma. Am J Respir Crit Care Med 1996; 153(2):530–534.
52. Gan WQ, Man SF, Senthilselvan A, et al. Association between chronic obstructive pulmonary disease and systemic inflammation: a systematic review and a meta-analysis. Thorax 2004; 59(7):574–580.
53. Vernooy JH, Kucukaycan M, Jacobs JA, et al. Local and systemic inflammation in patients with chronic obstructive pulmonary disease: soluble tumor necrosis factor receptors are increased in sputum. Am J Respir Crit Care Med 2002; 166(9):1218–1224.
54. Churg A, Wang RD, Tai H, et al. Macrophage metalloelastase mediates acute cigarette smoke-induced inflammation via tumor necrosis factor-alpha release. Am J Respir Crit Care Med 2003; 167(8):1083–1089.
55. Huang SL, Su CH, Chang SC. Tumor necrosis factor-α gene polymorphism in chronic bronchitis. Am J Respir Crit Care Med 1997; 156(5):1436–1439.
56. Sakao S, Tatsumi K, Igari H, et al. Association of tumor necrosis factor alpha gene promoter polymorphism with the presence of chronic obstructive pulmonary disease. Am J Respir Crit Care Med 2001; 163(2):420–422.
57. Sakao S, Tatsumi K, Igari H, et al. Association of tumor necrosis factor-α gene promoter polymorphism with low attenuation areas on high-resolution CT in patients with COPD. Chest 2002; 122(2):416–420.

58. Ishii T, Matsuse T, Teramoto S, et al. Neither IL-1β, IL-1 receptor antagonist, nor TNF-α polymorphisms are associated with susceptibility to COPD. Respir Med 2000; 94(9):847–851.

59. Hegab AE, Sakamoto T, Saitoh W, et al. Polymorphisms of TNFalpha, IL1beta, and IL1RN genes in chronic obstructive pulmonary disease. Biochem Biophys Res Commun 2005; 329(4):1246–1252.

60. Kucukaycan M, Van Krugten M, Pennings HJ, et al. Tumor necrosis factor-alpha +489G/A gene polymorphism is associated with chronic obstructive pulmonary disease. Respir Res 2002; 3(1):29.

61. Higham MA, Pride NB, Alikhan A, et al. Tumour necrosis factor-alpha gene promoter polymorphism in chronic obstructive pulmonary disease. Eur Respir J 2000; 15(2):281–284.

62. Keatings VM, Cave SJ, Henry MJ, et al. A polymorphism in the tumor necrosis factor-alpha gene promoter region may predispose to a poor prognosis in COPD. Chest 2000; 118(4):971–975.

63. Patuzzo C, Gile LS, Zorzetto M, et al. Tumor necrosis factor gene complex in COPD and disseminated bronchiectasis. Chest 2000; 117(5):1353–1358.

64. Sandford AJ, Chagani T, Weir TD, et al. Susceptibility genes for rapid decline of lung function in the Lung Health Study. Am J Respir Crit Care Med 2001; 163(2):469–473.

65. Ferrarotti I, Zorzetto M, Beccaria M, et al. Tumour necrosis factor family genes in a phenotype of COPD associated with emphysema. Eur Respir J 2003; 21(3):444–449.

66. Lappalainen U, Whitsett JA, Wert SE, et al. Interleukin-1beta causes pulmonary inflammation, emphysema, and airway remodeling in the adult murine lung. Am J Respir Cell Mol Biol 2005; 32(4):311–318. Epub 2005, Jan 2024.

67. Hurme M, Santtila S. IL-1 receptor antagonist (IL-1RA) plasma levels are co-ordinately regulated by both IL-1RA and IL-1β genes. Eur J Immunol 1998; 28(8):2598–2602.

68. Joos L, McIntyre L, Ruan J, et al. Association of IL-1β and IL-1 receptor antagonist haplotypes with rate of decline in lung function in smokers. Thorax 2001; 56(11):863–866.

69. Zheng T, Zhu Z, Wang Z, et al. Inducible targeting of IL-13 to the adult lung causes matrix metalloproteinase- and cathepsin-dependent emphysema. J Clin Invest 2000; 106(9):1081–1093.

70. van der Pouw Kraan TC, Kucukaycan M, Bakker AM, et al. Chronic obstructive pulmonary disease is associated with the -1055 IL-13 promoter polymorphism. Genes Immun 2002; 3(7):436–439.

71. He JQ, Connett JE, Anthonisen NR, et al. Polymorphisms in the IL13, IL13RA1, and IL4RA genes and rate of decline in lung function in smokers. Am J Respir Cell Mol Biol 2003; 28(3):379–385.

72. Hegab AE, Sakamoto T, Saitoh W, et al. Polymorphisms of IL4, IL13, and ADRB2 genes in COPD. Chest 2004; 126(6):1832–1839.

73. Lanone S, Zheng T, Zhu Z, et al. Overlapping and enzyme-specific contributions of matrix metalloproteinases-9 and -12 in IL-13-induced inflammation and remodeling. J Clin Invest 2002; 110(4):463–474.

74. Takanashi S, Hasegawa Y, Kanehira Y, et al. Interleukin-10 level in sputum is reduced in bronchial asthma, COPD and in smokers. Eur Respir J 1999; 14(2):309–314.

75. Eskdale J, Gallagher G, Verweij CL, et al. Interleukin 10 secretion in relation to human IL-10 locus haplotypes. Proc Natl Acad Sci USA 1998; 95(16): 9465–9470.

76. Seifart C, Dempfle A, Plagens A, et al. TNF-alpha-, TNF-beta-, IL-6-, and IL-10-promoter polymorphisms in patients with chronic obstructive pulmonary disease. Tissue Antigens 2005; 65(1):93–100.

77. Burgess JL, Fierro MA, Lantz RC, et al. Longitudinal decline in lung function: evaluation of interleukin-10 genetic polymorphisms in firefighters. J Occup Environ Med 2004; 46(10):1013–1022.

78. Wert SE, Yoshida M, LeVine AM, et al. Increased metalloproteinase activity, oxidant production, and emphysema in surfactant protein D gene-inactivated mice. Proc Natl Acad Sci USA 2000; 97(11):5972–5977.

79. Hawgood S, Ochs M, Jung A, et al. Sequential targeted deficiency of SP-A and -D leads to progressive alveolar lipoproteinosis and emphysema. Am J Physiol Lung Cell Mol Physiol 2002; 283(5):L1002–L1010.

80. Glasser SW, Detmer EA, Ikegami M, et al. Pneumonitis and emphysema in sp-C gene targeted mice. J Biol Chem 2003; 278(16):14291–14298. Epub 12003, Jan 14297.

81. Guo X, Lin HM, Lin Z, et al. Surfactant protein gene A, B, and D marker alleles in chronic obstructive pulmonary disease of a Mexican population. Eur Respir J 2001; 18(3):482–490.

82. Bartram U, Speer CP. The role of transforming growth factor beta in lung development and disease. Chest 2004; 125(2):754–765.

83. Morris DG, Huang X, Kaminski N, et al. Loss of integrin alpha(v)beta6-mediated TGF-beta activation causes Mmp12-dependent emphysema. Nature 2003; 422(6928):169–173.

84. de Boer WI, van Schadewijk A, Sont JK, et al. Transforming growth factor β1 and recruitment of macrophages and mast cells in airways in chronic obstructive pulmonary disease. Am J Respir Crit Care Med 1998; 158(6):1951–1957.

85. Celedon JC, Lange C, Raby BA, et al. The transforming growth factor-beta1 (TGFβ1) gene is associated with chronic obstructive pulmonary disease (COPD). Hum Mol Genet 2004; 13(15):1649–1656. Epub 2004, Jun 1642.

86. Wu L, Chau J, Young RP, et al. Transforming growth factor-beta1 genotype and susceptibility to chronic obstructive pulmonary disease. Thorax 2004; 59(2):126–129.

87. Su ZG, Wen FQ, Feng YL, et al. Transforming growth factor-beta1 gene polymorphisms associated with chronic obstructive pulmonary disease in Chinese population. Acta Pharmacol Sin 2005; 26(6):714–720.

88. Philipson K, Falk R, Camner P. Long-term lung clearance in humans studied with Teflon particles labeled with chromium-51. Exp Lung Res 1985; 9(1–2): 31–42.

89. Camner P, Philipson K, Friberg L. Tracheobronchial clearance in twins. Arch Environ Health 1972; 24(2):82–87.

90. Poller W, Faber JP, Scholz S, et al. Sequence analysis of the cystic fibrosis gene in patients with disseminated bronchiectatic lung disease. Application in the identification of a cystic fibrosis patient with atypical clinical course. Klinische Wochenschrift 1991; 69(14):657–663.

91. Gervais R, Lafitte JJ, Dumur V, et al. Sweat chloride and ΔF508 mutation in chronic bronchitis or bronchiectasis. Lancet 1993; 342(8877):997.

92. Pignatti PF, Bombieri C, Benetazzo M, et al. CFTR gene variant IVS8–5T in disseminated bronchiectasis. Am J Hum Genet 1996; 58(4):889–892.

93. Bombieri C, Benetazzo M, Saccomani A, et al. Complete mutational screening of the CFTR gene in 120 patients with pulmonary disease. Hum Genet 1998; 103(6):718–722.

94. Tzetis M, Efthymiadou A, Strofalis S, et al. CFTR gene mutations—including three novel nucleotide substitutions—and haplotype background in patients with asthma, disseminated bronchiectasis and chronic obstructive pulmonary disease. Hum Genet 2001; 108(3):216–221.

95. Divac A, Nikolic A, Mitic-Milikic M, et al. High frequency of the R75Q CFTR variation in patients with chronic obstructive pulmonary disease. J Cyst Fibros 2004; 3(3):189–191.

96. Matsushita I, Hasegawa K, Nakata K, et al. Genetic variants of human beta-defensin-1 and chronic obstructive pulmonary disease. Biochem Biophys Res Commun 2002; 291(1):17–22.

97. Ioannidis JP, Ntzani EE, Trikalinos TA, et al. Replication validity of genetic association studies. Nat Genet 2001; 29(3):306–309.

98. Foster MW, Sharp RR. Beyond race: towards a whole-genome perspective on human populations and genetic variation. Nat Rev Genet 2004; 5(10):790–796.

99. Claverie JM. Fewer genes, more noncoding RNA. Science 2005; 309(5740): 1529–1530.

15

β_2-Adrenergic Receptor Polymorphisms and Asthmatic Phenotypes

STEPHEN B. LIGGETT

Departments of Medicine and Physiology,
University of Maryland School of
Medicine,
Baltimore, Maryland, U.S.A.

IAN P. HALL

Division of Therapeutics and Molecular
Medicine, University Hospital of
Nottingham,
Nottingham, U.K.

I. Introduction

β-Agonists are the most often utilized therapeutics for treating asthma, both in the setting of acute bronchoconstriction and as a controller agent to minimize asthma exacerbations. These agents activate β_2-adrenergic receptors (β_2AR) localized to various cell-types in the airway and are a mainstay of treatment based on their bronchodilating effects. Nevertheless, there is extensive inter-individual variability in the response to a β-agonist, of which genetics is thought to account for as much as 50% (1). Furthermore, even in the absence of β-agonist treatment per se, β_2ARs are activated by the endogenous agonist epinephrine, and their expression is altered by pathophysiologic events and other drugs (i.e., corticosteroids). Thus, not withstanding pharmacogenomic considerations, genetic variation of the β_2AR may have impact on asthma, asthma phenotypes and pulmonary function. In this chapter the localization, structure and function of the β_2AR is briefly presented, the known genetic variations and their phenotypes in cells are discussed, and the results of clinical studies ascertaining disease relevance presented.

II. β₂-AR Localization, Structure, and Function

In the lung, β₂AR are localized on airway epithelium, airway smooth muscle, alveolar walls, pulmonary vasculature, and resident and transitory immune cells (2). Clearly relevant to asthma, is the presence of these receptors on airway smooth muscle, where activation evokes relaxation of bronchi that are constricted by virtually any stimuli. Also likely relevant to asthma is epithelial expression where fluid and electrolytic flux and ciliary beat frequency is, in part, regulated by β₂AR. Like other members of the G-protein coupled receptor superfamily, the β₂AR (a member of the large "A group" of receptors) is a membrane bound receptor with its amino-terminus on the exterior of the cell, its carboxy-terminus on the interior, and seven transmembrane spanning (TMS) domains which appear to be α-helices (Fig. 1). Connecting each TMS domain are extracellular and intracellular loops as shown, with a "fourth" loop localized in the cell beginning at the carboxy-terminus of the seventh TMS domain and terminating at a membrane anchoring palmitoylated cysteine. The receptor has three N-linked glycosylation sites: two in the amino-terminus, and one in the second extracellular loop of the receptor, the latter found only in higher order primates (3). Ligand binding (agonist or antagonist) occurs via interactions at specific amino acids in the "core" of the TMS domains. Signaling to the cell interior involves coupling to a G-protein (classically the stimulatory G-protein, G_s) which then acts on effectors such as adenylyl cyclase. β₂AR-G-protein interaction occurs in the cell interior, at intracellular TMS domains 2, 3 and part of the carboxy-tail. In the above scenario, then, β-agonist activation leads to activation of adenylyl cyclase, which converts adenosine tri phosphate to cyclic adenosine mono phosphate (cAMP), the latter activating protein

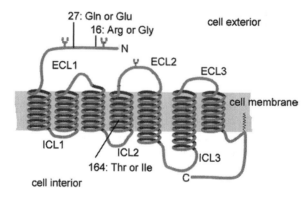

Figure 1   Pictorial representation of the β₂-adrenergic receptors. The extracellular loops, intracellular loops and the α-helices of the transmembrane spanning domains are shown. The approximate location, and the alleles, of the human polymorphisms are indicated.

kinase A (PKA). PKA phosphorylates many intracellular proteins, which in cardiac muscle evokes contractions and in smooth muscle relaxation.

An early model concerning agonist-receptor interaction was a simple lock-and-key switch concept: the receptor was dormant until an agonist fitted perfectly, which then turned-on the receptor by inducing a fixed conformation change. Two newer concepts are relevant in terms of β_2AR polymorphisms and asthma (Fig. 2). First, it is now clear that β_2AR oscillate, in the absence of agonist, to the "active" state (sometimes denoted R*). Agonists serve to stabilize the receptor in R*, neutral antagonists have minimal effect, and inverse agonists move the equilibrium towards the inactive R conformation. It also now appears that receptor conformation(s) "held" by the agonist (denoted here R^{*1}, R^{*2}, etc.) can differ based on the structure of the agonist (4,5). Subtle interactions of drug with the sensitive binding pocket residues can thus potentially provide different stabilized conformations of the receptor. Furthermore, the nature of the conformation does not readily conform to the traditional characterization of agents as full or partial agonists (4,5). A second important concept relevant to pharmacogenetics is that an agonist may stabilize more than one conformation of the β_2AR. As such, a given agonist might evoke several downstream signals, some being advantageous for asthma treatment and others deleterious or limiting bronchodilator efficacy (Fig. 2). Some of these other pathways known to be activated by β_2AR include coupling to G_i, activation of G-protein coupled receptor kinases (GRKs) and mitogen activated protein kinases (MAP kinases), phosphodiesterase redistribution, and β-arrestin recruitment (see below).

Once bound by agonist, most G-protein coupled receptors display a waning of the initial signal over time, which has by consensus been denoted by the term "desensitization" (as opposed to "downregulation"). A very early event in desensitization is phosphorylation of the receptor by GRKs that are substrates for the binding of β-arrestins to the complex, serving to physically impair receptor G-protein interaction. [β-arrestin recruitment is also a "signal" itself, as it serves as a scaffold to bring other proteins into

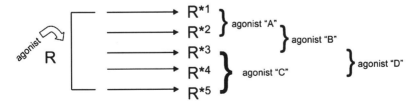

Figure 2   Pleotropic signaling by β-agonists. The unbound receptor (R) is shown to be stabilized by various agonists (denoted A, B, C, D) into various activated conformations (R^{*1}, R^{*2}, etc.). These various states have different downstream effects in the cell.

the microdomain participating in activation of pathways such as activation of MAP kinases (6).] PKA also phosphorylates β_2AR, causing a decrease in G_s coupling and an increase in G_i coupling (7). These early events (fully implemented after < 30 minutes of agonist exposure) may be acting so quickly that the "initial, non-desensitized" physiologic response is never appreciated. However, continued phosphorylation of the receptors by the above two mechanisms does impact the agonist response that is observed even hours after initial exposure (8). Two other processes, though, are at play as agonist exposure reaches approximately two hours and longer: decreased mRNA and degradation of receptor protein. These latter two processes ultimately lead to a loss of net cellular expression of the receptor in the cell, which has been termed "downregulation." Receptor protein degradation involves complex trafficking processes that are dependent on receptor conformation, GRK and β-arrestin action, and other intracellular events that are influenced by the initial trigger, which is agonist occupancy. mRNA changes appear to be somewhat cell-type dependent, but include changes in the rate of transcription, and mRNA stability (9,10). The rate of translation is also affected by the intracellular milieu, and binding proteins to an A/U rich region of the 3'UTR of the gene have been shown to be an important determinant of this process (11).

III. Genetic Variation of the Human β_2-AR

A. Features of the β_2-AR Gene

The β_2AR gene is intronless, localized to chromosome 5q31. The full length of the 5' promoter sequence is not fully appreciated, but likely does not extend past ~3000 bp. Its features are somewhat like those of weak "housekeeping genes," which is consistent with the near ubiquitous expression of the β_2AR on most cell types in the body. The 5'UTR is ~250 bp in length and reporter gene assays have indicated significant control of expression is influenced by this region and adjacent 5' flanking sequences (12). The polyadenylation site of the 3'UTR occurs ~500 bp from the last base of the terminal codon. No alternative start sites or splice variants have been identified, i.e., transcription and subsequent translation of the β_2AR gene produces one receptor. However, a short open reading frame (ORF) within a 5' leader cistron is co-transcribed, resulting in a 19 amino acid peptide, termed the β_2AR upstream peptide (BUP), that partially regulates β_2AR translation (13,14). The human ORF produces a protein of 413 amino acids.

B. β_2-Adrenergic Receptors Variants

Early interrogations of the gene for polymorphisms concentrated on this coding region (15), where three nonsynonymous single nucleotide polymorphisms (SNPs) and five synonymous SNPs were found as compared to a reference DNA sequence. Table 1 shows the location and frequency of the individual polymorphisms and the common diplotypes by ethnic group. The nonsynonymous SNPs correspond to amino acid positions 16 (Arg or Gly), 27 (Gln or Glu) and 164 (Thr or Ile). While there have been some other reports of variations (as abstracts or found in various databases), some have been found only once, and many have not been replicated or verified. Amino acid positions 16 and 27 are in the amino-terminus of the receptor, while 164 is in TMS domain 4 (Fig. 1).

C. In Vitro Effects of β₂-AR Polymorphisms and Haplotypes

The initial approach (16,17) to investigate the relevance of β₂AR polymorphisms and their haplotypes was to build these polymorphic receptors by site-directed mutagenesis and to recombinantly express them in a cell with no background β₂AR (the CHW Chinese hamster fibroblast cell line). Agonist and antagonist binding, coupling to adenylyl cyclase, and cellular trafficking was assessed. This recombinant system was recognized as somewhat artificial, but nevertheless allowed for a direct comparison between the receptors, expressed at the same levels, without the possibility of polymorphisms of other elements of the signal transduction system since the host cell was the same for each stably transfected line. As noted already (Table 1), the positions 16 and 27 SNPs are common, while the 164 is rare. Interestingly, the Arg16/Gln27 was considered the "wild-type" receptor because it was the originally cloned receptor; however, Gly at position 16 is more common, particularly in whites. In these early recombinant studies, all four combinations of these two common SNPs were studied. Subsequently, it was noted that the Arg16/Glu27 variant is very uncommon, so three diplotypes are relevant concerning these amino-terminal polymorphisms. These variations had no effect on ligand affinity or coupling to Gs. However, long-term exposure to the agonist isoproterenol revealed enhanced downregulation (due to enhanced receptor degradation) with diplotypes having Gly at position 16 compared to Arg (17). This was true regardless of the position of 27 allele. The Ile164 polymorphism had decreased agonist-stimulated coupling to Gs and agonist-promoted internalization (16), and a more rapid release of the long-acting β-agonist salmeterol (18) [which binds in TMS domain 4 as well as other regions (19)] under washout conditions. Of note, there were no 5′ or 3′ flanking sequences utilized in these constructs, so any polymorphisms in these regions that occur in the population were not at play. Subsequent studies of human airway smooth muscle cells in primary culture (20) generally recapitulated these downregulation phenotypes, although there was greater variability, some heterozygous genotypes had to be utilized, and undoubtedly polymorphisms in other β₂AR-related genes confounded interpretation. It should also be noted that using airway smooth muscle cells, or mast cells, that others have found somewhat different

Table 1 Localization, Allele Frequencies, and In Vitro Phenotypes of β2-Adrenergic Receptors Coding Block Polymorphism

Nucleotide no.	Alleles	Amino acid no.	Alleles	Frequency %			
				Ca	A-A	As	Allele
46	A or G	16	Arg or Gly	40	50	60	Arg
79	C or G	27	Gln or Glu	40	27	20	Gln
491	C or T	164	Thr or Ile	—	5[a]	—	Ile
Diplotype		*Diplotype*					
	A+C	Arg+Gln		33	55	57	
	A+G	Arg+Glu		<2	<2	<2	
	G+C	Gly+Gln		13	31	30	
	G+G	Gly+Glu		48	6	10	

[a]Heterozygous frequency with likely similar ethnic distribution.

phenotypes, which may be due to the technical aspects of the studies or the cell-type. In human lung mast cells, agonist-promoted functional desensitization of the cAMP response was not different between homozygous Arg16 and homozygous Gly16 cells after 24 hours of exposure to isoproterenol (21). In contrast, like in the recombinant CHW cell system, the Glu27 receptor underwent less desensitization that the Gln27 receptor. Receptor downregulation (i.e., a decrease in receptor expression) was not quantitated. In a study of human airway smooth muscle cells, Shore and colleagues (22) showed that cells expressing at least one Glu27 allele had *enhanced* acute and chronic desensitization of cAMP responses and cell relaxation (measured by magnetic twisting cytometry). There were no differences in the groups when cells were stratified by genotype at position 16. This phenotype was observed with agonist exposures as short as one hour, which is a time point where little downregulation occurs, but other events such as phosphorylation and intracellular trafficking are well underway. Thus the basis for the phenotype observed by magnetic twisting cytometry, with this extent of agonist exposure, is not clear. In a study of human lymphocytes, $β_2$AR signaling was stratified by a 3-locus haplotype, at position 19 of the BUP, and positions 16 and 27 of the receptor (23). The polymorphism at amino acid position 19 of BUP (nucleotide -47 from the $β_2$AR ORF) is in 100% linkage-disequilibrium with the polymorphism at amino acid position 27 of the receptor; so in essence this represented a 2-locus haplotype. Desensitization (cAMP production) to a two-hour exposure to isoproterenol was found to be greatest for Gly16/Gln27 lymphocytes. Of note, no haplotype-specific desensitization differences were noted with a 30 minutes exposure to isoproterenol. It is unclear what additional desensitization process(es) are underway after two hours of exposure that are not present after 30 minutes of exposure; so the mechanism of this haplotype-dependent phenotype is not readily apparent.

The 5′ flanking region to −1023 has been interrogated along with the ORF and 12 SNPs were found, organized into 13 haplotypes (24). Some SNPs and/or haplotypes had frequencies that were much greater in one ethnic group versus others (Table 2). Some haplotypes "partitioned" the previously defined amino acid position 16 and 27 SNPs into various subgroups. This provided evidence that genetic control of $β_2$AR expression (and ultimately the physiologic response) was likely to be more complex than initially expected. A relationship between these $β_2$AR haplotypes and the acute force expiratory volume in one second (FEV₁) response to albuterol in asthmatics was found (24). And furthermore, when two of the common haplotypes that had differential responses in vivo were studied in a recombinant expression system (which included the 5′ promoter and 5′UTR as well as the coding region), $β_2$AR mRNA and protein expression was different between the two haplotypes, in a magnitude and direction similar to that of the human in vivo studies. No studies of a similar nature have been

Table 2 Haplotypes of the Human β₂-Adrenergic Receptors

Nucleotide: Alleles:	-1023 G/A	-709 C/A	-654 G/A	-468 C/G	-406 C/T	-367 T/C	-47 T/C	-20 T/C	46 G/A	79 C/G	252 G/A	491 C/T	523 C/A	Frequency (%) Ca	A-A	Aa
Haplotype																
1	A	C	G	C	C	T	T	T	A	C	G	C	C	0.7	25.0	12.5
2	A	C	G	G	C	C	C	C	G	C	G	C	C	48.3	6.3	10.0
3	G	A	A	C	C	T	T	T	A	G	G	C	C	0.7	0.0	0.0
4	G	C	A	C	C	T	T	T	A	C	G	C	C	33.0	29.7	45.0
5	G	C	A	C	C	T	T	T	G	C	G	C	C	1.4	0.0	0.0
6	G	C	G	C	C	T	T	T	G	C	A	C	A	13.2	31.3	30.0
7	G	C	A	C	C	T	T	T	G	C	A	T	A	1.0	1.6	0.0
8	G	C	G	C	C	T	T	T	A	C	A	C	A	0.7	0.0	0.0
9	A	C	G	C	T	T	T	T	A	C	G	C	C	0.0	4.7	0.0
10	G	C	G	C	C	T	T	T	G	C	A	C	C	0.7	0.0	0.0
11	G	C	G	C	C	T	T	T	G	C	G	C	C	0.3	0.0	2.5
12	A	C	G	G	G	T	T	T	A	C	G	C	C	0.0	1.6	0.0

published as of this writing, but there is evidence from clinical studies and other resequencing efforts that there is additional genetic variability in the gene. Importantly, these various haplotypes of the β_2AR may affect different phenotypes relevant to asthma. One can readily envision, for example, that the following physiologic responses are in some way related to β_2AR expression/function: bronchial hyperreactivity, β-agonist protection from a constrictive challenge, acute bronchodilation, lung development, airway responses and symptom control over prolonged β-agonist use, and adverse affects. And, given what we know about the differences in pharmacologic properties (in vitro and in vivo) of the β-agonists in use, the β-agonist employed in pharmacogenetic studies, as well as the concomitantly adminis-tered other drugs, are likely to affect phenotype. So, depending on the SNPs/ haplotypes that are chosen for a human study, the therapeutic agents, and the outcome measures, it is not surprising that there have been some discordant results reported to date on the effects of genetic variability of the β_2AR gene and asthma phenotypes. In the subsequent section, we discuss several studies in detail so as to provide examples of the aforementioned issues. Given the number of clinical studies to date, it is not possible to discuss them all, but several other reviews have provided summaries of additional studies (25–29).

IV. Clinical Studies of β₂-AR Variants in Asthma

A. Disease Risk

Following the initial identification of polymorphic variation in the human β_2AR, it was suggested that these polymorphisms might account in part for the risk of developing asthma (15). Although the initial study (which involves small numbers) did suggest a possible role perhaps in determining severity, subsequent studies involving moderate numbers (generally <300) failed to show convincing effects [see for example (30)]. One difficulty in evaluating these studies is the problem of "drifting phenotype": for example in one study we were able to demonstrate association between the Gln27Glu polymorphism and total IgE (31) but no effect on asthma risk per se, while in another study involving a younger population, there appeared to be an association of this polymorphism with asthma risk in children (32) which disappeared in adults. Interpretation of these studies is complicated to some extent by the identification of suggestive linkage in the region of 5q31 con-taining the human β_2AR gene for other sub-phenotypes of atopy. This may be, in part, related to the presence of other potential candidate genes within this region. The region of 5q23–31 contains many interesting candidate genes for asthma sub-phenotypes, including a cluster of cytokine genes (IL4, IL5, IL9, IL13), the glucocorticoid receptor, platelet derived growth factor receptor and the calcium activated potassium channel β-subunit. While link-age disequilibrium is less strong across this part of chromosome 5q than in some other regions, some extended linkage disequilibrium blocks do exist and it is conceivable that some of the reported data in association studies on the β_2AR gene are due to linkage disequilibrium effects with other candidate genes in the region.

In an attempt to resolve the issue of potential contribution to disease risk, there have been two recent meta-analyses examining risk of asthma with the polymorphisms within the coding region (for which most data exist). The recent meta-analysis undertaken by Thakkinstian et al. (33) identified a total of 67 studies from which allele frequencies could potentially be estimated; of which 26 studies contained information on allele frequencies for both the codon 16 and 27 polymorphisms. However when study quality was assessed objectively, the total number of studies available to examine asthma related phenotypes was markedly reduced: five studies were able to provide estimates of association in children for the position 16 polymorphism and seven studies in adults. The same number of studies were available for examining the effects of the position 27 polymorphism. Overall the main conclusion was that there was no significant effect of the position 16 polymorphism in adults but there appeared to be a possible recessive protective effect of Gly16 in children (odds ratio 0.71, 95% CI = 0.53–0.96). Heterozygotes at the position 27 locus appear to be at decreased risk of asthma (odds ratio 0.73, 95% CI = 0.62–0.87) in adults whereas children homozygous for the Glu27 polymorphism appeared to have a decreased risk of asthma (odds ratio 0.6, 95% CI = 0.35–0.99). These effects are relatively small and despite including over 1000 subjects and controls in the meta-analysis the confidence intervals around most of these effects were broad. A position 16/27 diplotype analysis suggested Glu27 was protective and that this was modified by the allele at position 16. Taken together, for the β_2AR polymorphisms examined to date, this meta-analysis indicates only a small contribution to asthma risk.

The second meta-analysis was performed by Contopoulos-Ioannidis et al. (34): this included 28 studies, but all studies with contributing data were included without an initial screen for quality (as was performed in the aforementioned analysis). Overall the main conclusion was that no major contribution was likely to exist between these polymorphisms and risk of asthma. The difference in conclusion between the two meta-analyses is likely to be due to the inclusion of a quality threshold cut off in the first of the studies described. Interestingly, a strong association between Gly16 homozygosity and nocturnal asthma was noted (odds ratio 5.15, 95% CI = 2.4–10.84) and asthma severity (odds ratio 2.84, 95% CI = 1.62–4.96).

B. Response to β-Agonist

There has been concern since the 1960s that high doses, or the regular administration of short acting β-agonists may give rise to adverse effects in asthmatic (and other) subjects [see for example (35,36)]. Asthma exacerbations and sudden death, while rare, were linked to the prescribing of isoprenaline and fenoterol in early studies: these studies were published before the potential importance of β_2AR polymorphisms became apparent. Defining the mechanism underlying rare adverse effects to β-agonists has become increasingly important given the recent Food and Drug Administration warnings on the prescribing of long acting β-agonists partly as a result of the Salmeterol Multi-center Asthma Research Trial (SMART) study in which a small excess of deaths was seen in the group receiving salmeterol. Whether or not β_2AR polymorphisms contribute to these rare adverse effects has not been adequately studied. There have, however, been a number of studies looking at efficacy and β_2AR polymorphisms. Effects of β_2AR polymorphisms can be demonstrated both on bronchodilator responses and on broncho-protective responses (i.e., the ability to protect against non-specific airway challenge). In general these studies have shown enhanced acute bronchodilator responses in individuals homozygous for Arg16 (37) but greater loss of bronchoprotection or broncho-dilator desensitization with this genotype (38–41). In a retrospective study of 190 asthmatics receiving placebo or albuterol for 16 weeks, genotyping was performed at the position 16 and 27 loci (42). Arg16 homozygous subjects who received regularly scheduled albuterol had a decline in morning and evening peak expiratory flow rate (PEFR). In contrast, when using albuterol on an as-needed basis, there was no change in these parameters for Arg individuals. Gly16 homozygotes had no change in PEFRs when receiving regularly-scheduled albuterol. There was no position 27-associated phenotype. Baseline pulmonary function was not associated with genotype. These results thus suggested that Arg16 subjects may not benefit from regular short-acting β-agonists. It is intriguing to note that the Arg16 receptor in transfected CHW cells (17) and human airway smooth muscle cells (20) appears to undergo less agonist-promoted downregulation compared to the Gly16 variant. We have hypothesized a "dynamic" model of β_2AR regulation that may explain why the Arg16 patients appear to have a greater loss of agonist-promoted PEFRs compared to the Gly16 patients (43). In essence, the notion is based on "pre-regulation" of the sensitive Gly16 receptor by endogenous epinephrine. So, subsequent chronic albuterol has little *additional* downregulation and thus Gly16 appears as the more physiologically "stable" receptor. In contrast, Arg16 is less regulated by epinephrine, and thus displays the labile downregulatory events from chronic albuterol observed in the study.

Another trial of similar design retrospectively genotyped 108 subjects who received regularly scheduled albuterol or salmeterol (44). For the albuterol groups, the total, major and minor exacerbations were greater for Arg16 homozygous subjects compared to those who were homozygous for Gly16 (Fig. 3). The homozygous Arg16 exacerbation rate was also greater than those with the same genotype receiving placebo. The change in PEFRs qualitatively showed a decrease for the Arg homozygotes during the

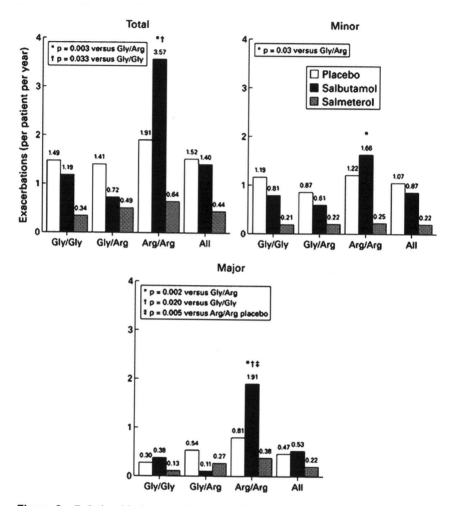

Figure 3 Relationship between β₂-adrenergic receptors genotype, β-agonist treatment, and asthma exacerbation rates. The genotype is at amino acid position 16 of the receptor. *Source*: From Ref. 44.

25-week albuterol treatment period, but this did not quite reach statistical significance. In the salmeterol groups there were much fewer exacerbations, and little PEFR variability, thus the study could not adequately assess the effect of β₂AR genotype on the response to salmeterol. Nevertheless, the Arg16 variant again appears to impart a less favorable clinical response.

The above results prompted a prospective study of albuterol in a genotype-stratified, randomized placebo-controlled cross-over trial in patients with mild asthma, termed Beta-Adrenergic Response by Genotype (BARGE) (45). Because the Arg16 genotype is less common than Gly, recruitment proceeded so as to have approximately equal number of homozygous Arg and homozygous Gly patients (37 and 41, respectively). Regularly scheduled albuterol or placebo was given for 16 weeks, then an eight-week washout, followed by a cross-over to the other agent. Ipratropium bromide was provided for rescue. The findings are summarized in Figure 4. During the randomization period, patients who were homozygous for Gly16, who were treated with albuterol, had an increase in morning PEFR compared to placebo of the same genotype. However, patients who were

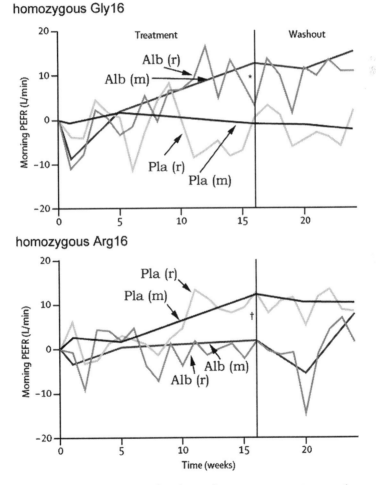

Figure 4 Relationship between β₂-adrenergic receptors genotype and morning peak expiratory flow rate during chronic treatment with albuterol or placebo. *Abbreviations*: Al, albuterol; Pl, placebo; r, raw mean data; m, modeled data; $^{*}p = 0.017$ vs. placebo; $^{†}p = 0.020$ vs. placebo. *Source*: From Ref. 45.

homozygous for Arg16 had no significant improvement in PEFR while on albuterol, and indeed had a significantly increased PEFR response while receiving placebo. This latter finding actually suggests that withdrawal of albuterol in Arg16 homozygous patients has a beneficial effect. This deleterious physiologic observation also paralleled symptom scores and the need for supplementary β-agonist. From this study, and the two prior retrospective studies (42,44), there appears to be a growing body of evidence that Arg16 patients not only do not benefit, but may deteriorate, while being treated with regularly scheduled albuterol. And, they may improve when withdrawn from chronic albuterol treatment (45). This genotype occurs in ~20% of the world's population. The variability in the response attributed to this genotype is probably $< 25\%$. Nevertheless, this single position polymorphism appears to be one part of the pharmacogenetic profile of β-agonists in the treatment of asthma.

As indicated above, there are a number of other polymorphisms in the 5′ flanking region, such that there are multiple β$_2$AR haplotypes. In one study (24), these haplotypes were associated with the acute bronchodilator response to two puffs of albuterol. There were a number of limitations to this study of extended β$_2$AR haplotypes. These include a relatively simple phenotype (change in FEV$_1$ from the pretreatment value), the lack of other ethnic groups (only whites were studied for the physiologic tests), possible confoundment from other drugs, potentially incomplete haplotypes since the 3′UTR was not resequenced for polymorphisms, and the relatively small subpopulation of homozygous haplotypes. Interestingly, one of the haplotypes (haplotype 4) had the smallest increase in FEV$_1$ (and the lowest in vitro expression), and is the major haplotype that includes Arg16 (Table 2). This might imply that this polymorphism or haplotype is "hyporesponsive," although baseline bronchodilator response in BARGE was not different by genotype. Nevertheless, it is noteworthy that those with this genotype (and thus haplotype) had the least favorable improvement in PEFR during long-term β-agonist treatment, suggesting some link between polymorphism/haplotype-directed expression, acute bronchodilator response, and long-term bronchodilator response. In another study of β$_2$AR haplotypes (46), some participants in the CAMP study (47) were genotyped as well as their parents. A family-based analysis showed that the post-bronchodilator FEV$_1$ (both as a quantitative and qualitative trait) was associated with the -654 and $+46$ position polymorphisms. Of particular interest was the finding that the nonsynonymous $+523$ polymorphism in the coding region was associated with bronchodilator responsiveness. Given that this polymorphism does not change the aminoacid in the protein, and indeed defines a haplotype, the implication of this finding is that other polymorphisms of the β$_2$AR, in strong linkage-disequilibrium with $+523$, are affecting phenotype. The 3′UTR is a likely region for such variation and is currently under study.

V. Limitations of Current Studies and Future Directions

Common polymorphisms of genes that control airway caliber and responsiveness relative to asthma undoubtedly involve a host of receptors, effectors and elements deep within multiple signal transduction pathways. The β_2AR was a natural first choice as a candidate gene for risk, disease modification, and pharmacogenetics. Despite intense efforts, there are a number of critical issues that remain unaddressed. First, it is clear that if multiple ethnic groups, and multiple polymorphisms or haplotypes are to be utilized, then large populations will need to be studied. In addition, from a public health standpoint, moderate and severe asthmatics must also be included. Indeed, findings from mild asthmatics are not necessarily relevant to those who have the greatest need for individualized therapy. It is also unclear as to whether other drugs used for the treatment of asthma can alter genotype-phenotype relationships. This effect could be direct (i.e., corticosteroids increase β_2AR expression), or indirect (i.e., another agent obfuscates the phenotype by acting at another point in the signaling network). Studies need to be designed either to directly address this with multiple groups, or, a standard regimen including corticosteroids is maintained for all subjects. Even among the available β-agonists, there is a paucity of data on whether the observed phenotypes represent a class effect, or whether certain properties of these drugs (such as those of salmeterol or formoterol) have specific phenotypes associated with β_2AR genotype. It is also noteworthy that very few of the published studies examine the same phenotypes. In some cases, the investigators' are indeed interested in a specific phenotype, such as airway hyperresponsiveness as opposed to acute bronchodilator response. Yet, even when the goals appear to be similar, protocols differ enough that when discrepancies arise, it is unclear what role the study design played in the outcome. Finally, it is now clear that other immediate partners of the β_2AR, such as adenylyl cyclase, are also polymorphic, with in vitro and in vivo phenotypes (48,49). Thus these other genes must be considered with various epistatic interactions in order to fully appreciate the predictiveness of β_2AR polymorphisms.

Acknowledgments

The authors thank Esther Moses for manuscript preparation. Funded by NIH grants HL045967 and HL065899.

References

1. Drazen JM, Silverman EK, Lee TH. Heterogeneity of therapeutic responses in asthma. Br Med Bull 2000; 56(4):1054–1070.
2. Green SA, Liggett SB. G protein coupled receptor signalling in the lung. 1996; (4):67–90.

3. Mialet-Perez J, Green SA, Miller WE, et al. A primate-dominant third glycosylation site of the β2-adrenergic receptor routes receptors to degradation during agonist regulation. J Biol Chem 2004; 279(37):38,603–38,607.

4. Jewell-Motz EA, Small KM, Liggett SB. α_{2A}/α_{2C}-adrenergic receptor third loop chimera show that agonist interaction with receptor-subtype backbone establishes G protein-coupled receptor kinase phosphorylation. J Biol Chem 2000; 275:28,989–28,993.

5. Kobilka BK. Agonist-induced conformational changes in the beta2 adrenergic receptor. J Pept Res 2002; 60(6):317–321.

6. Lefkowitz RJ, Shenoy SK. Transduction of receptor signals by beta-arrestins. Science 2005; 308(5721):512–517.

7. Daaka Y, Luttrell LM, Lefkowitz RJ. Switching of the coupling of the β_2-adrenergic receptor to different G proteins by protein kinase A. Nature 1997; 390:88–91.

8. McGraw DW, Donnelly ET, Eason MG, et al. Role of βARK in long-term agonist-promoted desensitization of the β_2-adrenergic receptor. Cell Signal 1998; 10(3):197–204.

9. Hosoda K, Fitzgerald LR, Vaidya VA, et al. Regulation of beta 2-adrenergic receptor mRNA and gene transcription in rat C6 glioma cells: effects of agonist, forskolin, and protein synthesis inhibition. Mol Pharmacol 1995; 48:206–211.

10. Hadcock JR, Wang H, Malbon CC. Agonist-induced destabilization of β-adrenergic receptor mRNA. Attenuation of glucocorticoid induced upregulation of β-adrenergic receptors. J Biol Chem 1992; 267:4740–4746.

11. Kandasamy K, Joseph K, Subramaniam K, et al. Translational control of beta2-adrenergic receptor mRNA by T-cell-restricted intracellular antigen-related protein. J Biol Chem 2005; 280(3):1931–1943.

12. Scott MGH, Swan C, Wheatley AP, et al. Identification of novel polymorphisms within the promoter region of the human beta2 adrenergic receptor gene. Br J Pharmacol 1999; 126(4):841–844.

13. Parola AL, Kobilka BK. The peptide product of a $5'$ leader cistron in the beta 2 adrenergic receptor mRNA inhibits receptor synthesis. J Biol Chem 1994; 269(6):4497–4505.

14. McGraw DW, Forbes SL, Kramer LA, et al. Polymorphisms of the $5'$ leader cistron of the human β_2-adrenergic receptor regulate receptor expression. J Clin Invest 1998; 102:1927–1932.

15. Reihsaus E, Innis M, MacIntyre N, et al. Mutations in the gene encoding for the β_2-adrenergic receptor in normal and asthmatic subjects. Am J Resp Cell Mol Biol 1993; 8:334–339.

16. Green SA, Cole G, Jacinto M, et al. A polymorphism of the human β_2-adrenergic receptor within the fourth transmembrane domain alters ligand binding and functional properties of the receptor. J Biol Chem 1993; 268:23,116–23,121.

17. Green S, Turki J, Innis M, et al. Amino-terminal polymorphisms of the human β_2-adrenergic receptor impart distinct agonist-promoted regulatory properties. Biochemistry 1994; 33:9414–9419.

18. Green SA, Rathz DA, Schuster AJ, et al. The Ile164 β_2-adrenoceptor polymorphism alters salmeterol exosite binding and conventional agonist coupling to G_s. Eur J Pharmacol 2001; 421:141–147.

19. Green SA, Spasoff AP, Coleman RA, et al. Sustained activation of a G protein coupled receptor via "anchored" agonist binding: molecular localization of the salmeterol exosite within the β₂-adrenergic receptor. J Biol Chem 1996; 271:24,029–24,035.

20. Green SA, Turki J, Bejarano P, et al. Influence of β₂-adrenergic receptor genotypes on signal transduction in human airway smooth muscle cells. Am J Resp Cell Mol Biol 1995; 13:25–33.

21. Chong LK, Chowdry J, Ghahramani P, et al. Influence of genetic polymorphisms in the β₂-adrenoceptor on desensitization in human lung mast cells. Pharmacogenetics 1999; 10:153–162.

22. Moore PE, Laporte JD, Abraham JH, et al. Polymorphism of the β₂-adrenergic receptor gene and desensitization in human airway smooth muscle. Am J Respir Crit Care Med 2000; 162:2117–2124.

23. Oostendorp J, Postma DS, Volders H, et al. Differential desensitization of homozygous haplotypes of the beta2-adrenergic receptor in lymphocytes. Am J Respir Crit Care Med 2005; 172(3):322–328.

24. Drysdale CM, McGraw DW, Stack CB, et al. Complex promoter and coding region β₂-adrenergic receptor haplotypes alter receptor expression and predict in vivo responsiveness. Proc Natl Acad Sci USA 2000; 97:10, 483–10,488.

25. Liggett SB. Pharmacogenetics of relevant targets in asthma. Clin Exp Allergy 1998; 28:77–79.

26. Small KM, McGraw DW, Liggett SB. Pharmacology and physiology of human adrenergic receptor polymorphisms. Annu Rev Pharmacol Toxicol 2003; 43:381–411.

27. Rana BK, Shiina T, Insel PA. Genetic variations and polymorphisms of G protein-coupled receptors: functional and therapeutic implications. Annu Rev Pharmacol Toxicol 2001; 41:593–624.

28. Fenech A, Hall IP. Pharmacogenetics of asthma. Br J Clin Pharmacol 2002; 53(1):3–15.

29. Hall IP. Pharmacogenetics, pharmacogenomics and airway disease. Respir Res 2002; 3(1):10.

30. Dewar JC, Wheatley AP, Venn A, et al. β₂-adrenoceptor polymorphisms are in linkage disequilibrium, but are not associated with asthma in an adult population. Clin Exp Allergy 1998; 28:442–448.

31. Dewar JC, Wilkinson J, Wheatley A, et al. The glutamine 27 β₂ adrenoceptor polymorphism is associated with elevated immunoglobulin E levels in asthmatic families. J Allergy Clin Immunol 1997; 100:261–265.

32. Hopes E, McDougall C, Christie G, et al. Association of glutamine 27 polymorphism of β₂ adrenoceptor with reported childhood asthma: population based study. BMJ 1998; 316:664–664.

33. Thakkinstian A, McEvoy M, Minelli C, et al. Systematic review and meta-analysis of the association between beta2-adrenoceptor polymorphisms and asthma: a HuGE review. Am J Epidemiol 2005; 162(3):201–211.

34. Contopoulos-Ioannidis DG, Manoli EN, Ioannidis JP. Meta-analysis of the association of beta2-adrenergic receptor polymorphisms with asthma phenotypes. J Allergy Clin Immunol 2005; 115(5):963–972.

35. Sears MR, Taylor DR, Print CG, et al. Regular inhaled beta-agonist treatment in bronchial asthma. Lancet 1990; 336:1391–1396.
36. Van Schayck CP, Dompeling E, Van Herwaarden CL, et al. Bronchodilator treatment in moderate asthma or chronic bronchitis: continuous or on demand? A randomised controlled study. BMJ 1991; 303(6815):1426–1431.
37. Martinez FD, Graves P, Baldini M, et al. Association between genetic poly-morphisms of the beta2-adrenoceptor and response to albuterol in children with and without a history of wheezing. J Clin Invest 1997; 100(12):3184–3188.
38. Tan S, Hall IP, Dewar J, et al. Association between beta 2-adrenoceptor poly-morphism and susceptibility to bronchodilator desensitisation in moderately severe stable asthmatics. Lancet 1997; 350(9083):995–999.
39. Turki J, Pak J, Green S, et al. Genetic polymorphisms of the β_2-adrenergic receptor in nocturnal and non-nocturnal asthma: evidence that Gly16 correlates with the nocturnal phenotype. J Clin Invest 1995; 95:1635–1641.
40. Lima JJ, Thomason DB, Mohamed MHN, et al. Pharmacodynamics and drug action: impact of genetic polymorphisms of the β_2-adrenergic receptor on albuterol bronchodilator pharmacodynamics. Clin Pharmacol Ther 1999; 65:519–525.
41. Hancox RJ, Sears MR, Taylor DR. Polymorphism of the β_2-adrenoceptor and the response to long-term β_2-agonist therapy in asthma. Eur Respir J 1998; 11:589–593.
42. Israel E, Drazen JM, Liggett SB, et al. The effect of polymorphisms of the β_2-adrenergic receptor on the response to regular use of albuterol in asthma. Am J Respir Crit Care Med 2000; 162(1):75–80.
43. Liggett SB. Polymorphisms of the β_2-adrenergic receptor. N Engl J Med 2002; 346(7):536–538.
44. Taylor DR, Drazen JM, Herbison GP, et al. Asthma exacerbations during long term β agonist use: influence of β_2 adrenoceptor polymorphism. Thorax 2000; 55:762–767.
45. Israel E, Chinchilli VM, Ford JG, et al. Use of regularly scheduled albuterol treatment in asthma: genotype-stratified, randomised, placebo-controlled cross-over trial. Lancet 2004; 364(9444):1505–1512.
46. Silverman EK, Kwiatkowski DJ, Sylvia JS, et al. Family-based association analysis of beta2-adrenergic receptor polymorphisms in the childhood asthma management program. J Allergy Clin Immunol 2003; 112(5):870–876.
47. The Childhood Asthma Management Program Research Group. Long-term effects of budesonide or nedocromil in children with asthma. N Engl J Med 2000; 343(15):1054–1063.
48. Small KM, Brown KM, Theiss CT, et al. An Ile to Met polymorphism in the catalytic domain of adenylyl cyclase type 9 confers reduced β_2-adrenergic recep-tor stimulation. Pharmacogenetics 2003; 13(9):535–541.
49. Tantisira KG, Small KM, Litonjua AA, et al. Molecular properties and pharma-cogenetics of a polymorphism of adenylyl cyclase 9 in asthma: interaction between β-agonist and corticosteroid pathways. Hum Mol Genet 2005; 14(12):1671–1677.

16

Interleukin-13

DONATA VERCELLI

Arizona Respiratory Center and Department of Cell Biology, University of Arizona,
Tucson, Arizona, U.S.A.

I. Introduction

Few genes appear to be as critical for the pathogenesis of allergic inflammation in humans and animal models as interleukin (IL)-13, and even fewer
appear to determine susceptibility to allergy and asthma across human
populations as consistently as IL-13. The reason behind the central role
of this cytokine in disease pathogenesis probably lies in the properties of
IL-13, the frequency with which the human IL-13 locus is targeted by natural genetic variation, and the functional consequences of this variation.
Here we will discuss the properties of IL-13 relevant to allergic lung inflammation; we will review the results of genetic association studies investigating
the relationship between IL-13 polymorphisms and allergic phenotypes;
and we will propose a blueprint for functional studies of genetic variation
based on the experience gained through the analysis of a common IL-13
coding variant.

II. IL-13: The Central Mediator of Allergic Lung Inflammation

IL-13, a cytokine typically produced during Th2 cell responses, is a central mediator of allergic inflammation and is sufficient to induce most, if not all of the key features of experimental asthma (1,2). Several studies have established that IL-13 promotes bronchial hyperresponsiveness (BHR) in response to allergen challenge. Indeed, IL-13 knock-out (KO) mice failed to develop allergen-induced BHR, despite the presence of vigorous Th2-biased, eosinophilic pulmonary inflammation. However, BHR was restored by the administration of recombinant IL-13. Moreover, adoptive transfer of allergen-specific Th2 cells generated from T-cell receptor-transgenic IL-13 KO mice failed to induce BHR in recipient mice with severe combined immunodeficiency, although such Th2 cells produced high levels of IL-4 and IL-5 and induced significant airway inflammation (3). These studies demonstrated that IL-13 is necessary and sufficient for the induction of BHR, and that eosinophilic airway inflammation in the absence of IL-13 is inadequate for the induction of this phenotype. Interestingly, allergen challenge of transgenic mice selectively lacking eosinophils demonstrated that these cells are required for asthma-associated BHR and mucus accumulation in the lung (4). These results raise the possibility that eosinophil-derived IL-13 may contribute to Th2-like inflammation in these mouse models and/or eosinophils may play an important role in Th2-derived IL-13 production (5).

Because IL-13 induces phenotypic features of asthma in mice deficient in T- and B-lymphocytes (1), the contribution of this cytokine to the development of asthma is most likely mediated by direct effects on resident airway cells. Despite activating a common signaling pathway, IL-13 induced dramatically different patterns of gene expression in airway epithelial cells, airway smooth muscle cells, and lung fibroblasts (6). IL-13 has pronounced and direct effects on smooth muscle, inducing calcium fluxes and augmenting the calcium and contractile responses of these cells to leukotriene D4 (7). The airway epithelium also undergoes dramatic structural and secretory changes in response to IL-13, including a characteristic structural derangement and downregulation of tight-junction proteins, leading to diminished epithelial barrier capacity (8). Microarray studies have shown that epithelial cells upregulate a variety of intracellular and surface molecules in response to IL-13, including transforming growth factor (TGF)-β, IL-8, granulocyte macrophage–colony stimulating factor, IL-13Rα2 (9) and CC-chemokine receptor 3 (6). Epithelial cells stimulated with IL-13 secrete large quantities of eosinophil and basophil chemoattractants, such as eotaxin-1/CCL11 (10), eotaxin-2/CCL24, eotaxin-3/CCL26, monocyte chemoattractant protein-4/CCL13 (11) and thymus-and activation-regulated chemokine/CCL17 (12). Release of these chemokines by IL-13–activated epithelial cells may be critical for the amplification and maintenance of allergic inflammation, because it can induce influx of IL-4/IL-13–producing cells, such as eosinophils, basophils, and Th2 cells. Interestingly, IL-13 induces proliferation of well-differentiated normal human bronchial epithelial cells. This effect of IL-13 is mediated through the epidermal growth factor receptor (EGFR) and TGF-α, a potent ligand for EGFR, which is rapidly released from epithelial cells in response to IL-13 (13). These results are consistent with a mechanism whereby IL-13 induces epithelial cells to release TGF-α, which in turn binds via an autocrine/paracrine-type action to the EGFR, initiating proliferation. IL-13–induced airway remodeling in vivo may involve this epithelium-driven response.

Mucus overproduction is consistently linked to asthma symptoms and morbidity, and IL-13 is now thought to be especially critical for allergen-induced mucus production. Mice lacking STAT6, the main mediator of IL-13 and IL-4 signaling (14), were protected from all pulmonary effects of IL-13. Selective reconstitution of STAT6 in epithelial cells was sufficient for IL-13–induced mucus production in the absence of inflammation, fibrosis or other lung pathology, demonstrating the importance of direct effects of IL-13 on epithelial cells in causing a central feature of asthma (15). Consistent results were obtained in a model in which in vitro-generated T-cell receptor transgenic Th2 cells were transferred into recipient mice and activated in the respiratory tract with inhaled antigen. In this model, CD4 Th cells could stimulate mucus only through a common, IL-13–mediated pathway. All Th cytokines depended on IL-13 for this effect and IL-13 acted on structural cells within the lung, not through intermediate inflammatory cells (16). Interestingly, IL-13 was solely responsible for goblet cell metaplasia in vascular endothelial growth factor (VEGF) transgenic mice (17). VEGF and IL-13 appear to be involved in amplificatory feedback circuits, because while VEGF works in part through IL-13, IL-13 increases VEGF release (18) and VEGF expression by acting at the post-transcriptional level (19).

IL-13 also appears to control fibrosis through a TGF-β1–mediated pathway. Experiments with transgenic mice that overexpress IL-13 in the lung showed that IL-13 is a potent inducer of matrix metalloproteinase (MMP)-9 and TGF-β1 expression, and that the activation of TGF-β1 is mediated by a MMP-9-dependent mechanism (20). Collagen deposition in the lungs of IL-13 transgenic mice was substantially decreased when TGF-β activity was neutralized. Of note, studies on liver fibrosis caused by Schistosoma mansoni infection pointed to the existence of another pro-fibrotic pathway that is IL-13–dependent but TGF-β1–independent (21).

IL-13–dependent inflammation is amplified by local effector molecules, such as acidic mammalian chitinase. Chitin is a surface component of parasites and insects, and chitinases are induced in lower life forms during infections with these agents. Although chitin itself does not exist in humans, chitinases are present in the human genome. It was recently shown that acidic mammalian chitinase is induced via a Th2-specific, IL-13–mediated pathway in epithelial cells and macrophages in an aeroallergen asthma model, and is expressed in exaggerated quantities in human asthma. Acidic mammalian chitinase neutralization improved Th2 inflammation and BHR, in part by inhibiting IL-13 pathway activation and chemokine induction. Chitinase may thus be an important mediator of IL-13–induced responses in Th2 inflammation (22).

Human allergic inflammation and experimental asthma share several IL-13–related signatures (23). However, IL-13 induces class switch recombination to immunoglobulin (Ig)E in human but not murine B-cells (24) and upregulates the expression of CD23, an IgE receptor, on human B-cells and monocyte/macrophages (25). Since events mediated by the binding of IgE to its receptors are integral effectors of allergic reactions in tissues (26), induction of IgE synthesis and IgE receptors is likely to be critical for the pro-inflammatory role played by human IL-13 in allergy and asthma.

III. IL-13 Regulation in Early Life

It is now well recognized that immunological events in early life—particularly, unbalanced T-helper responses—are likely to play an essential role in shaping allergic inflammation in adults (27,28). Compared to adult cells, human neonatal T-cells are deficient in their ability to mount Th1 responses (29,30), a feature dependent on epigenetic programs intrinsic to immune cells, which limit interferon (IFN)-γ (31) and IL-12 (32) expression. Importantly, reduced IFN-γ production after birth is a strong predictor of wheezing by one year of age (33) and atopy in early life (34).

The immune deficit at birth is not restricted to Th1 responses; IL-4 and IL-5 secretion by human neonatal T-cells is also drastically reduced. IL-13, on the other hand, is readily and vigorously expressed upon T-cell activation, even in the absence of Th2 polarizing stimuli (35,36). Furthermore, IL-13 is readily detectable in the human placenta (37). While the molecular mechanisms responsible for the unique propensity of neonatal CD4+ T-cells to selectively express IL-13 remain unknown, robust correlations exist between IL-13 expression at birth or within the first years of life and subsequent susceptibility to atopy and elevated IgE levels (36,38–41).

A fundamental question raised by the propensity of human neonatal CD4+ T-cells to express IL-13 pertains to the role of this cytokine in the evolution of immunity. Vigorous, rapid antigen-driven IL-13 responses may have been highly adaptive because of the dominant role IL-13 plays in resistance to pathogens, particularly the parasites most abundant in the environments our species originally encountered (42,43). Indeed, IL-13 regulates epithelial cell turnover in the gut, which is critical for parasite expulsion (44). Consistent with this hypothesis, IL13–1112CT, an IL-13 promoter polymorphism associated with increased IL-13 expression (Cameron et al., submitted for publication), is also associated with protection from Schistosoma hematobium infection (45) and severe malaria (46), and recent evidence suggests the IL-13 locus is under positive selection (47). During more recent times, environmental and hygienic conditions typical of western lifestyles may have led to a dysfunction of the regulatory interface necessary to balance T-helper effector responses, resulting in the current association between levels of IL-13 expression in early life and allergic phenotypes in adults and more generally, in the striking increase in the incidence of allergic disease observed over the last few decades (48,49).

IV. IL-13 Association Studies

The IL-13 locus on chromosome 5q31 contains a block of common single nucleotide polymorphisms (SNPs) in virtually complete linkage disequilibrium (LD) which spans the third intron (+1923CT), the fourth exon (+2044GA) and the 3' untranslated region of the gene (+2525GA, +2580CA, and +2749CT) (50). Two SNPs in the promoter (−1512AC and -1112CT) are also in strong, albeit not complete, LD with the distal polymorphisms. In view of the critical role played by genetic factors in determining susceptibility to allergic inflammation, and the central role of IL-13 in the pathogenesis of this process, the robust associations found between genetic variation in IL-13 and allergic/asthmatic phenotypes are not surprising. In fact, IL-13 is among the genes for which associations with allergic disease phenotypes have been replicated most often (51).

The association studies published so far have focused mostly on IL13+2044GA in the coding region and IL13–1112CT in the promoter. IL13+2044GA is strongly associated with increased total serum IgE, (50,52–55) asthma (56), atopy (57), atopic dermatitis (52,57,58) and a grouped phenotype including eosinophilia, IgE, and positive skin tests (59). IL13–1112CT (aka-1055) is associated with asthma, BHR and skin test responsiveness (60,61), total IgE (62), sensitization to food and outdoor allergens (62,63) and latex allergy (64). Most of these associations were found in Caucasian and/or Asian populations. More recently, IL13–1112CT was found to be associated with asthma/atopy in a small African-American population sample (65). Interestingly, a significant gene–gene interaction was detected between an IL-4Rα coding variant (S478P) and IL13–1112CT. Individuals with the risk genotype for both genes had increased risk to develop asthma (66) and food sensitization (67) compared to individuals with both non-risk genotypes.

V. A Corollary: IL-13 and Chronic Obstructive Pulmonary Disease

A discussion of the role of IL-13 in lung disease would not be complete if we did not mention emerging data reinforcing the possibility that the pulmonary consequences of genetic IL-13 dysregulation may reach beyond allergic inflammation. As discussed elsewhere in this book, the various forms of airway obstruction have been proposed to be different expressions of a single disease entity. Intrinsic factors (e.g., BHR and atopy), endogenous factors (e.g., sex and age), and exogenous factors (e.g., allergens, infections, and smoking) would all play a role in the pathogenesis of chronic nonspecific lung disease. This view has come to be widely known as the Dutch hypothesis (68). Needless to say, genetic evidence will be essential to prove or disprove this hypothesis. Indeed, the finding of genetic pathways common to asthma and chronic obstructive pulmonary disease (COPD) would lend strong support to the single-disease view of lung inflammation.

Cigarette smoke exposure is the major cause of COPD. However, only a minority of smokers develops significant COPD, and patients with asthma or asthma-like BHR or eosinophilia experience accelerated loss of lung function after cigarette smoke exposure. While lung inflammation is a characteristic feature of patients with COPD, the mediators of this inflammation and their contributions to the pathogenesis and varied natural history of COPD are only incompletely defined. Recent studies in mice and humans suggest IL-13 may be a major mediator of inflammation in COPD. Indeed, inducible overexpression of IL-13 in the lung was shown to cause emphysema with enhanced lung volumes and compliance, mucus metaplasia, and inflammation (69). MMP-2, -9, -12, -13, and -14 and several cathepsins were induced by IL-13 in this setting. In addition, treatment with MMP or cysteine proteinase antagonists significantly decreased emphysema and inflammation, but not mucus, in these animals. These studies demonstrated that IL-13 is a potent stimulator of MMP and cathepsin-based proteolytic pathways in the lung. Most importantly, these studies highlighted pathways that may underlie both COPD and asthma.

Based on these findings, it was hypothesized that variants in the IL-13, IL-13Rα1, and IL-4Rα genes would be associated with an accelerated rate of decline of lung function among smokers. Although the IL-4RA551RR genotype was the only one found to be associated with this phenotype, the association became more significant in subjects who also had the IL13−1112TT genotype (70). Another study, from the Netherlands, recently reported an increased frequency of the IL13−1112 T-allele in COPD patients compared to both healthy controls and smoking individuals with normal lung function (71). Notably, IL13+2044A, although closely linked to IL13−1112T, was present at normal allelic frequencies. Finally, no significant difference in the frequencies of the IL13−1112TT genotype was found between Han Chinese patients with COPD and controls, but IL13 – 1112T was associated with increased risk of COPD among smokers (72). Overall, these data suggest that natural variation in IL-13 may provide a mechanistic bridge between asthma and COPD.

VI. IL-13+2044GA: Functional Studies

Although the overall association between allergic inflammation and SNPs in IL-13 was replicated in several ethnically diverse populations (51) and is extremely robust, the extensive LD found in the IL-13 locus prevents the tools of genetic epidemiology from deciphering the contribution of individual polymorphisms to increased disease risk. Functional studies are required to determine which polymorphisms within a complex haplotype affect gene expression and/or function, and characterize the molecular mechanisms by which genetic variation in IL-13 increases susceptibility to allergic disease.

IL13+2044GA is of particular interest because this SNP is found in approximately 25% of the general population (50) and is expected to result in the non-conservative replacement of a positively charged arginine (R) with a neutral glutamine (Q) at position 130 (numbering including the signal peptide; also referred to as position 110 when numbering does not include the signal peptide) (54,56,73,74). Because the R130Q substitution occurs in α-helix D, the region of IL-13 that is thought to interact with IL-4Rα/IL-13Rα1 heterodimers (75), IL13+2044GA has the potential to affect IL-13–dependent signaling events.

We examined the impact of IL13+2044GA on the functional properties of IL-13 by directly comparing the activity of recombinant wild type (WT) IL-13 and IL-13R130Q on primary human cells involved in the effector mechanisms of allergic inflammation. Our results showed that IL-13R130Q is significantly more active than WT IL-13 in all the models that were tested: induction of STAT6 phosphorylation and CD23 expression in monocytes, hydrocortisone-dependent IgE switching in B-cells. Moreover, IL-13R130Q was neutralized less effectively than WT IL-13 by an IL-13Rα2 decoy, a property that could contribute to enhanced activity of the minor variant in vivo. Neither IL-13 variant was able to engage T-cells, suggesting increased allergic inflammation in carriers of IL13+2044A 44A depends on enhanced IL-13–mediated Th2 effector functions rather than increased Th2 differentiation (76). Collectively our data indicate that natural variation in the coding region of IL13 may be an important genetic determinant of susceptibility to allergy.

Performing these functional studies taught us several things. One hurdle related to the biological activity of the recombinant IL-13 protein variants. Native IL-13 is glycosylated (77), a post-translational modification commonly missing in prokaryotic expression systems. Furthermore,

C-terminal truncation immediately downstream of R130 appeared to occur in *Escherichia coli*–expressed IL-13 (76). Because we found eukaryotic IL-13 to be significantly more active than prokaryotic IL-13 over the physiologic range, all functional studies were performed using recombinant IL-13 variants expressed in eukaryotic cells, even though this approach was much more cumbersome and time consuming. In addition, because the R130Q substitution appeared to affect the recognition of IL-13 epitopes by the available enzyme-linked immunosorbent assay (ELISA) antibodies, resulting in underestimation of the minor variant, concentrations of eukaryotic IL-13R130Q were adjusted using a correction factor developed through a combination of in vitro translation and western blotting analysis. We expect that many other studies of protein variants expressed as a result of naturally occurring nonsynonymous polymorphisms will encounter similar difficulties. Our experience suggests that bacterially expressed recombinant proteins should be chosen for these experiments only if they fully recapitulate the activity of native molecules. ELISAs will also have to be validated for their ability to recognize different protein variants with comparable efficiency.

The results of functional studies are not always straightforward. Another group recently compared the activities of WT IL-13 and IL-13R130Q (73) and found them to be indistinguishable. The discrepancies between these results and ours are likely to reflect significant differences in the experimental design. Arima et al. used recombinant IL-13 expressed in a prokaryotic system and a target B-cell line overexpressing IL-13Rα1. Utilization of target cells overexpressing a receptor is likely to mask subtle differences in the affinity of its ligand, because the overall strength of ligand/receptor interactions will be dictated by the artificially increased number of receptors rather than by the affinity of individual ligand binding events. Furthermore, as mentioned above, bacterially expressed IL-13 molecules are unstable and undergo rapid degradation at the C-terminus, the same region that contains the R130Q substitution under investigation. Reliance on eukaryotic IL-13 proteins and primary human cells therefore provides a more sensitive approach to detect subtle differences in the properties of the natural IL-13 variants.

VII. Conclusions

The importance of genetic factors in influencing the risk to develop allergic inflammation is well established (78,79). Polymorphisms that may dysregulate the function and/or expression of IL-13 occur frequently in the population and have been consistently associated with allergic phenotypes (51). However, these polymorphisms are linked with one another in extended haplotype blocks which can mask the effects of individual SNPs. Therefore the mechanisms underlying the association between allergic disease and variation in IL-13 will remain unclear unless multiple functional facets of the genotype/phenotype association are explored and dissected in depth.

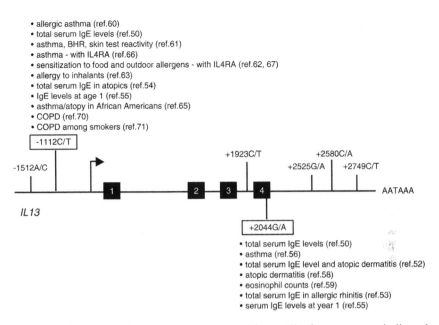

• allergic asthma (ref.60)
• total serum IgE levels (ref.50)
• asthma, BHR, skin test reactivity (ref.61)
• asthma - with IL4RA (ref.66)
• sensitization to food and outdoor allergens - with IL4RA (ref.62, 67)
• allergy to inhalants (ref.63)
• total serum IgE in atopics (ref.54)
• IgE levels at age 1 (ref.55)
• asthma/atopy in African Americans (ref.65)
• COPD (ref.70)
• COPD among smokers (ref.71)

-1112C/T
+1923C/T
+2580C/A
-1512A/C
+2525G/A
+2749C/T
1
2 3 4
AATAAA
IL13

+2044G/A

• total serum IgE levels (ref.50)
• asthma (ref.56)
• total serum IgE level and atopic dermatitis (ref.52)
• atopic dermatitis (ref.58)
• eosinophil counts (ref.59)
• total serum IgE in allergic rhinitis (ref.53)
• serum IgE levels at year 1 (ref.55)

Figure 1   Genetic variation at the human IL13 locus. The four exons are indicated by black boxes. The transcription start site is marked by a right pointing arrow. The position of common SNPs is noted (numbering is from the ATG). The main phenotypes associated with individual SNPs are shown. *Abbreviations*: SNPs, single nucleotide polymorphisms; BHR, bronchial hyperresponsiveness; IL, interleukin; COPD, chronic obstructive pulmonary disease; IgE, immunoglobulinE.

SNPs in coding regions constitute the majority of disease alleles in Mendelian disorders (80), and a recent analysis suggests common disease variants are likely to show a similar trend (81). Our results show IL-13R130Q, a common variant encoded by IL13+2044A and associated with elevated serum IgE levels and other allergy-related phenotypes in individuals of multiple ethnic backgrounds (51), is significantly more active than WT IL-13 in enhancing essential effector pathways of allergic inflammation in primary human cells.

Structure/function analyses provide mechanistic insights into the increased activity of IL-13R130Q. The replacement of R130 with a glutamine occurs in α-helix D, a region of the molecule critical for its interactions with IL-13 receptors. Alanine scanning mutagenesis recently revealed R130 to be important for IL-13 binding to IL-13Rα2 (75), the decoy receptor expressed both on cells and as a soluble protein, which binds IL-13 with high affinity but does not signal (82). IL-13Rα2 is a key negative regulator of IL-13 responses in vivo (83) and its expression is strongly enhanced by IL-13 itself (9), pointing to the existence of complex feedback loops designed to tightly control IL-13–dependent events. Consistent with this scenario, IL-13R130Q was neutralized by a soluble IL-13Rα2-Fc chimera much less effectively than WT IL-13, suggesting the minor IL-13 variant might to some extent escape the dampening mechanisms that normally restrain the activity of WT IL-13 in vivo.

In comparison with the drastic effects often obtained by genetic manipulation in animal models, the functional differences between the common and the minor IL-13 variant may appear too modest to influence disease susceptibility. Several considerations argue against this conclusion. Our results are quantitatively in line with those recently obtained in several other functional studies of human polymorphic genes, such as CD14 (84), IL-3 (85), SLC22A4 (86), TGF-β (87), LGALS2 (88) and LTA (89), all of which show subtle effects of individual common risk alleles. Furthermore, functional differences between the IL-13 variants became manifest within a physiologically relevant concentration range. Finally, IL13+2044GA is in strong LD with a promoter SNP, IL13−1112CT, which results in increased IL-13 transcription in CD4+ Th2 cells (Cameron et al., submitted for publication). The transcriptional enhancement conferred by IL13-1112T is relatively modest as well, but the increase in IL-13 activity caused by the RQ replacement, combined with the concomitant increase in IL-13 transcription associated with the -1112T allele, may effectively synergize to amplify IL-13– dependent events. The functional impact of SNP–SNP interactions within the same gene could be further amplified by gene–gene interactions along the same pathway (90), e.g., when IL13R130Q is expressed in carriers of the gain-of-function IL4RV50R551 variant (74).

The lesson that emerges from these studies is somewhat sobering. Experimental strategies that are successful in classical immunology may not be readily applicable to functional genomics work, whose targets are inherently elusive. When studying the effects of human genetic variation, we actually explore complex interactions between polymorphic genes (and their products) and the cellular milieu: nothing less than a gene-environment interaction in the nucleus (91). Both genes and environments need to be faithfully modeled, because the effects of genetic variation are likely to be context-dependent. Thus, functional studies need to recreate the specific biological conditions under which natural genetic variation exerts its subtle effects, and these conditions may be different for different polymorphisms. Therefore, even at this early stage of functional genomics studies, it is clear that unraveling the molecular mechanisms whereby natural genetic variation shapes the pathogenesis of complex diseases will require more adequate conceptual frameworks as well as novel experimental and analytical tools (92).

References

1. Grünig G, Warnock M, Wakil AE, et al. Requirement for IL-13 independently of IL-4 in experimental asthma. Science 1998; 282:2261–2263.

2. Wills-Karp M, Luyimbazi J, Xu X, et al. Interleukin-13: central mediator of allergic asthma. Science 1998; 282:2258–2261.

3. Walter DM, McIntire JJ, Berry G, et al. Critical role for IL-13 in the development of allergen-induced airway hyperreactivity. J Immunol 2001; 167:4668–4675.

4. Lee JJ, Dimina D, Macias MP, et al. Defining a link with asthma in mice congenitally deficient in eosinophils. Science 2004; 305:1773–1776.

5. Mattes J, Yang M, Mahalingam S, et al. Intrinsic defect in T-cell production of IL-13 in the absence of both IL-5 and eotaxin precludes the development of eosinophilia and airways hyperreactivity in experimental asthma. J Exp Med 2002; 195:1433–1444.

6. Lee JH, Kaminski N, Dolganov G, et al. Interleukin-13 induces dramatically different transcriptional programs in three human airway cell types. Am J Respir Cell Mol Biol 2001; 25:474–485.

7. Eum SY, Maghni K, Tolloczko B, Eidelman DH, Martin JG. IL-13 may mediate allergen-induced hyperresponsiveness independently of IL-5 or eotaxin by effects on airway smooth muscle. Am J Physiol Lung Cell Mol Physiol 2005; 288:L576–L584.

8. Ahdieh M, Vandenbos T, Youakim A. Lung epithelial barrier function and wound healing are decreased by IL-4 and IL-13 and enhanced by IFN-γ. Am J Physiol Cell Physiol 2001; 281:C2029–C2038.

9. Zheng T, Zhu Z, Liu W, et al. Cytokine regulation of IL-13Rα2 and IL-13Rα1 in vivo and in vitro. J Allergy Clin Immunol 2003; 111:720–728.

10. Lilly CM, Nakamura H, Kesselman H, et al. Expression of eotaxin by human lung epithelial cells: induction by cytokines and inhibition by glucocorticoids. J Clin Invest 1997; 99:1767–1773.

11. Ying S, Meng Q, Zeibecoglou K, et al. Eosinophil chemotactic chemokines [eotaxin, eotaxin-2, RANTES, monocyte chemoattractant protein-3 (MCP-3), and MCP-4], and C-C chemokine receptor 3 expression in bronchial biopsies from atopic and nonatopic (intrinsic) asthmatics. J Immunol 1999; 163:6321–6329.

12. Sekiya T, Miyamasu M, Imanishi M, et al. Inducible expression of a Th2-type CC chemokine thymus- and activation-regulated chemokine by human bronchial epithelial cells. J Immunol 2000; 165:2205–2213.

13. Booth BW, Adler KB, Bonner JC, Tournier F, Martin LD. Interleukin-13 induces proliferation of human airway epithelial cells in vitro via a mechanism mediated by transforming growth factor-α. Am J Respir Cell Mo Biol 2001; 25:739–743.

14. Kaplan MH, Schindler U, Smiley ST, Grusby MJ. Stat6 is required for mediating responses to IL-4 and for the development of Th2 cells. Immunity 1996; 4:313–319.

15. Kuperman DA, Huang X, Koth LL, et al. Direct effects of interleukin-13 on epithelial cells cause airway hyperreactivity and mucus overproduction in asthma. Nat Med 2002; 8:885–889.

16. Whittaker L, Niu N, Temann UA, et al. Interleukin-13 mediates a fundamental pathway for airway epithelial mucus induced by CD4 T cells and interleukin-9. Am J Respir Cell Mol Biol 2002; 27:593–602.

17. Lee CG, Link H, Baluk P, et al. Vascular endothelial growth factor (VEGF) induces remodeling and enhances TH2-mediated sensitization and inflammation in the lung. Nat Med 2004; 10:1095–1103.

18. Corne J, Chupp G, Lee CG, et al. IL-13 stimulates vascular endothelial cell growth factor and protects against hyperoxic acute lung injury. J Clin Invest 2000; 106:783–791.

19. Faffe DS, Flynt L, Bourgeois K, Panettieri RA, Shore SA. IL-13 and IL-4 induce VEGF release from airway smooth muscle cells: role of VEGF genotype. Am J Respir Cell Mol Biol 2005. (E-published Oct 6).

20. Lee C, Homer R, Zhu Z, et al. Interleukin-13 induces tissue fibrosis by selectively stimulating and activating transforming growth factor β-1. J Exp Med 2001; 194:809–821.

21. Kaviratne M, Hesse M, Leusink M, et al. IL-13 activates a mechanism of tissue fibrosis that is completely TGF-β independent. J Immunol 2004; 173:4020–4029.

22. Zhu Z, Zheng T, Homer RJ, et al. Acidic mammalian chitinase in asthmatic Th2 inflammation and IL-13 pathway activation. Science 2004; 304:1678–1682.

23. Cohn L, Elias JA, Chupp GL. Asthma: mechanisms of disease persistence and progression. Annu Rev Immunol 2004; 22:789–815.

24. Punnonen J, Aversa G, Cocks BJ, et al. Interleukin 13 induces interleukin 4–independent IgG4 and IgE synthesis and CD23 expression by human B cells. Proc Natl Acad Sci USA 1993; 90:3730–3734.

25. Cosentino G, Soprana E, Thienes CP, Siccardi AG, Viale G, Vercelli D. IL-13 downregulates CD14 expression and TNF-α secretion in human monocytes. J Immunol 1995; 155:3145–3151.

26. Gould HJ, Sutton BJ, Beavil AJ, et al. The biology of IgE and the basis of allergic disease. Annu Rev Immunol 2003; 21:579–628.

27. Martinez FD. What have we learned from the Tucson children's respiratory study? Paediatr Respir Rev 2002; 3:193–197.

28. Martinez FD. Toward asthma prevention—does all that really matters happen before we learn to read? N Engl J Med 2003; 349:1473–1475.

29. Siegrist CA. Neonatal and early life vaccinology. Vaccine 2001; 19:3331–3346.

30. Adkins B, Leclerc C, Marshall-Clarke S. Neonatal adaptive immunity comes of age. Nat Rev Immunol 2004; 4:553–564.

31. White GP, Watt PM, Holt BJ, Holt PG. Differential patterns of methylation of the IFN-gamma promoter at CpG and non-CpG sites underlie differences in IFN-gamma gene expression between human neonatal and adult CD45RO- T-cells. J Immunol 2002; 168:2820–2827.

32. Goriely S, Van Lint C, Dadkhah R, et al. A defect in nucleosome remodeling prevents IL-12(p35) gene transcription in neonatal dendritic cells. J Exp Med 2004; 199:1011–1016.

33. Guerra S, Lohman IC, Halonen M, Martinez FD, Wright AL. Reduced interferon-γ production and soluble CD14 levels in early life predict recurrent wheezing by 1 year of age. Am J Respir Crit Care Med 2004; 169:70–76.

34. Martinez FD, Stern DA, Wright AL, Holberg CJ, Taussig LM, Halonen M. Association of interleukin-2 and interferon-γ production by blood mononuclear cells in infancy with parental allergy skin tests and with subsequent development of atopy. J Allergy Clin Immunol 1995; 96:652–660.

35. Ribeiro-do-Couto LM, Boeije LC, Kroon JS, et al. High IL-13 production by human neonatal T-cells: neonate immune system regulator? Eur J Immunol 2001; 31:3394–3402.

36. Neaville W, Tisler C, Bhattacharya A, et al. Developmental cytokine response profiles and the clinical and immunologic expression of atopy during the first year of life. J Allergy Clin Immunol 2003; 112:740–746.

37. Williams TJ, Jones CA, Miles EA, Warner JO, Warner JA. Fetal and neonatal IL-13 production during pregnancy and at birth and subsequent development of atopic symptoms. J Allergy Clin Immunol 2000; 105:951–959.

38. van der Velden VH, Laan MP, Baert MR, de Waal Malefyt R, Neijens HJ, Savelkoul HF. Selective development of a strong Th2 cytokine profile in high-risk children who develop atopy: risk factors and regulatory role of IFN-gamma, IL-4 and IL-10. Clin Exp Allergy 2001; 31:997–1006.

39. Ohshima Y, Yasutomi M, Omata N, et al. Dysregulation of IL-13 production by cord blood CD4+ T Cells is associated with the subsequent development of atopic disease in infants. Pediatr Res 2002; 51:195–200.

40. Lange J, Ngoumou G, Berkenheide S, et al. High interleukin-13 production by phytohaemagglutinin- and Der p 1–stimulated cord blood mononuclear cells is associated with the subsequent development of atopic dermatitis at the age of 3 years. Clin Exp Allergy 2003; 33:1537–1543.

41. Ly NP, Li Y, Sredl DL, et al. Elevated allergen-induced IL-13 secretion predicts IgE elevation in children ages 2–5 years. J Clin Immunol 2005; 25:314–320.

42. Turner JD, Faulkner H, Kamgno J, et al. Th2 cytokines are associated with reduced worm burdens in a human intestinal helminth infection. J Infect Dis 2003; 188:1768–1775.

43. Jackson JA, Turner JD, Rentoul L, et al. T helper cell type 2 responsiveness predicts future susceptibility to gastrointestinal nematodes in humans. J Infect Dis 2004; 190:1804–1811.

44. Cliffe LJ, Humphreys NE, Lane TE, Potten CS, Booth C, Grencis RK. Accelerated intestinal epithelial cell turnover: a new mechanism of parasite expulsion. Science 2005; 308:1463–1465.

45. Kouriba B, Chevillard C, Bream J, et al. Analysis of the 5q31–q33 locus shows an association between IL13–1055C/T IL-13–591A/G polymorphisms and Schistosoma haematobium infections. J Immunol 2005; 174:6274–6281.

46. Ohashi J, Naka I, Patarapotikul J, Hananantachai H, Looareesuwan S, Tokunaga K. A single-nucleotide substitution from C to T at position -1055 in the IL-13 promoter is associated with protection from severe malaria in Thailand. Genes Immun 2003; 4:528–531.

47. Zhou G, Zhai Y, Dong X, et al. Haplotype structure and evidence for positive selection at the human IL13 locus. Mol Biol Evol 2004; 21:29–35.

48. Wills-Karp M, Santeliz J, Karp CL. The germless theory of allergic disease: revisiting the hygiene hypothesis. Nat Rev Immunol 2001; 1:69–75.

49. Vercelli D. Innate immunity: sensing the environment and regulating the regulators. Curr Op Allergy Clin Immunol 2003; 3:343–346.

50. Graves PE, Kabesch M, Halonen M, et al. A cluster of seven tightly linked polymorphisms in the IL-13 gene is associated with total serum IgE levels in three populations of white children. J Allergy Clin Immunol 2000; 105: 506–513.

51. Hoffjan S, Nicolae D, Ober C. Association studies for asthma and atopic diseases: a comprehensive review of the literature. Respir Res 2003; 4:14.

52. Liu X, Nickel R, Beyer K, et al. An IL13 coding region variant is associated with a high total serum IgE level and atopic dermatitis in the German multicenter atopy study (MAS-90). J Allergy Clin Immunol 2000; 106:167–170.
53. Wang M, Xing Z, Lu C, et al. A common IL-13 Arg130Gln single nucleotide polymorphism among Chinese atopy patients with allergic rhinitis. Hum Genet 2003; 113:387–390.
54. Heinzmann A, Jerkic SP, Ganter K, et al. Association study of the IL13 variant Arg110Gln in atopic diseases and juvenile idiopathic arthritis. J Allergy Clin Immunol 2003; 112:735–739.
55. Hoffjan S, Ostrovnaja I, Nicolae D, et al. Genetic variation in immunoregulatory pathways and atopic phenotypes in infancy. J Allergy Clin Immunol 2004; 113:511–518.
56. Heinzmann A, Mao X, Akaiwa M, et al. Genetic variants of IL-13 signalling and human asthma and atopy. Hum Mol Genet 2000; 9:549–559.
57. He JQ, Chan-Yeung M, Becker AB, et al. Genetic variants of the IL13 and IL4 genes and atopic diseases in at-risk children. Genes Immun 2003; 4:385–389.
58. Tsunemi Y, Saeki H, Nakamura K, et al. Interleukin-13 gene polymorphism G4257A is associated with atopic dermatitis in Japanese patients. J Dermatol Sci 2002; 30:100–107.
59. DeMeo D, Lange C, Silverman E, et al. Univariate and multivariate family-based association analysis of the IL-13 ARG130GLN polymorphism in the Childhood Asthma Management Program. Genet Epidemiol 2002; 23:335–348.
60. van der Pouw Kraan TCTM, van Veen A, Boeije LCM, et al. An IL-13 promoter polymorphism associated with increased risk of allergic asthma. Genes Immun 1999; 1:61–65.
61. Howard TD, Whittaker PA, Zaiman AL, et al. Identification and association of polymorphisms in the Interleukin-13 gene with asthma and atopy in a Dutch population. Am J Respir Cell Mol Biol 2001; 25:377–384.
62. Liu X, Beaty T, Deindl P, et al. Associations between total serum IgE levels and the 6 potentially functional variants within the genes IL4, IL13, and IL4RA in German children: the German Multicenter Atopy Study. J Allergy Clin Immunol 2003; 112:382–388.
63. Hummelshoj T, Bodtger U, Datta P, et al. Association between an interleukin-13 promoter polymorphism and atopy. Eur J Immunogenet 2003; 30:355–359.
64. Brown RH, Hamilton RG, Mintz M, Jedlicka AE, Scott AL, Kleeberger SR. Genetic predisposition to latex allergy: role of interleukin 13 and interleukin 18. Anesthesiology 2005; 102:496–502.
65. Moissidis I, Chinoy B, Yanamandra K, et al. Association of IL-13, RANTES, and leukotriene C4 synthase gene promoter polymorphisms with asthma and/or atopy in African Americans. Genet Med 2005; 7:406–410.
66. Howard TD, Koppelman GH, Xu J, et al. Gene-gene interaction in asthma: IL4RA and IL13 in a Dutch population with asthma. Am J Hum Genet 2002; 70:230–236.
67. Liu X, Beaty TH, Deindl P, et al. Associations between specific serum IgE response and 6 variants within the genes IL4, IL13, and IL4RA in German children: the German Multicenter Atopy Study. J Allergy Clin Immunol 2004; 113:489–495.

68. Postma DS, Boezen HM. Rationale for the Dutch hypothesis. Allergy and airway hyperresponsiveness as genetic factors and their interaction with environment in the development of asthma and COPD. Chest 2004; 126(2 suppl): 96S–104S.

69. Zheng T, Zhu Z, Wang Z, et al. Inducible targeting of IL-13 to the adult lung causes matrix metalloproteinase- and cathepsin-dependent emphysema. J Clin Invest 2000; 106:1081–1093.

70. He JQ, Connett JE, Anthonisen NR, Sandford AJ. Polymorphisms in the IL13, IL13RA1, and IL4RA genes and rate of decline in lung function in smokers. Am J Respir Cell Mol Biol 2003; 28:379–385.

71. Van der Pouw Kraan TC, Kucukaycan M, Bakker AM, et al. Chronic obstructive pulmonary disease is associated with the -1055 IL-13 promoter polymorphism. Genes Immun 2002; 3:436–439.

72. Jiang L, He B, Zhao MW, Ning LD, Li XY, Yao WZ. Association of gene polymorphisms of tumour necrosis factor-alpha and interleukin-13 with chronic obstructive pulmonary disease in Han nationality in Beijing. Chin Med J (Engl) 2005; 118:541–547.

73. Arima K, Umeshita-Suyama R, Sakata Y, et al. Upregulation of IL-13 concentration in vivo by the IL13 variant associated with bronchial asthma. J Allergy Clin Immunol 2002; 109:980–987.

74. Chen W, Ericksen MB, Levin LS, Khurana Hershey GK. Functional effect of the R110Q IL13 genetic variant alone and in combination with IL4RA genetic variants. J Allergy Clin Immunol 2004; 114:553–560.

75. Madhankumar AB, Mintz A, Debinski W. Alanine-scanning mutagenesis of alpha-helix D segment of interleukin-13 reveals new functionally important residues of the cytokine. J Biol Chem 2002; 277:43194–43205.

76. Vladich FD, Brazille SM, Stern D, Peck ML, Ghittoni R, Vercelli D. IL-13 R130Q, a common variant associated with allergy and asthma, enhances effector mechanisms essential for human allergic inflammation. J Clin Invest 2005; 115:747–754.

77. Minty A, Chalon P, Derocq J-M, et al. Interleukin-13 is a new human lymphokine regulating inflammatory and immune responses. Nature 1993; 362: 248–250.

78. Cookson WO, Moffatt MF. Genetics of asthma and allergic disease. Hum Mol Genet 2000; 9:2359–2364.

79. Vercelli D. Genetic polymorphism in allergy and asthma. Curr Op Immunol 2003; 15:609–613.

80. Carlson CS, Eberle MA, Kruglyak L, Nickerson DA. Mapping complex disease loci in whole-genome association studies. Nature 2004; 429:446–452.

81. Botstein D, Risch N. Discovering genotypes underlying human phenotypes: past successes for Mendelian disease, future approaches for complex disease. Nat Genet 2003; 33(suppl):228–237.

82. Donaldson DD, Whitters MJ, Fitz LJ, et al. The murine IL-13 receptor α2: molecular cloning, characterization and comparison with murine IL-13 receptor α1. J Immunol 1998; 161:2317–2324.

83. Wood N, Whitters MJ, Jacobson BA, et al. Enhanced Interleukin-13 responses in mice lacking IL-13 receptor α2. J Exp Med 2003; 197:703–709.

84. LeVan TD, Bloom JW, Bailey TJ, et al. A common single nucleotide polymorphism in the CD14 promoter decreases the affinity of Sp protein binding and enhances transcriptional activity. J Immunol 2001; 167:5838–5844.
85. Schweiger A, Stern D, Lohman IC, Baldini M, Martinez FD, Halonen M. Differences in proliferation of the hematopoietic cell line TF-1 and cytokine production by peripheral blood leukocytes induced by 2 naturally occurring forms of human IL-3. J Allergy Clin Immunol 2001; 107:505–510.
86. Tokuhiro S, Yamada R, Chang X, et al. An intronic SNP in a RUNX1 binding site of SLC22A4, encoding an organic cation transporter, is associated with rheumatoid arthritis. Nat Genet 2003; 35:341–348.
87. Silverman ES, Palmer LJ, Subramaniam V, et al. Transforming growth factor-β1 promoter polymorphism C-509T is associated with asthma. Am J Respir Crit Care Med 2004; 169:214–219.
88. Ozaki K, Inoue K, Sato H, et al. Functional variation in LGALS2 confers risk of myocardial infarction and regulates lymphotoxin-α secretion in vitro. Nature 2004; 429:72–75.
89. Knight JC, Keating BJ, Kwiatkowski DP. Allele-specific repression of lymphotoxin-α by activated B cell factor-1. Nat Genet 2004; 36:394–399.
90. Lohmueller KE, Pearce CL, Pike M, Lander ES, Hirschhorn JN. Meta-analysis of genetic association studies supports a contribution of common variants to susceptibility to common disease. Nat Genet 2003; 33:177–182.
91. Vercelli D. The functional genomics of CD14 and IgE-mediated disease: An integrated view. J Allergy Clin Immunol 2002; 109:14–21.
92. Vercelli D. Genetic regulation of IgE responses: Achilles and the tortoise. J Allergy Clin Immunol 2005;116:60–64.

17

CD14 and Toll-Like Receptors

STEFANO GUERRA

Arizona Respiratory Center and Mel and
Enid Zuckerman College of Public
Health, University of Arizona,
Tucson, Arizona, U.S.A.

FERNANDO D. MARTINEZ

Arizona Respiratory Center and Department
of Pediatrics, University of Arizona,
Tucson, Arizona, U.S.A.

I. Introduction

In the last decade, extraordinary progress has been made in characterizing at the molecular and genetic level the components of the human immune system that mediate the innate response to microbial organisms and products. Among these components are CD14 and the family of toll-like receptors (TLRs). CD14 interacts with TLR4 and at least another protein, MD-2, to form a receptor complex with specificity for endotoxin [lipopolysaccharide, (LPS)—a component of gram-negative bacteria]. The TLR family includes at least 10 transmembrane proteins (TLR1-10) that recognize a large variety of viral and bacterial constituents and are essential for an effective host defense against microbes. The sequencing of the human genome has revealed substantial interindividual variation in the genes encoding CD14 and TLRs, and functional studies have shown that some of these genetic variants have a significant impact on gene expression and/or protein function (1).

Because of the postulated role of microbial exposure in the inception and clinical progression of asthma and chronic obstructive pulmonary disease (COPD), CD14 and TLRs have been proposed as candidate genes for these diseases. Findings from several association studies (reviewed later in this chapter and summarized in Table 1) support a significant effect of some variants of these genes, particularly on allergies and asthma. However, findings have not been consistent across different studies and different populations and, to date, our understanding of these genetic associations remains limited. A possible reason for these inconsistencies is that the effect of genetic variants on disease susceptibility is not consistent itself, being influenced by the level and time of exposure to environmental stimuli (i.e., microbial organisms and products), which can largely vary across different populations. The existence and nature of such gene-by-environment interactions is receiving growing attention and recent evidence suggests that innate immunity genes can indeed play a "non-unidirectional" or even ambivalent role in asthma and atopy, conferring protection or risk according to the environment and the time in life at which they exert their effects. In this chapter, we will review the biological rationale and the experimental and epidemiological evidence for the interplay between genetic variation in CD14/TLRs and microbial exposures in affecting risk and severity of asthma and COPD.

II. Biology and Genetic Variation of CD14 and Toll-Like Receptors

CD14 is a pattern recognition receptor with specificity for endotoxin and—in conjunction with TLR4 and MD-2—is part of the LPS receptor complex. CD14 is expressed both anchored on the membrane (mCD14) of several cell types, particularly mature myeloid cells (47), and in soluble form (sCD14) in human fluids, including blood. TLRs are recently identified transmembrane proteins that recognize different microbial conserved structures. Specific ligands have been identified for most TLRs present in humans (48–50). They include products derived from both bacteria (LPS for TLR4; various lipoproteins for TLR1, 2, and 6; unmethylated CpG DNA for TLR9) and viruses (double stranded RNA for TLR3; G- and U-rich single-stranded RNA for TLR8) (48,49). Some TLRs operate in heterodimeric forms. For example, TLR2 may form heterodimers with TLR1 and TLR6 in order to recognize specific lipoproteins derived from gram-positive bacteria (51). Other TLRs require collaborating innate proteins to respond to their ligands (51). The most illustrative case is represented by the interaction between TLR4 and CD14/MD-2 to obtain efficient binding to LPS and signal transduction (52,53).

CD14 and TLRs are central molecules of the innate immune system and are expressed in many cell types involved in the first line of defense of the organism against pathogens, both at the systemic and local level. In the lung, these receptors are expressed by some of the major cell types

Table 1 Functional Single Nucleotide Polymorphisms in the CD14 and Toll-Like Receptor Genes That Have Been Most Extensively Investigated in Relation to Asthma and Chronic Obstructive Pulmonary Disease

Gene	Functional SNPs	Genetic associations with phenotypes related to asthma and COPD
CD14	−159C→T: Affects affinity of Sp protein binding (2); Regulates sCD14 levels (3–11) and monocyte membrane expression of CD14 (12,13); Affects bacteria-induced cytokine production (12,14)	T-allele ↓ Atopy/IgE (3,6,10,15–20) ↑ Atopy in populations presumably exposed to high levels of endotoxin (21,22) ↑ Eczema/IgE in families with positive history of asthma (23) ↓ Early-onset airway hyperresponsiveness (18) and atopic asthma (20) ↑ Nonatopic asthma and food allergy (24) ↓ Or ↑ atopy, IgE, eczema, and asthma depending on the level of environmental exposure (25–28) ↓ Lung function and ↑ respiratory symptoms among farmers (29) ↑ *Chlamydia pneumoniae* infection (30,31)
	−1619A→G: regulates sCD14 levels (4)	G-allele: ↓ lung function and ↑ respiratory symptoms among farmers (29)
TLR4	+896A→G: Asp→Gly at amino acid position 299; Hyporesponsiveness to endotoxin (32,33); Decreased LPS-induced cytokine production (32,34); Decreased systemic inflammatory response to LPS (33)	G-allele In the general population: ↑ asthma risk (34), ↓ atopy among subjects exposed to high levels of endotoxin (35) Among asthmatics: ↑ atopy (36), ↓ severity of asthma (19), ↓ bronchial hyperresponsiveness among asthmatic exposed to high levels of endotoxin (37) ↓ COPD (inconsistent results) (38,39) ↑ Severe respiratory syncytial virus infection (40) ↑ Infection by gram-negative bacteria (41,42)

(Continued)

Table 1 Functional Single Nucleotide Polymorphisms in the CD14 and Toll-Like Receptor Genes That Have Been Most Extensively Investigated in Relation to Asthma and Chronic Obstructive Pulmonary Disease (*Continued*)

Gene	Functional SNPs	Genetic associations with phenotypes related to asthma and COPD
TLR2	−16934T→A:	A-allele
	Regulates expression of membrane TLR2 on monocytes (43)	↑ Atopy, hay fever, and asthma among farmers (35)
TLR6	+744C→T	T-allele
	Pro→Ser at amino acid position 249	↓ Asthma in African-Americans (44);
	Functional impact unknown	↑ Asthma in Caucasians of German origin (45)
TLR10	+2322A→G	G-allele
	Ile→Val at amino acid position 775	↑ Asthma in two independent samples (46)
	Functional impact unknown	

Abbreviations: COPD, chronic obstructive pulmonary disease; TLR, toll-like receptor; LPS, lipopoly saccharide; SNPs, single nucleotide polymorphisms.

involved in the pathogenesis of asthma and COPD: macrophages, neutrophils, and epithelial cells (54,55). Engagement of CD14 and TLRs with specific ligands initiates complex intracellular signaling cascades that result in the NF-κB–mediated expression of immune molecules, such as inflammatory cytokines and inducible nitric oxide synthase (56). These molecular events are important for clearing infection, but they can also lead to host-tissue damage and airway reactivity when the inflammatory response is intense and/or persistently upregulated.

CD14 and TLRs show substantial interindividual genetic variation, mainly in the form of single nucleotide polymorphisms (SNPs). Within the collaborative Innate Immunity Programs for Genomic Applications, CD14 and TLRs have been resequenced and a large number of SNPs have been identified in these genes (1,57). However, the majority of these SNPs are infrequent (frequency of minor allele is less than 10%). In addition, by using an algorithm developed within the Seattle SNPs Program (58), a substantially lower number of SNPs (TagSNPs) can be selected that are sufficient to efficiently describe all common patterns of variation in each gene within most ethnic groups (59). Although this is not always the case for the ethnic group of African-Americans, in other ethnic groups for each gene a relatively small number of haplotypes (usually lower than 10) is carried by at least 80% of the chromosomes (1). These data have important implications for genetic association studies because they provide the rationale for using a limited number of carefully selected SNPs—considered both individually and in combination in their chromosomal sequence (haplotype)—in order to describe most of the genetic variation of interest.

Some of the genetic variants identified in CD14 and TLRs have been shown to have a functional impact on gene expression and/or protein function and to affect cytokine production after microbial exposure (Table 1) (12,14,32,34). Of these genetic variants, the SNP at position-159 (also referred to as—260 depending on the position from which the nucleotides are counted) in the 5' flanking region of the CD14 gene has been one of the most extensively studied for three main reasons. First, this common C→T transition has been known since 1999 (3), when our group screened the CD14 gene for polymorphisms and found no SNPs of any significance in the coding region, but several SNPs in the 5' genomic region. Second, subsequent functional studies (2) have elucidated the functional impact of this SNP on CD14 gene expression rates and transcription factor interactions. In these studies, in a relevant cell type (MonoMac cells), a luciferase reporter assay showed that the T-allele was associated with higher transcription rates than the C-allele. Electromobility shift assays showed that these modifications in transcription rates could potentially be attributed to alterations caused by CD14/-159 in the complex interactions between this genomic region and the SP1 and SP3 transcription factors (2). Finally, the presence of detectable levels of sCD14 in several human fluids, including serum and breast milk (4,60), has provided an easily identifiable intermediate phenotype to study potential effects of the CD14/-159 SNP on gene expression and/or protein production. The CD14/-159T-allele has been consistently found to be associated with increased sCD14 levels in human plasma in independent populations (3–10) and as early as three months of age (11). Recent studies have suggested that additional SNPs in the 5' flanking region of the CD14 gene are associated with sCD14 levels in plasma (4,11) and breast milk (4) and that the combination of alleles at multiple polymorphic sites (haplotype) in the CD14 promoter region may represent a better model than single SNPs considered individually to study the functional impact of CD14 genetic variation (4).

Of note, in addition to representing an intermediate phenotype in the relation of CD14 genetic variation to disease, sCD14 levels in plasma have been directly linked to human disease. Elevated levels of sCD14 in serum have been associated with the clinical progression and/or prognosis in septic shock (61) as well as in several infectious and autoimmune diseases (62–64). At the same time, adequate levels of sCD14 in plasma at birth and in amniotic fluid during gestation appear required to confer protection against early recurrent wheezing (65) and atopy (66), suggesting an important role of this molecule in influencing the maturation of immune responses (65).

The missense mutation Asp→Gly in codon 299 of the TLR4 gene (a component of the receptor complex that binds endotoxin) represents another example of an innate immunity genetic variant for which functionality has been demonstrated. Seminal work in mice showed that missense mutations in the coding region of the TLR4 gene rendered the animals resistant to endotoxin but highly susceptible to gram-negative infections (67). Later work by Arbour et al. (32) confirmed hyporesponsiveness to inhaled endotoxin in humans carrying the two cosegregating missense mutations in codons 299 and 399 (Asp299Gly and Thr399Ile) of the TLR4 receptor. Subjects heterozygous for Asp299Gly and Thr399Ile had less steep dose-response slopes in decline of forced expiratory volume in one second (FEV_1) when exposed to inhaled LPS than subjects homozygous for the wild type (because of the low frequency of the minor allele, subjects homozygous for these genetic variants are very rare). In addition, increase in production of interleukin (IL)-1α by airway epithelial cells after stimulation with LPS was present among homozygotes for the wild type, but abolished in heterozygotes. Of note, transfection of THP-1 cells demonstrated that the Asp299Gly mutation, but not the Thr399Ile mutation, interrupted TLR4-mediated LPS signaling, implicating the former as a functionally relevant variant. A subsequent study showed that the Asp299Gly mutation was also responsible for a blunted systemic responsiveness to inhaled endotoxin (33). After LPS inhalation, in fact, subjects heterozygous for Asp299Gly had significantly lower numbers of white blood cell counts and lower levels of C-reactive protein and LPS-binding protein compared with homozygotes for the common allele (33).

III. Marginal and Interactive Effects of CD14 Genetic Variation on Atopic Phenotypes

Since the late 1980s (68), a series of epidemiological observations suggested the idea (later dubbed the hygiene hypothesis) that exposure to microbial products, such as endotoxin, early in life could confer protection against asthma and allergy by triggering precoded maturational mechanisms of the immune system and influencing the type of immune responses mounted against allergens (69). Children presumably more heavily exposed to microbial products (such as those with older siblings or attending day care) were found less likely to develop allergies and asthma (68,70) and studies in rural communities demonstrated that the likelihood of becoming sensitized against aeroallergens and of having atopic asthma was inversely proportional to the concentration of endotoxin present in home dust (71).

It is thus not surprising that the effects of CD14 genetic variation on allergic sensitization and asthma were studied since the very first description of the CD14/-159 SNP. In that original report (3), our group found children homozygous for the-159T-allele to have higher levels of plasma sCD14 and to be less atopic (as determined by the number of positive skin tests against allergens) than peers carrying the C-allele. The association between the CD14/-159T-allele and increased plasma levels of sCD14 has been subsequently replicated (4–11) and subjects homozygous TT have been also shown to have increased mCD14 expression on antigen presenting cells as compared with carriers of the other genotypes (12,13). However, the relationship between the CD14/-159 SNP and atopic sensitization (leaving asthma aside) has been—at first disappointedly—inconsistent across different studies.

Three paradigmatic examples of inconsistent findings in well-designed studies aimed at replicating the association between CD14/-159 and atopy come from the Netherlands, Germany, and a rural community in the northern United States. In the first of these studies, in a Dutch urban adult population Koppelman et al. found that carriers of the T-allele had on average a lower number of positive skin tests and lower total serum immunoglobulin (Ig)E levels and were less likely to report allergic symptoms than subjects homozygous for the C-allele (15). These findings were quite consistent with those reported by our group in the above-mentioned report in 1999 (3). However, two subsequent large epidemiological studies from Germany—including a longitudinal study from the multicenter allergy study cohort—failed to find any association between CD14/-159 and IgE levels or the prevalence of atopic diseases (9,72). To complicate things even more, reports regarding subjects supposedly heavily exposed to endotoxin emerged that questioned even the direction of the association between CD14/-159T and atopy. Ober et al. studied allergic sensitization among the Hutterites, a rural population living in a communal setting in the northern United States, and found that, contrary to findings in urban populations, the CD14/-159T-allele was associated with an increased risk of sensitization in these subjects (21). Similar findings were reported by Amelung et al. among workers in the animal facilities of the Jackson laboratories, presumably heavily exposed to endotoxin (22).

Several possible explanations may be proposed for these unexpected results, including simple random variations around the null. However, an alternative explanation is that the effects of CD14/-159 on atopic disease are dependent upon the level of environmental exposure, namely endotoxin load. In other words, inconsistencies in previous studies on CD14/-159 may reflect underlying gene-by-environment interactions. In epidemiological terms, an interaction between two different factors *A* and *B* is present when the main effect of factor *A* on disease risk differs significantly across different levels of exposure to factor *B*. Most often, interactions are quantitative, meaning that the association between factor *A* and disease risk has different magnitude—*but the same direction*—across different levels of exposure to factor *B* (Fig. 1A and B). Namely, the association between

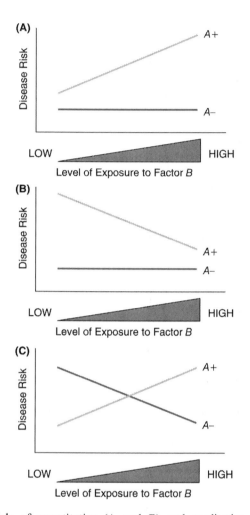

Figure 1   Models of quantitative (**A** and **B**) and qualitative (**C**) interactions between factors *A* and *B* in affecting disease risk. If we assume that factor *A* represents a dichotomous genetic factor (*A*+, allele A present; *A*-, allele A absent) and factor *B* an environmental factor measured on a continuous scale then (**A**) Illustrates the case in which genetic effects of factor *A* will be stronger at high levels of exposure to the environmental factor *B*. Larger sample sizes and lower measurement errors will be required in epidemiological studies to detect the association between factor *A* and disease risk in populations exposed to low levels of factor *B*. (**B**) Illustrates the case in which genetic effects of factor *A* will be stronger at low levels of exposure to the environmental factor *B*. Larger sample sizes and lower measurement errors will be required in epidemiological studies to detect the association between factor *A* and disease risk in populations exposed to high levels of factor *B*. (**C**) Illustrates the case in which genetic effects of factor *A* will be opposite at low and high levels of exposure to the environmental factor *B*. At middle ranges of exposure to environmental factor *B*, factor *A* has no effects on disease risk.

factor A and disease can be stronger at high levels of exposure to factor B (Fig. 1A) or at low levels of exposure to factor B (Fig. 1B). If the interaction between CD14/-159 and endotoxin load in affecting atopy risk were of the type depicted in Figure 1B, one of the implications of this quantitative interaction would be that even well-designed replication studies that use populations with high levels of exposure to endotoxin may not be able to replicate the significant association between CD14/-159 and atopic disease that was found in previous studies among populations with lower levels of exposure to endotoxin. This is especially true for replication studies that do not have sufficiently large sample sizes or sufficiently low misclassification rates. However, in the presence of a quantitative interaction, in no case other than Type 1 error (i.e., an association is detected as significant simply by chance when in fact no true association exists) one would expect a replication study to find an association between factor A and disease with opposite direction as compared with previous studies. As seen above, that appears to be the case for the relationship between CD14/-159 and atopy, as the C-allele was associated with increased risk of atopy in some studies and decreased risk of atopy in others, with some studies in yet other populations showing no association between CD14/-159 and atopy at all. This type of interaction is known as qualitative (as contrasted with quantitative interaction), because the same factor A is associated with increased or decreased risk of disease according to the level of exposure to factor B (Fig. 1C). In other words, the direction itself of the association between factor A and disease risk is dependent upon factor B. In the case of CD14/-159, it is tempting to speculate that the opposite effects of the T-allele found in different populations may be dependent upon the different endotoxin loads to which the study populations are exposed.

Two recent studies have provided important new information in support of this scenario (25,26). Zambelli-Weiner et al. (25) studied the association between prevalence of asthma and CD14/-159 in a population of African descent in the island of Barbados. Contrary to other studies, concentration of endotoxin in house dust was also measured, and the effects of CD14/-159 were assessed at different levels of exposure. The authors found that, at low levels of exposure to endotoxin, the T-allele was protective, whereas at high levels of exposure the C-allele was protective. They could not distinguish between the effects on asthma and those on atopic sensitization, because most subjects with asthma were atopic. A similar pattern was observed among children in rural communities in central Europe, where— much like in the study in Barbados—the T-allele of CD14/-159 was protective against atopy at low levels of endotoxin exposure, unrelated to it at intermediate levels, and a risk factor for allergic sensitization at high levels of exposure (26). This study confirmed also the previous finding by Gern et al. (27) of a significant interaction between dog ownership and CD14/-159 SNP in affecting risk of atopic disease and serum IgE levels. However, this effect seemed to be independent of the concentration of endotoxin measured in house dust. Previously, Litonjua et al. (73) had also found the negative associations between exposures to dog and cat allergen and wheeze to be independent of the effects of endotoxin. It is thus likely that having a pet in the home may have effects on allergic sensitization that are only partially explained by the concomitant increased exposure to endotoxin.

Whether the presented findings on CD14/-159 and atopy are related to underlying gene-by-environment interactions as well as the exact nature (quantitative vs. qualitative) of these interactions remain to be determined. However, these findings have an immediate and critical implication for studies of genetic epidemiology addressing the relation of innate immunity genes (and possibly other genetic variants as well) to asthma. Dissecting the complex interplay between genetic variants and environmental factors will not be possible by studying either of these main effects independent of the other and future genetic association studies will increasingly need to include assessments of environmental exposures as an essential part of their design. Most likely, this will prove a challenging task because of ethical and practical difficulties in measuring exposures with acceptable accuracy in studies on humans.

IV. The Relation of Microbial Exposure to Asthma and Chronic Obstructive Pulmonary Disease

In the case of genetic variants that affect susceptibility to asthma and COPD by mediating response to microbial organisms and products, not only the level but also the timing of exposure to environmental stimuli needs to be taken into account, adding a further layer of complexity to the study of these genetic associations. In addition, the same genetic variants can have substantially different effects on susceptibility to disease and severity of disease. For example, microbial exposure early in life may be linked to reduced risk of atopic sensitization and asthma, and studies in animal models have shown that exposure to endotoxin prior to (but not after) sensitization abolishes Th2-type responses linked to asthma phenotypes (74). However, once asthma has occurred, viral infections and endotoxin exposure are well-established triggers of disease symptoms and exacerbations and aggravating factors of disease severity (75). These results suggest that activation of the endotoxin receptor system (and/or other innate immunity receptors) needs to occur at the right time during the sensitization process to exert its protective effects on asthma risk and—in adult age or after the onset of asthma—it may rather represent a deleterious exposure for disease progression.

In relation to COPD, there is a strong rationale for expecting direct deleterious effects of infections and endotoxin exposure on both the development and the clinical progression of the disease.

There are at least two lines of evidence that suggest that these exposures may affect susceptibility to COPD. First, exposure to CD14/TLRs ligands has been shown to lead to airway inflammation and lung damage. In the lungs of smokers and in those of patients with COPD, macrophages and neutrophils tend to accumulate in the alveoli, bronchioli, and small airways (76). Among patients with COPD, the degree of infiltration of the airways with macrophages correlates inversely with the severity of the disease (77). Macrophages express CD14 and TLRs (54). Some of these receptors are also expressed by neutrophils (55) and airway epithelial cells (78). Inflammatory mediators that are produced in response to binding of CD14 and TLRs to microbial ligands in the lung are important for clearing infection, but they can also lead to host-tissue damage when the inflammatory response is persistently upregulated. Exposure to microbial products may directly induce an increased release of matrix metalloproteinases from macrophages, as shown in vitro in humans (79) and in vivo in animal models (80). Alternatively, endotoxin via NF-κB can induce the release of proinflammatory cytokines, including chemokines such as IL-8, which in turn may attract neutrophils and provoke the release of their proteinases (81,82). Indeed, the possibility of targeting TLRs and/or the related cytokine-driven inflammation is being currently studied as a potentially innovative therapeutic approach in inflammatory diseases (54), including chronic airway diseases (83).

Second, endotoxin is a known component of noxious agents associated with COPD. Endotoxin inhalation is a potent inflammatory stimulus in both animal models and humans (84). Among farmers and workers exposed to organic dusts, the rate of decline of lung function correlates directly with the level of exposure to endotoxin (85–87). Endotoxin is also an active component of cigarette smoke (88,89) and smoking one pack of cigarettes per day delivers a dose of respirable endotoxin comparable to that associated with cotton textile work (88).

In addition to COPD susceptibility, microbial exposures may be also involved in the clinical progression of this disease. Infections are, in fact, a major cause of acute exacerbations and a determinant of acceleration of FEV_1 decline in COPD patients. The majority (up to 80%) of COPD exacerbations are infectious in origin (90,91). Elegant studies have shown that acute exacerbations are frequently associated with the isolation of a new strain of a bacterial pathogen (92). The bacterial species most commonly isolated from sputum during exacerbations are nontypable *Hemophilus influenzae*, *Moraxella catarrhalis*, and *Streptococcus pneumoniae* (90,93), but viruses have been also shown to play an important role (91). Apart from acute exacerbations, bacteria can be isolated from patients with COPD also during stable periods. The biological meaning of this colonization has not been conclusively understood (94,95), but several lines of evidence support the hypothesis that chronic lower airway bacterial colonization is not an "innocent bystander" and might be directly related to the progression of the disease (93,94,96). Among patients with COPD, frequency and severity of acute exacerbations as well as FEV_1 decline are directly correlated with airway bacterial colonization (97,98). Airway bacterial loads appear also to be related to airway inflammation in patients with stable chronic bronchitis (99). Recently, progression of COPD has been linked to the infiltration of the wall of small airways by innate and adaptive inflammatory immune cells (77). This might represent a possible histological hallmark of the immune response to chronic airway colonization in COPD patients. The TLR family, in conjunction with CD14, assures recognition of pathogen-associated patterns (48) borne by bacteria and viruses, including those involved in COPD exacerbations and airway colonization.

V. Genetic Variation in Toll-Like Receptors and Asthma

In addition to the above-mentioned studies on CD14, genetic variants of several TLRs have been also investigated in relation to asthma risk and severity. The missense mutation Asp299Gly in the TLR4 gene reportedly associated with hyporresponsiveness to inhaled endotoxin represents an interesting candidate genetic marker for asthma (32,33). Associations of this mutation with susceptibility to asthma have been to date inconsistent (34,100) and evidence is emerging that this polymorphism—rather than being associated with asthma per se—might affect disease severity and/or modify the effects of endotoxin on asthma and atopy at high levels of exposure. Children with asthma carrying the Gly299 allele were found to be more atopic than asthmatics carrying the AA genotype (36), but this variant was also found to be protective against bronchial hyperresponsiveness and atopy among subjects exposed to high levels of endotoxin (35,37).

Other four TLRs that have recently received some attention in relation to susceptibility to asthma are TLR2 (35), TLR6 (44,45), TLR9 (101–103), and TLR10 (46). TLR2 is a receptor with specificity for a wide variety of components of the cell membrane of gram-positive and gram-negative bacteria. Much like in the case of CD14, recent evidence suggests the existence of important gene-by-environment interactions in modulating the effects of genetic variation of TLR2 on asthma and atopy (35). In European rural communities of farmers, children carrying at least one copy of the T-allele at position -16934 in the first intron of TLR2 were found to be protected against development of asthma, hay fever, and atopy as compared with children carrying the AA genotype (35). However, these associations were not present among children from the same communities who were not living at farms and supposedly were exposed to lower levels of the microbial products that are abundant in the animal-farming environment. Findings from subsequent in vitro studies have shown that monocytes from healthy adult volunteers carrying the TLR2/-16934TT genotype express significantly more membrane TLR2 than monocytes from carriers of the A-allele, suggesting a functional role of TLR2/-16934 that may contribute toward susceptibility for asthma and allergy (43).

TLR6 is structurally related to TLR2, with which it can form heterodimers for recognition of bacterial lipopeptides. A missense mutation in codon 249 (Ser249Pro) has been identified in the extracellular domain of the protein and has been associated—with opposite directions—in two independent studies with asthma, but not COPD (44,45). Although the Ser249Pro mutation results in a nonconservative amino acid change, the impact of this polymorphism on protein function remains to be determined.

TLR9 recognizes unmethylated CpG-rich DNA, a motif far more common in bacterial than in mammalian DNA. In preliminary analyses, the C-allele at position -1237 of the 5' flanking region of TLR9 was associated with asthma in a small case-control study (101). However, two subsequent larger studies failed to find any relation of TLR9 polymorphisms/haplotypes to asthma and total and specific IgE levels in serum (102,103).

Finally, a recent report has provided support for TLR10 genetic variation affecting asthma risk (46). The specific ligands and functions of TLR10 have not been determined yet, but Lazarus et al. found the SNPs + 1031G→A and +2322A→G to be associated with physician-diagnosed asthma both in a large case-control study and in a family-based cohort (46). Both mutations are in the coding region of TLR10, with the polymorphism +1031 being a synonymous SNP and the polymorphism +2322 being a missense mutation that introduces a change from Isoleucine to Valine at amino acid position 775 of the protein. To date, no replication study on these associations between TLR10 genetic variants and asthma has been conducted yet.

VI. CD14/TLR4 Genetic Variation and Chronic Obstructive Pulmonary Disease

Despite the strong scientific rationale for expecting a direct link between interindividual variation in innate immunity genes and COPD susceptibility and clinical progression, to date studies on this topic have been scanty. Because of the possible harmful effects of endotoxin exposure on lung health, one would expect the CD14 alleles associated with increased plasma sCD14 levels and, possibly, endotoxin hyperresponsiveness to be linked to low lung function among workers who are occupationally exposed to high levels of endotoxin. Consistent with this scenario, in a recent study LeVan et al. found farmers homozygous for CD14/-159T to have lower levels of FEV_1 and forced expiratory flow (FEF) during the middle half of the forced vital capacity (FEF_{25-75}) than farmers carrying the other genotypes (29). Farmers carrying the TT genotype were also at increased risk of wheezing. The same associations were replicated with the G-allele at position -1619, a SNP in strong but not complete linkage disequilibrium with CD14/-159, which had been also previously associated with increased plasma sCD14 levels (4). Findings from this study, together with those from previous functional studies, suggest a hypothetical causal pathway in endotoxin-induced airflow limitation: "CD14 polymorphisms→increased gene expression→ increased sCD14 levels→hyperresponsiveness to inhaled endotoxin→ increased airway inflammation→airflow limitation." Future empirical demonstration will be required to determine whether the underlying mechanisms of these genetic associations are indeed part of this causal pathway.

As mentioned above, subjects carrying the missense mutation Asp299Gly in the TLR4 gene have been shown to be less responsive to reduction of FEV_1 (32) and increase of markers of systemic inflammation (33), following endotoxin challenge. Therefore, the Gly299 allele should be also expected to be protective against development of airflow limitation among subjects exposed to endotoxin. In the above-mentioned study among farmers (29), no effect of Gly299 on lung function or respiratory symptoms was found. However, the Gly299 allele is quite rare in the general population (100) and studies aimed at detecting its effects on disease risk will need to be accordingly powered in terms of sample size. In a recent study from Germany (38), 7% of 152 hospitalized COPD patients were found to carry at least one copy of Gly299 as compared with 14% of 444 ethnically matched controls. Previously, Sabroe et al. had found no effect of Asp299Gly on lung function in a group of 289 smokers (39).

The effects of Asp299Gly on COPD may not be related only to endotoxin responsiveness. The same polymorphism has been, in fact, linked to susceptibility to viral and bacterial infections. Although endotoxin is the major ligand of TLR4, the innate immune responses to the fusion protein of the most important wheezing-related virus [namely, the respiratory syncytial virus (RSV)] were shown to be mediated by TLR4 and RSV was shown to persist longer in the lungs of TLR4-deficient mice (104). Subsequently, the Gly299 polymorphism was found to be overrepresented among infants hospitalized with severe RSV bronchiolitis, as compared with infants with mild RSV bronchiolitis or healthy adults (40). In addition to RSV infections, the TLR4 missense mutation at codon 299 appears to confer susceptibility to gram-negative infections (41,42). Lorenz et al. found patients with septic shock to carry the Gly299 allele more frequently than control blood donors (41). The authors also found that, among patients with septic shock, those carrying the alleles Gly299 and/or Ile399 had a higher prevalence of gram-negative infections (41). Similarly, Agnese et al. found that, in an intensive care unit population at risk for sepsis, 79% of patients carrying the cosegregating TLR4 mutations Gly299 and Ile399 had gram-negative infections, as compared with only 17% of patients who carried the wild type alleles (42). In a subsequent study, other rare TLR4 coding variants were found to be overrepresented among patients with systemic meningococcal infections (105). Given these findings, the impact of TLR4 coding variants on acute exacerbations and disease progression in patients with

COPD appears to be a very promising—yet to date largely unexplored—area of research. Gram-negative bacteria, in fact, play a central role in airway colonization and infections in patients with COPD and TLR4 signaling is likely to be an essential part in clearing the lungs from gram-negative bacteria, including nontypable *H. influenzae* (106) a species commonly isolated from COPD patients both during acute exacerbations and in stable conditions.

VII. Conclusions

The relation of genetic variation of CD14/TLRs to asthma and COPD holds remarkable scientific interest and promising public health implications, but it also offers a clear indication of the complexity of the gene-by-environment interactions involved in these multifactorial, polygenic diseases and of the challenges that scientists face to capture this complexity. In this chapter, we have mainly discussed the marginal and interactive effects of functional SNPs of the two major components of the endotoxin receptor system (i.e., CD14 and TLR4). This is consistent with the large number of studies conducted on atopy, asthma, and COPD involving these two genes, as contrasted with the fewer studies that addressed the role of other TLRs in these diseases. There are several reasons why scientists have focused mainly on CD14 and TLR4 to date. First, endotoxin has been long known to be linked to occupational decline of lung function. Second, within the frame of the hygiene hypothesis, endotoxin represents an easily detectable indicator of microbial exposure. Finally, functional studies have shown that genetic variation in CD14 and TLR4 can affect gene expression and protein function, providing the rationale for expecting an effect of these SNPs on human disease. Because of the potential role of other microbial components (such as those derived from gram-positive bacteria or viruses) in asthma and COPD, most likely polymorphisms in other TLRs will be also increasingly explored in relation to these diseases in future studies. It is also likely that future studies will increasingly use systematic approaches to describe genetic variation within genes by targeting TagSNPs that identify blocks of linkage disequilibrium and by using these TagSNPs to construct haplotypes and study the combined effects of polymorphisms at multiple loci (within and between genes) on disease risk.

   Although several arguments—including the unambiguous temporal relationship between exposure (i.e., genotype) and outcome (i.e., disease)— support the validity of the case-control study design for detecting genetic components of complex diseases (107), long-term longitudinal cohort studies will probably represent our best resource to dissect the specific interactions between innate immunity genes and microbial exposures in asthma and COPD. Longitudinal studies allow temporal assessment of environmental exposures and onset of disease (which cannot be resolved in cross-sectional studies) and identification of hypothetical windows of opportunity (i.e., critical periods in life in which exposures exert their effects on disease risk). In addition, they allow a longitudinal—and therefore insensitive to recall bias—characterization of different respiratory phenotypes that can recognize very different underlying genetic and environmental risk factors (e.g., nonfully reversible airflow limitation due to long-term asthma as contrasted with smoking-related COPD) (108–111). Finally, prospective data allow direct measurement of disease progression—such as slope of decline of FEV_1—and minimize the risk for survivor effects because at risk genotypes are determined before disease onset and, therefore, their carriers are not artificially removed from the pool of incident cases by mortality events, as it may happen with prevalent cases.

Regardless of the implemented study design and the gene under investigation, future genetic studies on asthma and COPD will need to take into account some important lessons from the inconsistent findings of previous studies on innate immunity genes. Discrepancies between well-designed genetic studies on CD14/-159 and allergies, for example, may be telling us something quite fundamental not only about how these diseases develop, but also how we can study and understand better their underlying mechanisms. Contrary to what has been the rule for monogenic diseases, the association between genetic variations and polygenic conditions such as asthma and COPD may not always be unidirectional; that is, not always will the same alleles be associated with the conditions under study, depending on the level and timing of exposure to environmental factors. The most important implication is that applying simple principles of fixed genetic penetrance, which work well for monogenic diseases, to the study of these complex diseases and ignoring the nonlinear influences of gene-by-environment interactions will not prove a successful strategy in genetic epidemiology studies. To capture the complexity of these interactions, future studies will need to face the challenges of seeking statistical detection of interactive effects, conducting assessments of environmental exposures in large samples of human populations, and centering criteria of study design selection (including estimation of statistical power, risk of bias, and adjustment for confounding) that have been traditionally used for detection of main effects, around detection of nonlinear effects.

References

1. Lazarus R, Vercelli D, Palmer LJ, et al. Single nucleotide polymorphisms in innate immunity genes: abundant variation and potential role in complex human disease. Immunol Rev 2002; 190:9–25.
2. LeVan TD, Bloom JW, Bailey TJ, et al. A common single nucleotide polymorphism in the CD14 promoter decreases the affinity of Sp protein binding and enhances transcriptional activity. J Immunol 2001; 167(10):5838–5844.

3. Baldini M, Lohman IC, Halonen M, Erickson RP, Holt PG, Martinez FD. A Polymorphism in the 5′ flanking region of the CD14 gene is associated with circulating soluble CD14 levels and with total serum immunoglobulin E. Am J Respir Cell Mol Biol 1999; 20(5):976–983.

4. Guerra S, Lohman CI, LeVan TD, Wright AL, Martinez FD, Halonen M. The differential effect of genetic variation on soluble CD14 levels in human plasma and milk. Am J Reprod Immunol 2004; 52(3):204–211.

5. Shimada K, Miyauchi K, Mokuno H, et al. Promoter polymorphism in the CD14 gene and concentration of soluble CD14 in patients with in-stent restenosis after elective coronary stenting. Int J Cardiol 2004; 94(1):87–92.

6. Leung TF, Tang NL, Sung YM, et al. The C-159T polymorphism in the CD14 promoter is associated with serum total IgE concentration in atopic Chinese children. Pediatr Allergy Immunol 2003; 14(4):255–260.

7. Koenig W, Khuseyinova N, Hoffmann MM, et al. CD14 C(-260)® T polymorphism, plasma levels of the soluble endotoxin receptor CD14, their association with chronic infections and risk of stable coronary artery disease. J Am Coll Cardiol 2002; 40(1):34–42.

8. Karhukorpi J, Yan Y, Niemela S, et al. Effect of CD14 promoter polymorphism and *H. pylori* infection and its clinical outcomes on circulating CD14. Clin Exp Immunol 2002; 128(2):326–332.

9. Kabesch M, Hasemann K, Schickinger V, et al. A promoter polymorphism in the CD14 gene is associated with elevated levels of soluble CD14 but not with IgE or atopic diseases. Allergy 2004; 59(5):520–525.

10. Takeuchi K, Suzuki S, Yagawa M, Yuta A, Majima Y. A CD14 gene polymorphism is associated with the IgE level for Dermatophagoides pteronyssinus. Acta Otolaryngol 2005; 125(9):966–971.

11. LeVan TD, Guerra S, Klimecki W, et al. The impact of CD14 polymorphisms on the development of soluble CD14 levels during infancy. Genes Immun 2006; 7(1):77–80.

12. Eng HL, Wang CH, Chen CH, Chou MH, Cheng CT, Lin TM. A CD14 promoter polymorphism is associated with CD14 expression and Chlamydia-stimulated TNF alpha production. Genes Immun 2004; 5(5):426–430.

13. Hubacek JA, Rothe G, Pit'ha J, et al. C(-260)®T polymorphism in the promoter of the CD14 monocyte receptor gene as a risk factor for myocardial infarction. Circulation 1999; 99(25):3218–3220.

14. Temple SE, Cheong KY, Almeida CM, Price P, Waterer GW. Polymorphisms in lymphotoxin alpha and CD14 genes influence TNFalpha production induced by gram-positive and gram-negative bacteria. Genes Immun 2003; 4(4):283–288.

15. Koppelman GH, Reijmerink NE, Colin Stine O, et al. Association of a promoter polymorphism of the CD14 gene and atopy. Am J Respir Crit Care Med 2001; 163(4):965–969.

16. Buckova D, Holla LI, Schuller M, Znojil V, Vacha J. Two CD14 promoter polymorphisms and atopic phenotypes in Czech patients with IgE-mediated allergy. Allergy 2003; 58(10):1023–1026.

17. Gao PS, Mao XQ, Baldini M, et al. Serum total IgE levels and CD14 on chromosome 5q31. Clin Genet 1999; 56(2):164–165.

18. O'Donnell AR, Toelle BG, Marks GB, et al. Age-specific relationship between CD14 and atopy in a cohort assessed from age 8 to 25 years. Am J Respir Crit Care Med 2004; 169(5):615–622.

19. Sackesen C, Karaaslan C, Keskin O, et al. The effect of polymorphisms at the CD14 promoter and the TLR4 gene on asthma phenotypes in Turkish children with asthma. Allergy 2005: 60(12):1485–1495.

20. Sharma M, Batra J, Mabalirajan U, et al. Suggestive evidence of association of C-159T functional polymorphism of the CD14 gene with atopic asthma in northern and northwestern Indian populations. Immunogenetics 2004; 56(7): 544–547.

21. Ober C, Tsalenko A, Parry R, Cox NJ. A second-generation genomewide screen for asthma-susceptibility alleles in a founder population. Am J Human Genet 2000; 67(5):1154–1162.

22. Amelung PJ, Weisch DG, Xu J, Paigen B, Meyers DA, Bleecker ER. A polymorphism in CD14 is associated with high IgE levels in a population with laboratory animal allergy. Am J Respir Crit Car Med 2000; 161(3):A927.

23. Litonjua AA, Belanger K, Celedon JC, et al. Polymorphisms in the 5' region of the CD14 gene are associated with eczema in young children. J Allergy Clin Immunol 2005; 115(5):1056–1062.

24. Woo JG, Assa'ad A, Heizer AB, Bernstein JA, Hershey GK. The -159 C®T polymorphism of CD14 is associated with nonatopic asthma and food allergy. J Allergy Clin Immunol 2003; 112(2):438–444.

25. Zambelli-Weiner A, Ehrlich E, Stockton ML, et al. Evaluation of the CD14/-260 polymorphism and house dust endotoxin exposure in the Barbados Asthma Genetics Study. J Allergy Clin Immunol 2005; 115(6):1203–1209.

26. Eder W, Klimecki W, Yu L, et al. Opposite effects of CD 14/-260 on serum IgE levels in children raised in different environments. J Allergy Clin Immunol 2005; 116(3):601–607.

27. Gern JE, Reardon CL, Hoffjan S, et al. Effects of dog ownership and genotype on immune development and atopy in infancy. J Allergy Clin Immunol 2004; 113(2):307–314.

28. Choudhry S, Avila PC, Nazario S, et al. CD14 tobacco gene-environment interaction modifies asthma severity and immunoglobulin E levels in Latinos with asthma. Am J Respir Crit Care Med 2005; 172(2):173–182.

29. LeVan TD, Von Essen S, Romberger DJ, et al. Polymorphisms in the CD14 gene associated with pulmonary function in farmers. Am J Respir Crit Care Med 2005; 171(7):773–779.

30. Rupp J, Goepel W, Kramme E, Jahn J, Solbach W, Maass M. CD14 promoter polymorphism -159C > T is associated with susceptibility to chronic Chlamydia pneumoniae infection in peripheral blood monocytes. Genes Immun 2004; 5(5):435–438.

31. Eng HL, Chen CH, Kuo CC, Wu JS, Wang CH, Lin TM. Association of CD14 promoter gene polymorphism and Chlamydia pneumoniae infection. J Infect Dis 2003; 188(1):90–97.

32. Arbour NC, Lorenz E, Schutte BC, et al. TLR4 mutations are associated with endotoxin hyporesponsiveness in humans. Nat Genet 2000; 25(2):187–191.

33. Michel O, LeVan TD, Stern D, et al. Systemic responsiveness to lipopolysaccharide and polymorphisms in the toll-like receptor 4 gene in human beings. J Allergy Clin Immunol 2003; 112(5):923–929.

34. Fageras Bottcher M, Hmani-Aifa M, Lindstrom A, et al. A TLR4 polymorphism is associated with asthma and reduced lipopolysaccharide-induced interleukin-12(p70) responses in Swedish children. J Allergy Clin Immunol 2004; 114(3): 561–567.

35. Eder W, Klimecki W, Yu L, et al. Toll-like receptor 2 as a major gene for asthma in children of European farmers. J Allergy Clin Immunol 2004; 113(3): 482–488.

36. Yang IA, Barton SJ, Rorke S, et al. Toll-like receptor 4 polymorphism and severity of atopy in asthmatics. Genes Immun 2004; 5(1):41–45.

37. Werner M, Topp R, Wimmer K, et al. TLR4 gene variants modify endotoxin effects on asthma. J Allergy Clin Immunol 2003; 112(2):323–330.

38. Rohde G, Klein W, Arinir U, et al. Association of the ASP299GLY TLR4 polymorphism with COPD. Respir Med 2006; 100(5):892–896.

39. Sabroe I, Whyte MK, Wilson AG, Dower SK, Hubbard R, Hall I. Toll-like receptor (TLR) 4 polymorphisms and COPD. Thorax 2004; 59(1):81.

40. Tal G, Mandelberg A, Dalal I, et al. Association between common toll-like receptor 4 mutations and severe respiratory syncytial virus disease. J Infect Dis 2004; 189(11):2057–2063.

41. Lorenz E, Mira JP, Frees KL, Schwartz DA. Relevance of mutations in the TLR4 receptor in patients with gram-negative septic shock. Arch Intern Med 2002; 162(9):1028–1032.

42. Agnese DM, Calvano JE, Hahm SJ, et al. Human toll-like receptor 4 mutations but not CD14 polymorphisms are associated with an increased risk of gram-negative infections. J Infect Dis 2002; 186(10):1522–1525.

43. Dalvi MS, Halonen M. A polymorphism in TLR2 (-16934A®T) influences TLR2 surface expression on human monocytes. Proc Am Thorac Soc 2005; 2: A736.

44. Tantisira K, Klimecki WT, Lazarus R, et al. Toll-like receptor 6 gene (TLR6): single-nucleotide polymorphism frequencies and preliminary association with the diagnosis of asthma. Genes Immun 2004; 5(5):343–346.

45. Hoffjan S, Stemmler S, Parwez Q, et al. Evaluation of the toll-like receptor 6 Ser249Pro polymorphism in patients with asthma, atopic dermatitis and chronic obstructive pulmonary disease. BMC Med Genet 2005; 6:34.

46. Lazarus R, Raby BA, Lange C, et al. Toll-like receptor 10 genetic variation is associated with asthma in two independent samples. Am J Respir Crit Care Med 2004; 170(6):594–600.

47. Haziot A, Chen S, Ferrero E, Low MG, Silber R, Goyert SM. The monocyte differentiation antigen, CD14, is anchored to the cell membrane by a phosphatidylinositol linkage. J Immunol 1988; 141(2):547–552.

48. Akira S, Hemmi H. Recognition of pathogen-associated molecular patterns by TLR family. Immunol Lett 2003; 85(2):85–95.

49. Ulevitch RJ, Mathison JC, Correia JS. Innate immune responses during infection. Vaccine 2004; 22(suppl 1):S25–S30.

50. Heil F, Hemmi H, Hochrein H, et al. Species-specific recognition of single-stranded RNA via toll-like receptor 7 and 8. Sci 2004; 303(5663):1526–1529.

51. Mukhopadhyay S, Herre J, Brown GD, Gordon S. The potential for toll-like receptors to collaborate with other innate immune receptors. Immunol 2004; 112(4):521–530.

52. Cook DN, Pisetsky DS, Schwartz DA. Toll-like receptors in the pathogenesis of human disease. Nat Immunol 2004; 5(10):975–979.

53. Aderem A, Ulevitch RJ. Toll-like receptors in the induction of the innate immune response. Nature 2000; 406(6797):782–787.

54. Andreakos E, Foxwell B, Feldmann M. Is targeting toll-like receptors and their signaling pathway a useful therapeutic approach to modulating cytokine-driven inflammation? Immunol Rev 2004; 202:250–265.

55. Hayashi F, Means TK, Luster AD. Toll-like receptors stimulate human neutrophil function. Blood 2003; 102(7):2660–2669.

56. Basu S, Fenton MJ. Toll-like receptors: function and roles in lung disease. Am J Physiol Lung Cell Mol Physiol 2004; 286(5):L887–L892.

57. http://www.innateimmunity.net

58. http://pga.mbt.washington.edu

59. Carlson CS, Eberle MA, Rieder MJ, Yi Q, Kruglyak L, Nickerson DA. Selecting a maximally informative set of single-nucleotide polymorphisms for association analyses using linkage disequilibrium. Am J Hum Genet 2004; 74(1):106–120.

60. Labeta MO, Vidal K, Nores JE, et al. Innate recognition of bacteria in human milk is mediated by a milk-derived highly expressed pattern recognition receptor, soluble CD14. J Exp Med 2000; 191(10):1807–1812.

61. Landmann R, Zimmerli W, Sansano S, et al. Increased circulating soluble CD14 is associated with high mortality in gram-negative septic shock. J Infect Dis 1995; 171(3):639–644.

62. Lien E, Aukrust P, Sundan A, Muller F, Froland SS, Espevik T. Elevated levels of serum-soluble CD14 in human immunodeficiency virus type 1 (HIV-1) infection: correlation to disease progression and clinical events. Blood 1998; 92(6):2084–2092.

63. Nockher WA, Wick M, Pfister HW. Cerebrospinal fluid levels of soluble CD14 in inflammatory and non-inflammatory diseases of the CNS: upregulation during bacterial infections and viral meningitis. J Neuroimmunol 1999; 101(2): 161–169.

64. Egerer K, Feist E, Rohr U, Pruss A, Burmester GR, Dorner T. Increased serum soluble CD14, ICAM-1 and E-selectin correlate with disease activity and prognosis in systemic lupus erythematosus. Lupus 2000; 9(8):614–621.

65. Guerra S, Lohman IC, Halonen M, Martinez FD, Wright AL. Reduced interferon gamma production and soluble CD14 levels in early life predict recurrent wheezing by 1 year of age. Am J Respir Crit Care Med 2004; 169(1):70–76.

66. Jones CA, Holloway JA, Popplewell EJ, et al. Reduced soluble CD14 levels in amniotic fluid and breast milk are associated with the subsequent development of atopy, eczema, or both. J Allergy Clin Immunol 2002; 109(5):858–866.

67. Poltorak A, He X, Smirnova I, et al. Defective LPS signaling in C3H/HeJ and C57BL/10ScCr mice: mutations in TLR4 gene. Sci 1998; 282(5396): 2085–2088.

68. Strachan DP. Hay fever, hygiene, and household size. BMJ 1989; 299(6710): 1259–1260.
69. Martinez FD, Holt PG. Role of microbial burden in aetiology of allergy and asthma. Lancet 1999; 354(suppl 2):SII12–SII15.
70. Ball TM, Castro-Rodriguez JA, Griffith KA, Holberg CJ, Martinez FD, Wright AL. Siblings, day-care attendance, and the risk of asthma and wheezing during childhood. N Engl J Med 2000; 343(8):538–543.
71. Braun-Fahrlander C, Riedler J, Herz U, et al. Environmental exposure to endotoxin and its relation to asthma in school-age children. N Engl J Med 2002; 347(12):869–877.
72. Sengler C, Haider A, Sommerfeld C, et al. Evaluation of the CD14 C-159 T polymorphism in the German multicenter allergy study cohort. Clin Exp Allergy 2003; 33(2):166–169.
73. Litonjua AA, Milton DK, Celedon JC, Ryan L, Weiss ST, Gold DR. A longitudinal analysis of wheezing in young children: the independent effects of early life exposure to house dust endotoxin, allergens, and pets. J Allergy Clin Immunol 2002; 110(5):736–742.
74. Tulic MK, Wale JL, Holt PG, Sly PD. Modification of the inflammatory response to allergen challenge after exposure to bacterial lipopolysaccharide. Am J Respir Cell Mol Biol 2000; 22(5):604–612.
75. Liu AH. Endotoxin exposure in allergy and asthma: reconciling a paradox. J Allergy Clin Immunol 2002; 109(3):379–392.
76. Tetley TD. Macrophages and the pathogenesis of COPD. Chest 2002; 121 (suppl 5):156S–159S.
77. Hogg JC, Chu F, Utokaparch S, et al. The nature of small-airway obstruction in chronic obstructive pulmonary disease. N Engl J Med 2004; 350(26): 2645–2653.
78. Droemann D, Goldmann T, Branscheid D, et al. Toll-like receptor 2 is expressed by alveolar epithelial cells type II and macrophages in the human lung. Histochem Cell Biol 2003; 119(2):103–108.
79. Russell RE, Culpitt SV, DeMatos C, et al. Release and activity of matrix metalloproteinase-9 and tissue inhibitor of metalloproteinase-1 by alveolar macrophages from patients with chronic obstructive pulmonary disease. Am J Respir Cell Mol Biol 2002; 26(5):602–609.
80. Nevalainen M, Raulo SM, Brazil TJ, et al. Inhalation of organic dusts and lipopolysaccharide increases gelatinolytic matrix metalloproteinases (MMPs) in the lungs of heaves horses. Equine Vet J 2002; 34(2):150–155.
81. Martin TR, Mathison JC, Tobias PS, et al. Lipopolysaccharide binding protein enhances the responsiveness of alveolar macrophages to bacterial lipopolysaccharide. Implications for cytokine production in normal and injured lungs. J Clin Invest 1992; 90(6):2209–2219.
82. Rankin JA, Sylvester I, Smith S, Yoshimura T, Leonard EJ. Macrophages cultured in vitro release leukotriene B4 and neutrophil attractant/activation protein (interleukin 8) sequentially in response to stimulation with lipopolysaccharide and zymosan. J Clin Invest 1990; 86(5):1556–1564.
83. Barnes PJ. Cytokine-directed therapies for the treatment of chronic airway diseases. Cytokine Growth Factor Rev 2003; 14(6):511–522.

84. Rylander R. Endotoxin in the environment—exposure and effects. J Endotoxin Res 2002; 8(4):241–252.
85. Castellan RM, Olenchock SA, Kinsley KB, Hankinson JL. Inhaled endotoxin and decreased spirometric values. An exposure-response relation for cotton dust. N Engl J Med 1987; 317(10):605–610.
86. Vogelzang PF, van der Gulden JW, Folgering H, et al. Endotoxin exposure as a major determinant of lung function decline in pig farmers. Am J Respir Crit Care Med 1998; 157(1):15–18.
87. Iversen M, Dahl R. Working in swine-confinement buildings causes an accelerated decline in FEV1: a 7-yr follow-up of Danish farmers. Eur Respir J 2000; 16(3):404–408.
88. Hasday JD, Bascom R, Costa JJ, Fitzgerald T, Dubin W. Bacterial endotoxin is an active component of cigarette smoke. Chest 1999; 115(3):829–835.
89. Larsson L, Szponar B, Pehrson C. Tobacco smoking increases dramatically air concentrations of endotoxin. Indoor Air 2004; 14(6):421–424.
90. Wilson R. Bacteria, antibiotics and COPD. Eur Respir J 2001; 17(5):995–1007.
91. Soto FJ, Varkey B. Evidence-based approach to acute exacerbations of COPD. Curr Opin Pulm Med 2003; 9(2):117–124.
92. Sethi S, Evans N, Grant BJ, Murphy TF. New strains of bacteria and exacerbations of chronic obstructive pulmonary disease. N Engl J Med 2002; 347(7):465–471.
93. Sethi S. Infectious etiology of acute exacerbations of chronic bronchitis. Chest 2000; 117(5 suppl 2):380S–385S.
94. Wedzicha JA. Airway infection accelerates decline of lung function in chronic obstructive pulmonary disease. Am J Respir Crit Care Med 2001; 164(10 Pt 1): 1757–1758.
95. MacNee W. Airway infection does not accelerate decline in lung function in chronic obstructive pulmonary disease. Am J Respir Crit Care Med 2001; 164(10 Pt 1):1758–1760.
96. Sethi S. Bacterial infection and the pathogenesis of COPD. Chest 2000; 117 (5 suppl 1):286S–291S.
97. Patel IS, Seemungal TA, Wilks M, Lloyd-Owen SJ, Donaldson GC, Wedzicha JA. Relationship between bacterial colonisation and the frequency, character, and severity of COPD exacerbations. Thorax 2002; 57(9):759–764.
98. Wilkinson TM, Patel IS, Wilks M, Donaldson GC, Wedzicha JA. Airway bacterial load and FEV$_1$ decline in patients with chronic obstructive pulmonary disease. Am J Respir Crit Care Med 2003; 167(8):1090–1095.
99. Hill AT, Campbell EJ, Hill SL, Bayley DL, Stockley RA. Association between airway bacterial load and markers of airway inflammation in patients with stable chronic bronchitis. Am J Med 2000; 109(4):288–295.
100. Raby BA, Klimecki WT, Laprise C, et al. Polymorphisms in toll-like receptor 4 are not associated with asthma or atopy-related phenotypes. Am J Respir Crit Care Med 2002; 166(11):1449–1456.
101. Lazarus R, Klimecki WT, Raby BA, et al. Single-nucleotide polymorphisms in the toll-like receptor 9 gene (TLR9): frequencies, pairwise linkage disequilibrium, and haplotypes in three U.S. ethnic groups and exploratory case-control disease association studies. Genomics 2003; 81(1):85–91.

102. Berghofer B, Frommer T, Konig IR, et al. Common human toll-like receptor 9 polymorphisms and haplotypes: association with atopy and functional relevance. Clin Exp Allergy 2005; 35(9):1147–1154.

103. Noguchi E, Nishimura F, Fukai H, et al. An association study of asthma and total serum immunoglobin E levels for toll-like receptor polymorphisms in a Japanese population. Clin Exp Allergy 2004; 34(2):177–183.

104. Kurt-Jones EA, Popova L, Kwinn L, et al. Pattern recognition receptors TLR4 and CD14 mediate response to respiratory syncytial virus. Nat Immunol 2000; 1(5):398–401.

105. Smirnova I, Mann N, Dols A, et al. Assay of locus-specific genetic load implicates rare toll-like receptor 4 mutations in meningococcal susceptibility. Proc Natl Acad Sci USA 2003; 100(10):6075–6080.

106. Wieland CW, Florquin S, Maris NA, et al. The MyD88-Dependent, but Not the MyD88-Independent, Pathway of TLR4 Signaling Is Important in Clearing Nontypeable Haemophilus influenzae from the Mouse Lung. J Immunol 2005; 175(9):6042–6049.

107. Clayton D, McKeigue PM. Epidemiological methods for studying genes and environmental factors in complex diseases. Lancet 2001; 358(9290):1356–1360.

108. Guerra S. Overlap of asthma and chronic obstructive pulmonary disease. Curr Opin Pulm Med 2005; 11(1):7–13.

109. Silva GE, Sherrill DL, Guerra S, Barbee RA. Asthma as a risk factor for COPD in a longitudinal study. Chest 2004; 126:59–65.

110. Ulrik CS, Backer V. Nonreversible airflow obstruction in life-long nonsmokers with moderate to severe asthma. Eur Respir J 1999; 14(4):892–896.

111. Vonk JM, Jongepier H, Panhuysen CI, Schouten JP, Bleecker ER, Postma DS. Risk factors associated with the presence of irreversible airflow limitation and reduced transfer coefficient in patients with asthma after 26 years of follow up. Thorax 2003; 58(4):322–327.

18

Pharmacogenetics

KELAN TANTISIRA

Channing Laboratory and Pulmonary
Division, Brigham and Women's
Hospital, Harvard Medical School,
Boston, Massachusetts, U.S.A.

EUGENE BLEECKER

Division of Pulmonary and Critical Care
Medicine and Center for Human
Genomics, Wake Forest University
School of Medicine,
Winston-Salem, North Carolina, U.S.A.

Kuamon apechete.

—("Abstain from Beans") *Pythagoras* ~510 B.C.

I. Overview of Pharmacogenetics

A. Introduction

Individual response to pharmacologic agents varies tremendously. For example, the plasma level of a given medication may vary more than 1000-fold between two individuals having the same weight when treated with the same drug dosage (1). On average for a given drug, 30% of patients show beneficial effects, 30% fail to improve, 10% only experience side effects, and 30% are noncompliant (which may be related to either lack of efficacy or side effects) (2). Therefore, as many as 70% of all patients are using medications with no overt therapeutic benefit and are unnecessarily exposed to the potential to develop adverse drug reactions (ADRs) (3). In 1994, over 2 million "serious ADRs" and over 100,000 fatal ADRs were

357

noted, ranking ADRs between the fourth and the sixth leading cause of death in the United States (4). Overall, the cost of drug-related morbidity and mortality exceeded $177.4 billion in 2000 (5). As substantial as these figures are, the burden due to failure to respond therapeutically to drug therapy is likely to be much greater (6).

The ability to effectively prevent ADRs may lie in the recognition of genetic factors influencing these outcomes. Genetic factors also likely contribute to treatment response because the intraindividual response to a given therapeutic agent is highly repeatable (7). In fact, genetic variability in drug absorption, drug metabolism, and drug action at the receptor level is well known. Overall, an estimated from 20% to 95% of variability in drug disposition and effects may be attributable to genetics (8).

Pharmacogenetics is defined as the study of variability in drug response due to heritable factors. That is, pharmacogenetics seeks to determine the role of genetic determinants in an individual's response to therapy. Ideally, the field of pharmacogenetics will allow for "individualized therapy" based upon an individual's genetic makeup that will maximize the potential for therapeutic benefit, while minimizing the risk of adverse effects of a given drug. The potential for cost savings and for decreasing morbidity and mortality is immense.

This chapter provides a practical overview of the field of pharmacogenetics, with an emphasis on the genetics of drug-treatment response in asthma and chronic obstructive pulmonary disease (COPD). We begin with a description of the four major categories of pharmacogenetic response. The chapter continues with a review of the literature on the rationale behind pharmacogenetic testing and the pharmacogenetic associations that have been characterized in relation to asthma and COPD. We conclude with some thoughts on the future of pharmacogenetics in these two diseases.

B. Pharmacogenetic Categories

Pharmacogenetics has traditionally been divided into four categories based upon the effects of genetic variability on the pharmacologic properties of a drug. The categories include genetic variation related to pharmacokinetics, pharmacodynamics, idiosyncratic reactions, and disease pathogenesis (9). *Pharmacokinetics* studies the effect of the body upon an administered drug, including those related to the absorption, distribution, tissue localization, biotransformation, and excretion of drugs (10). The vast majority of pharmacogenetic investigations reported in the literature to date have been in this area. Interestingly, however, relatively few pharmacokinetic studies related to asthma and COPD pharmacogenetics have been performed. The major areas of pharmacokinetic investigations in the field of pharmacogenetics have been in the evaluation of genetic differences in drug metabolizing enzymes and drug transporters. The cytochrome P450

(CYP) enzymes are the most prevalent examples of drug metabolizing enzymes, while members of the adenosine triphosphate–binding cassette family of membrane transporters are among the most extensively studied transporters in terms of disposition and effects (8). Given the evolving knowledge of pharmacokinetic pharmacogenetics, preliminary dosing recommendations have been made based upon known genetic variations in drug metabolizing enzymes (6,11,12).

Pharmacodynamics is the study of the biochemical and physiological consequences of the administration of a drug and its mechanism of action (10), i.e., the effect of a drug at its therapeutic target. Genetic variation may lead to interindividual differences in response to a drug despite the presence of appropriate concentrations of the drug at its intended target. In this category, the genetic variation is typically present at the site of the target or one of the downstream participants in the target's mechanistic pathway, thereby modulating the effects of the drug. One example is the enhanced inhibition of platelets in subjects with the Pl^{A2} polymorphism, which encodes for Leu → Pro at position 33 of the GPIIIa subunit of the GPIIb-IIIa fibrinogen receptor (ITGB3) upon administration of aspirin (13). No differences in platelet aggregation are noted with this genetic variant in the absence of aspirin.

While studies of pharmacogenetic predictors of efficacy at therapeutic target sites are slated to eventually become the primary basis for "individualized therapy," to date there remain relatively few examples of replicable pharmacodynamic pharmacogenetic associations, compared with those related to pharmacokinetics (14). At least three reasons exist for the prominence of pharmacokinetic studies when compared to those fitting the pharmacodynamic category. The first is that the biology of drug metabolism and drug transport is relatively straightforward; each compound typically has one principal enzyme responsible for its metabolism. However, the physiology of most drug target pathways is fairly complex, providing multiple venues for investigation of the target pathway. The second is that genetic differences in drug metabolism can be as high as 10,000-fold, whereas such differences in target binding are generally less than 20-fold (15,16). The resultant ability (power) to detect differences in metabolism within a population given a compound is clearly far greater than the ability to detect variance in drug targets. Finally, the inheritance pattern underlying the pharmacogenetic effects related to differences in drug metabolism or transport can often be defined as Mendelian. In contrast, the inheritance patterns of pharmacodynamic pharmacogenetic relationships usually demonstrate relationships consistent with the complex traits underlying the purpose of the drug. Thus, these target responses tend to be determined by polygenic or gene–environment interactions, which are much more difficult to identify.

The *idiosyncratic* category of pharmacogenetic response to drugs includes the individuals that experience an ADR to a therapeutic agent that could not be anticipated based upon the known drug target. Examples of the idiosyncratic category include some compounds that are metabolized by arylamine-N-acetyltransferase 2 (*NAT2*), a phase II–drug metabolizing enzyme. Genetic differences in *NAT2* have been associated with predisposition to the development of peripheral neuropathy in certain individuals taking isoniazid (17) and hypersensitivity reactions to trimethoprim-sulfamethoxazole (including rash, granulocytopenia, and abnormal liver function tests) (17,18). Interestingly, the *NAT2* acetylator phenotype (based upon metabolized level of drugs) may correlate poorly with *NAT2* genotype (19,20), suggesting that factors other than drug level may explain these idiosyncratic reactions associated with genetic variation.

The final pharmacogenetic category is that of genetic factors influencing *disease pathogenesis*. Genetic variants that affect properties related to the mechanistic basis of disease, including those linked to disease susceptibility or disease progression, can also affect the ability of a therapeutic agent to treat the disease. This becomes apparent when one considers that the majority of medications are developed based upon knowledge of disease pathogenesis. The category can be exemplified by variation of the angiotensin converting enzyme (*ACE*) gene and its effect on the progression of disease related to systemic hypertension. The *ACE* gene carries a 287 nucleotide insertion/deletion polymorphism in intron 16; the deletion (D) allele has consistently been associated with higher ACE activity and higher angiotensin II levels (6,21). The prognosis of patients with systolic dysfunction is significantly worse in heterozygous and homozygous carriers of the *ACE D* allele than in *I* allele homozygotes (21). However, the *ACE D* allele also impacts therapeutic interactions on the converting enzyme itself. In a study comparing 12 homozygous *ACE DD* individuals with 11 homozygous for *ACE II*, enalapralat (an ACE inhibiting antihypertensive drug) had a significantly greater and longer lasting effect in subjects with the *ACE II* genotype than in those with the *ACE DD* genotype (22). Overall, *ACE* (*I/D*) genotype and plasma angiotensin II levels were predictive of >50% of the variation in response to ACE inhibition (22).

II. The Pharmacogenetics of Asthma

An estimated 300 million individuals worldwide are affected by asthma (23), a clinical disease characterized by inflammation, reversible airways obstruction, and bronchial hyperresponsiveness (24). Ninety percent of all asthma, including asthma in adults, has its origin in childhood. Of prevailing concern are the recent increases in asthma prevalence (23,25,26), hospitalization rates (27), and mortality (25,28). Between 1980 and 1994, the self-reported prevalence of asthma in the United States increased from 30.7 to 53.8 per 1000, an increase of 75% (25). An estimated $12.6 billion were spent on the diagnosis and management of asthma in the United States in 1998, of which 58% were direct medical expenditures (29). This represents over a doubling of costs compared to 1990. Medication costs are currently the largest component of these direct medical expenditures. Asthma therapy has been associated with ADRs, including serious and potentially fatal complications (30,31). Clearly, the ability to optimize asthma medications by maximizing response and minimizing side effects in a cost-effective manner would have tremendous global impact.

Asthma is a genetic disease, noted to cluster in families for over three centuries (32). Based on twin studies, the broad sense heritability estimates (proportion of the total variance of a trait due to genetic causes) of the diagnosis of asthma range from 36% (33) to 75% (34). Asthma is a complex disease, in that no single gene is causal by itself. Instead, it likely results from the influence of multiple genetic, environmental, and developmental factors. There are currently three major classes of therapeutic agents available for the treatment of asthma. Nevertheless, it has been estimated that as many as one-half of asthmatic patients do not respond to treatment with β_2-agonists, leukotriene antagonists, or inhaled corticosteroids (7,9). In evaluating asthma therapy response, measures of lung function, as manifested by the forced expiratory volume at one second (FEV_1), and of airway responsiveness, as measured by the provocative concentration of methacholine causing a 20% decrement in FEV_1 (PC_{20}), are commonly used. However, there are large interindividual variations in the FEV_1 and PC_{20} responses to asthma treatment (Fig. 1) (35,36). As the intraindividual response to treatment in patients with asthma is highly repeatable (7) and as both FEV_1 and PC_{20} are heritable traits (37,38), a genetic basis for the heterogeneity of this therapeutic response is plausible. Moreover, because asthma is a genetic disease, heritable factors that influence the natural history of asthma progression may also affect the ability of an individual to respond to therapy. Thus, the field of asthma is well suited to pharmacogenetic investigations.

A. Asthma Pharmacogenetic Phenotypes

Accurate phenotypic definition, including those pertaining to drug-treatment response, is crucial in genetic studies in order to avoid diagnostic misclassification (39,40). Examples of phenotypes that have been used or proposed in relation to asthma pharmacogenetics are listed in Table 1. However, as noted a quarter century ago, "asthma is like love. Everyone seems to know what it is, but no one can define it" (41). Given the limitations of the definition of asthma, it is not surprising that no one universally accepted, or optimal, definition of what constitutes a meaningful response to asthma therapy currently exists.

For pharmacokinetic studies, the measurement of drug levels is the normal focus of measurement, with the further assumption that drug levels

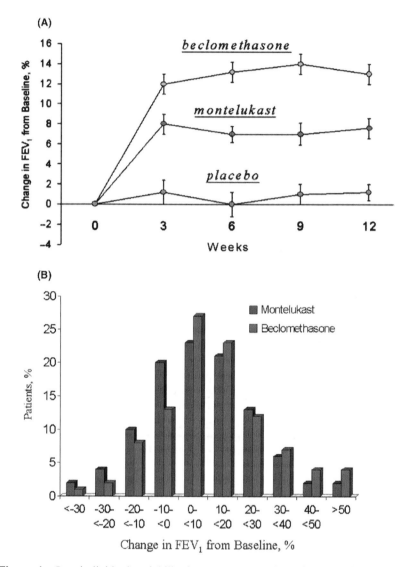

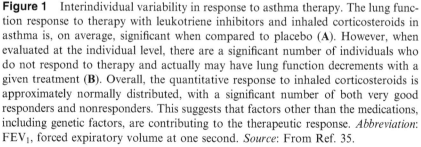

Figure 1   Interindividual variability in response to asthma therapy. The lung function response to therapy with leukotriene inhibitors and inhaled corticosteroids in asthma is, on average, significant when compared to placebo (**A**). However, when evaluated at the individual level, there are a significant number of individuals who do not respond to therapy and actually may have lung function decrements with a given treatment (**B**). Overall, the quantitative response to inhaled corticosteroids is approximately normally distributed, with a significant number of both very good responders and nonresponders. This suggests that factors other than the medications, including genetic factors, are contributing to the therapeutic response. *Abbreviation*: FEV_1, forced expiratory volume at one second. *Source*: From Ref. 35.

Table 1 Asthma Pharmacogenetic Phenotypes: Proposed and Used

Pharmacogenetic response class and measured phenotype	Applicable therapeutic pathway(s)
Pharmacokinetic	
Plasma/tissue β-agonist levels	β$_2$-Agonist
Plasma/tissue leukotriene levels	Leukotriene
Plasma/tissue cortisol levels	Corticosteroid
Hypokalemia/tachycardia	β$_2$-Agonist
Bone mineral density	Corticosteroid
Pharmacodynamic	
Measures of lung function	
FEV$_1$	*β$_2$-Agonist, leukotriene, corticosteroid*
Peak flow rates	*β$_2$-Agonist*, leukotriene, corticosteroid
Measures of airway tone	
Bronchodilator response	*β$_2$-Agonist*, ±leukotriene, *corticosteroid*
PC$_{20}$	β$_2$-Agonist, leukotriene, *corticosteroid*
Measures of atopy	
Eosinophil count	±β$_2$-Agonist, leukotriene, corticosteroid
IgE levels	±β$_2$-Agonist, leukotriene, corticosteroid
Other	
Health care utilization	β$_2$-Agonist, leukotriene, corticosteroid
Exhaled nitric oxide	±β$_2$-Agonist, *leukotriene*, corticosteroid
Disease modifying	
Asthma diagnosis	β$_2$-Agonist, leukotriene, corticosteroid
Basal lung function	β$_2$-Agonist, leukotriene, corticosteroid
Basal airway tone	β$_2$-Agonist, leukotriene, corticosteroid
Basal atopy measures	±β$_2$-Agonist, leukotriene, corticosteroid

Note: Phenotypes that have been used in association with a given therapeutic pathway and reported in the literature (see accompanying text) was mentioned in italics.
±, Role of phenotype in relationship to therapeutic drug class has yet to be fully determined.
Abbreviations: IgE, immunoglobulinE; FEV$_1$, forced expiratory volume at one second.

will subsequently correlate with both therapeutic success and medication side effects. Interestingly, while the pharmacokinetic profiles of the three major classes of asthma medications have been well characterized, pharmacogenetic studies evaluating the genetic basis for variability in drug metabolism of these agents have not been reported to date. All three of these types of asthma treatments are metabolized in the liver by well-known mechanisms; the β$_2$-agonists undergo sulfate conjugation (42), while both leukotriene antagonists and corticosteroids use the CYP system for a significant portion of their metabolism (43,44). Furthermore, each of these therapeutic medications demonstrates marked interindividual variability in drug metabolism, suggesting that genetics may play a role. In fact, in one study of the metabolism of the widely prescribed β$_2$-agonist albuterol (salbutamol), a classic bimodal peak in the rate of hepatic sulfation was noted [mean sulfation rates of 69.5 and 105 pmol/min/mg ($p < 0.05$)] (42). Additionally, while it may be argued that systemic pharmacokinetics has little to do with interindividual variation in response at the level of the therapeutic target, given that these medications are administered primarily through inhalation, a large percentage (approximately 40–90%) of drugs administered through metered dose inhalers is swallowed and available for systemic absorption (45). While the therapeutic benefit derived from this systemic absorption is unclear, systemic side effects that may be mediated in part due to genetic variation in drug metabolizing enzymes can clearly result. Finally, pharmacokinetic characteristics at or near the target receptor site can affect therapeutic efficacy. For instance, plasma protein binding, drug clearance, half-life, mean absorption time from the lungs to the systemic circulation, and lipid conjugation have all been related to target bioavailability in studies of inhaled corticosteroids (45). Similarly, all of the commonly prescribed β-agonist medications are racemic drugs, comprising a mixture of *R* and *S* isomers. While the *R* isomers mimic endogenous epinephrine in their action, producing bronchodilation and mast cell suppression, the *S* isomers have the potential to exacerbate airway reactivity (46). As the *S* isomer has a longer half-life, understanding the genetic determinants of its metabolism may shed light into the response to β-agonist medications. While we describe studies on theophylline as an example, pharmacogenetic studies directed toward exploring the genetic basis of the pharmacokinetics of the three major classes of asthma therapy are warranted.

In the case of pharmacodynamic studies of asthma therapies, intermediate phenotypes or measures of disease severity are often obtained preceding and following the administration of the drug, forming the basis of the measured therapeutic response. In the asthma pharmacogenetics literature to date, most of the quantitative intermediate phenotypes used to assess pharmacodynamic responses have focused on measures of lung function or airway tone. For example, in a study by Malmstrom et al. (35) comparing the efficacy of the inhaled steroid beclomethasone (200 µg bid) with the leukotriene antagonist montelukast (10 mg/qd), it is clear that both drugs are effective over a 12-week course of treatment with a mean increase in FEV_1 of 13.1% for the beclomethasone group and 7.4% for the montelukast group (Fig. 1A) (35). However, when these same data are viewed from a different perspective, focusing on the number of individuals as a function of percent change in FEV_1 from baseline, it is clear that many patients had little to no response (Fig. 1B). In fact, 22% of patients appear to have had an adverse response to treatment with a decline in FEV_1 at 12 weeks compared with baseline. The mean therapeutic improvement in FEV_1 for all patients is driven by a dramatic increase in FEV_1 in a minority of trial subjects. In a similar study, 38% of patients randomized to inhaled budesonide or fluticasone demonstrated improvements in FEV_1 of below 5% over the course of

24 weeks (47). Moreover, the FEV_1 correlates well with clinical asthma severity, degree of airways obstruction, and other physiologic markers of asthma severity and with response to treatment (48,49). Additionally, FEV_1 (48) and therapeutic change in FEV_1 (7) are highly reproducible for an individual. Each of these suggests the potential for a genetic contribution to change in FEV_1 in response to medications.

In addition to the FEV_1, both PC_{20} and bronchodilator response (the change in FEV_1 immediately following the administration of a short-acting β-agonist medication) have been frequently cited as response phenotypes. These are logical choices, because they are easily interpretable, correlate well with clinical disease, and demonstrate far greater interindividual variability than intraindividual variability (48,49). Other phenotypes, such as the peak expiratory flow rate (PEFR), have also been used. Clinically, increases in the variability of the PEFR have been used to suggest worsening asthma. However, while valid, PEFR variability as an outcome should be carefully scrutinized, because there is poor correlation of PEFR variability with symptoms or lung function (50), and PEFR measurements may have low reproducibility (51,52). Such poor repeatability for a phenotype may contribute to potential biases in pharmacogenetic study outcomes.

One qualitative asthma pharmacogenetic phenotype should be mentioned. Therapy in asthma is clearly not just directed toward the improvement of underlying lung function, but also toward the minimization of symptoms and avoidance of exacerbations, including those related to emergency room visits and hospitalizations (53). Asthma pharmacogenetic studies evaluating genetic predictors of health care utilization under asthma medications are underway.

A brief comment should be made with regard to phenotypes for the fourth category of pharmacogenetic response—genes that may influence the underlying pathogenesis or disease susceptibility to asthma. In general, these phenotypes should parallel the drug-treatment response phenotypes (e.g., FEV_1 or PC_{20} over time). However, as the genetic and molecular basis for asthma becomes clearer over time, novel phenotypes will become increasingly prominent. One example of this is the measurement of exhaled breath condensates for nitric oxide, which have been strongly clinically correlated with asthma diagnosis and severity, eosinophilia, and airway responsiveness (54). The production of exhaled nitric oxide is dependent on the presence of arginine via nitric oxide synthase; however arginase also competes for arginine as a substrate (55). Increased gene expression of arginase has been recently associated with the diagnosis of asthma (56). Given that dose-response relationships for changes in exhaled nitric oxide with inhaled corticosteroids have been established (54), the genetics of the arginase/nitric oxide synthase pathway would be of interest in elucidating mechanisms behind both the pathogenesis and drug-treatment response in asthma.

B. Pharmacokinetic Pharmacogenetics in Asthma

In this section, we highlight the features of the pharmacokinetic class of pharmacogenetics, focusing on drug metabolism by the CYP system. The CYPs are members of a superfamily of oxidative enzymes, sometimes also referred to as microsomal oxidative enzymes. This family forms the major system for oxidative metabolism of therapeutic substances (12). There are 58 different human CYP genes (1). Of these, *CYP2C9*, *CYP2D6*, and *CYP3A4* account for approximately 60% to 70% of all phase I–dependent metabolism of medications.

Theophylline Pharmacogenetics

Theophylline and related methylxanthine derivatives have weak bronchodilator and anti-inflammatory effects and are currently second-line agents for asthma management. Dose-related toxicities, such as tachycardia, headache, nausea, and seizures, are major problems that have limited their use (53). It has long been postulated that the variability in serum theophylline levels may be due to genetic factors. In a family-based study of theophylline metabolism, the heritability of rate constants of metabolite formation were 0.61, 0.84, 0.95, and 0.34 for 3-methylxanthine, 1-methyluric acid, 1,3-dimethyluric acid, and overall elimination rate, respectively (57), suggesting a strong genetic component. Recently, a common promoter polymorphism in the *CYP1A2* gene associated with altered clearance of theophylline was described (58). Specifically, the A allele of a G/A single nucleotide polymorphism (SNP) at position -2964 was associated with decreased clearance (increased serum levels) in a group of 75 Japanese asthmatics. These findings are biologically plausible because *CYP1A2* is known to degrade theophylline to 1,3-dimethyl uric acid before excretion in the urine, and poor metabolizers of theophylline are known to exist. This association is the first example of an asthma pharmacogenetic response that is caused by a polymorphism in the pharmacokinetic pathway of a drug. As mentioned, genetic investigations into the variability in drug metabolism of other asthma therapies are warranted.

C. The Pharmacogenetics of Asthma Drug Targets

In this section, we focus on the features of the drug-target response (pharmacodynamic) class of pharmacogenetics, concentrating on examples drawn from three therapeutic pathways in the management of asthma. These investigations have focused on the β_2-agonist, leukotriene antagonist, and corticosteroid pathways. Altogether, the data summarized below provide evolving evidence that response to asthma therapy is highly variable between individuals with asthma and genetic differences can help to predict the response to treatment in asthma.

The β_2-Adrenergic Receptor Pathway

β-adrenergic receptor agonists are the most commonly used class of medication in the treatment of asthma worldwide (59). Stimulation of the β_2-adrenergic receptor results in rapid and potent relaxation of airway smooth muscle. Interindividual variability in response to these agents has been recognized for over 60 years. For instance, the 1942 edition of Osler's *Principles and Practice of Medicine* noted, on the treatment of asthma, hypodermics of epinephrine, Mv to xv (0.3–1 cc) of a 1:1000 solution or of atropine, gr. 1/100 (0.6 mg), may give prompt relief, but individual cases vary greatly (60). Both short- and long-acting β-agonist agents are currently available and play distinct roles in the therapy of asthma (61). The literature on this class of medication dominates the field of asthma pharmacogenetics. This is likely related to the relatively early identification (62) and resequencing (63) of the gene encoding the primary receptor for this class of medications, the β_2-adrenergic receptor gene (*ADRB2*).

Two common (minor allele frequency 40–50%) nonsynonymous SNPs have been identified and well characterized in *ADRB2* (63). The first encodes for an amino acid change from arginine to glycine at position 16 (Arg16Gly), and the second for glutamic acid to glutamine at position 27 (Glu27Gln). The acute pharmacogenetic response to the administration of β-agonist medications has focused on the change in FEV_1 from before to immediately after the administration of the therapy [typically for a medication such as albuterol (salbutamol) the second measurement is performed 15–30 minutes after the therapy]. This change, known as the bronchodilator response, is a reasonable pharmacogenetic outcome, because these therapeutic agents are relied upon clinically to provide prompt relief to asthma symptoms. The bronchodilator response as a phenotypic outcome has been examined in multiple clinical trials. Many of the early studies differed substantially from one another with respect to study design, type of agonist utilized, and primary outcome assessed (59,64–66). Not surprisingly, there was marked inconsistency in results between trials.

Subsequently, other studies have demonstrated important associations of *ADRB2* variants with bronchodilator response. In a longitudinal birth cohort of 269 children (39.7% asthmatic), subjects who were Arg16 homozygous were 5.3 times more likely to show a significant bronchodilator response than Gly16 homozygotes (95% CI 1.6–17.7) (67). Heterozygotes showed intermediate response. Similarly, Lima et al. reported that bronchodilator responses were higher (18% vs. 4.9%, $p < 0.03$) and more rapid among Arg16 homozygotes as compared to Gly16 homozygotes and heterozygotes (68). Recently, *ADRB2* SNPs were genotyped in a comparative study of Mexican and Puerto Rican asthmatics (69). Strong associations of bronchodilator response to albuterol were noted with the Arg16 allele in the Puerto Rican population, with weaker associations noted with the

Gln27 allele in the Mexicans. Moreover, there was a strong interaction within the Puerto Ricans asthmatics and baseline level of FEV_1 in the genotypic relationship between Arg16Gly and acute bronchodilator change in FEV_1 upon administration of albuterol. The proportion of phenotypic variance explained by the FEV_1 level and position 16 genotype individually was reported to be 13.7% and 13.5%. However, the combination of FEV_1 level with position 16 genotype was reported to explain up to 44.4% of the genotypic variance (69). From these data, along with in vitro work, it appears that genetic variation in *ADRB2* does influence bronchodilator response, but the precise relationship between genotype, haplotype, and acute β-agonist response remains poorly understood.

The second phenotypic outcome evaluated has been the potential for downregulation of β-agonist receptor responsivity (tachyphylaxis) with the chronic administration of this class of therapy in association with *ADRB2* genetic variants. Two hundred fifty-five asthmatics of mild severity were randomized to either regular (180 μg QID) or as-needed albuterol use and were assessed over a 16-week period for evidence of tachyphylaxis and clinical deterioration (as measured by fall in AM PEFR). No difference in PEFR variation was observed between treatment groups (70). However, Arg16 homozygotes significantly decreased their PEFR with regular utilization of albuterol therapy, compared to both Arg16 homozygotes receiving as-needed albuterol and Gly16 homozygotes in either treatment group (71). The difference in evening PEFR between these groups was 31.6 ± 10.2 L/min comparing Arg16 homozygous regular users versus Gly16 homozygous regular users ($p = 0.002$) and 31.1 ± 13.0 L/min versus the Arg16 homozygous as-needed group ($p = 0.02$) (71). Similar differences in morning PEFR were noted (Fig. 2).

Further support for a correlation between Arg16 and increased in vivo beta-2 adrenergic receptor ($β_2AR$) desensitization (decreased response with continued/repeated agonist stimulation) was provided in a study examining the vascular response to intravenous $β_2$-agonist exposure. In this study of 26 healthy subjects, Arg16 homozygotes demonstrated almost complete physiologic desensitization within 90 minutes of constant infusion of isoproteronol, as compared to individuals with homozygous Gly16 receptors, who showed only 50% desensitization as late as 120 minutes ($p = 0.006$) (72).

$β_2AR$ desensitization was further evaluated in a prospective, genotype-stratified study of Arg16Gly on treatment-related changes in lung function. Israel et al. (73) matched homozygous Arg/Arg asthmatic individuals ($n = 37$) with homozygous Gly/Gly asthmatic individuals ($n = 41$), by level of FEV_1. The genotype-stratified individuals were then randomized in a double-blind, cross-over study of regularly scheduled albuterol therapy (four times daily) versus placebo over two 16-week periods with an intervening eight-week washout period. The major findings reasonably paralleled those previously reported for clinical trials genotyped retrospectively.

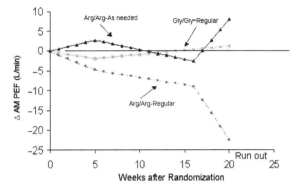

Figure 2 Response to chronic beta-agonist therapy in asthma, stratified by *ADRB2* genotype. Regular use of albuterol results in decrements in peak flow rates in asthmatics, when compared to as-needed therapy, but only in those homozygous for arginine at position 16 of the β_2-adrenergic receptor protein. *Source*: From Ref. 71.

Those Arg/Arg had lower morning peak flow rates during regularly scheduled treatment versus placebo (-10 L/min, $p = 0.02$), while those Gly/Gly had higher rates during those times (14 L/min, $p = 0.02$). The Arg/Arg minus Gly/Gly value was significant for morning PEFR (-24 L/min, $p = 0.0003$), evening PEFR, FEV_1, morning symptom score, and need for rescue medication.

The accompanying editorial to this manuscript pointed out three interesting data issues whose significance remains to be determined (74). First, improvement in the morning PEFR with regularly scheduled albuterol in the Gly/Gly group continued during the washout period. A similar improvement was noted during the washout period in a previous study as well (71). Next, no deterioration of the Arg/Arg individuals occurred while on regularly scheduled albuterol (74). Instead increases on placebo occurred after the run-in or washout periods. This is distinct from previously reported findings. Finally, the Arg/Arg group experienced a large increase in peak flow during the initial run-in period, despite averaging only one puff of β-agonist daily prior to the run-in (74). Clearly, these findings need to be replicated. That a common variant may portend to deterioration in PEFR of asthmatics given even minimal exposure to β-agonist medications may suggest huge implications. However, limitations, both those in the editorial and others, including the relatively small sample size, the use of multiethnic populations, and the very small percent of phenotypic variance explained argue against making broad generalizations from this data. Moreover, because regularly scheduled use of short-acting β-agonist medications is not a routine part of asthma management guidelines, the clinical relevance of this data remains uncertain.

Additional investigations into tachyphylaxis have focused on the relationship between *ADRB2* genotypes and rate of adverse outcome with regular β-agonist use. Upon regular usage of both short- and long-acting β-agonists, presence of at least one Gly16 allele is protective against exacerbations (75). Moreover in a meta-analysis evaluating long-acting β-agonist usage, subjects with at least one Arg allele demonstrated significant decrements in PC_{20} when compared to placebo, suggesting that the downregulation of the receptor accompanying tachyphylaxis may result in decreased bronchoprotection (76).

While most of the literature on the *ADRB2* gene has focused on the Arg16Gly and Gly27Gln, work has been performed into the investigation of the association of other portions of this gene with asthma therapeutic response. In a study of molecular haplotypes of *ADRB2*, the acute bronchodilator response to inhaled albuterol was approximately twice high in individuals homozygous for the most common haplotype than that in those homozygous for the second most common haplotype ($p = 0.046$) (77). Importantly, haplotypic analysis was more powerful in detecting associations compared to single SNP analyses (77). Nevertheless, a recent study of 176 Caucasians failed to confirm the association between any of the *ADRB2* haplotypes and bronchodilator response (78).

In a large family-based study involving the probands of the Childhood Asthma Management Program (CAMP), Silverman et al. (79) genotyped a subset of eight of the Drysdale *ADRB2* SNPs. A novel significant association of an SNP at position +523 with bronchodilator response to albuterol was noted. Given the proximity of this SNP to the true 3′ UTR, further work in better characterizing variation of the *ADRB2* 3′ UTR (and the promoter region) has occurred, with description of several novel variants (Fig. 3) (80). Of interest, a repeat region consisting of a variable number (9–14) of "C" alleles at position +1269 has now been identified. This poly-C track also contains additional SNP variation, adding to the complexity of the region. By imputing haplotypic substructure, it is clear that the poly-C region subdivides the aforementioned haplotypes further. Moreover, preliminary association studies of these subdivided haplotypes suggest that this region may influence both lung function and bronchodilator response. Confirmatory studies are underway.

Nearly all of the pharmacogenetic investigations into the β-agonist pathway to date have focused on the *ADRB2* gene. While some aspects of $β_2$-agonist pharmacogenetics have been ascertained, predictability remains low. Therefore, investigations into other candidate genes as determinants of $β_2$-agonist response have begun. Adenylate cyclase mediates signaling following activation of the $β_2AR$. A nonsynonymous polymorphism of the adenylate cyclase 9 gene (*ADCY9*) at amino acid 772 encoding an isoleucine to methionine substitution results in lower basal and $β_2AR$ mediated adenylyl cyclase activities (81). This nonsynonymous *ADCY9* SNP variant also

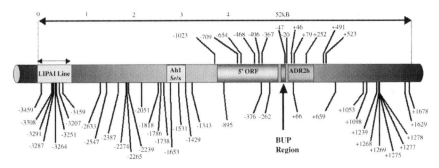

Figure 3 Novel variants identified via resequencing of ADRB2. New polymorphisms have now been identified in both the 5′ and 3′ UTR regions of ADRB2. In addition to the open reading frame in the 5′ end, there is a poly-C repeat track beginning at position +1269. This region is proximate to an antioxident response element (ARE) binding site. *Source*: From Hawkins GA, Tantisira K, Klanderman B, et al. Detailed sequence, haplotype, and association analysis of ADRB2 in a multi-ethnic asthma case and control population. Am J Respir Crit Care Med, submitted for publication.

demonstrates significantly greater albuterol-induced adenylyl cyclase activities in Met772 transfected lung cells compared to Ile772 (82). This effect is significantly enhanced upon the administration of exogenous corticosteroid. When genotyped in the CAMP clinical trial of 1041 childhood asthmatics, Met772 was associated with increased bronchodilator response, but only in those randomized to the inhaled corticosteroid arm of the trial (82). In further analyses of this *ADCY9* SNP in relationship to *ADRB2* haplotypes, *ADRB2* haplotypes were modestly associated with average bronchodilator response over the four-year clinical trial period, but this response was noted primarily in those subjects with at least one Met772 allele. Again, there was a significant interaction with the use of inhaled corticosteroids with those Met772 providing a very strong *ADRB2* haplotypic association with bronchodilator response when stratified by inhaled corticosteroid assignment (82).

In sum, studies on *ADRB2* provide evidence that the gene is likely associated with bronchodilator response, but that genetic prediction of this response may vary by ethnic group. Additionally, individuals homozygous for Arg16 demonstrate significant β_2AR desensitization, and these individuals (approximately 15% of population) are at risk of clinical deterioration with the regular use of β-agonists. This response does not appear to be predictable from currently available clinical or physiologic parameters and suggests that β_2AR genotyping may have a role in future clinical practice. Before this can be accomplished, however, better studies with standardized phenotypes in large populations need to be performed, because many of the described associations have not been replicated.

Emblematic of the problems with attempting broad generalizations about this gene at this time, a recent attempt at a meta-analysis of the pharmacogenetic effects of the *ADRB2* gene failed to reach convergence. These investigators cited that the literature review of this gene had noted *487 probed and reported outcomes* of which 95% were observed only once (83). Moreover, other β-adrenergic pathway genes appear to play roles in moderating response to β-agonist medications. Further work, including better characterization of these genes, their association with clinical outcomes, and their interactions with *ADRB2*, is underway.

The Leukotriene Antagonist Pathway

Leukotrienes are a family of eicosatetraenoic acids with profound effects on airway biology (84). The cysteinyl-leukotrienes (LTC_4, LTD_4, and LTE_4) are among the most potent bronchoconstrictors ever identified (85), and their effects are mediated by binding to the Cys-LT_1 receptor (86). LTB_4 is not a bronchoconstrictor but a chemotactic agent that attracts neutrophils, eosinophils, and monocytes (87). Asthmatics have increased levels of LTB_4 and cysteinyl-leukotrienes in their airways (88), and antileukotriene therapy has been associated with improvement in various types of asthma (89). Currently, two classes of antileukotriene drugs have been approved for asthma treatment, the leukotriene Cys-LT_1receptor antagonists (e.g., pranlukast, zafirlukast, and pranlukast) and the 5-lipoxygenase (5-LO) inhibitor (zileuton). Despite the overall improvement versus placebo with antileukotriene drugs, the interindividual response is highly variable (35); genetic factors may be responsible for some of this heterogeneity (7).

Expression of 5-LO protein is regulated at a number of levels (90). At the transcriptional level, binding of different transcription factors to specific consensus binding sites in the 5-LO gene (*ALOX5*) promoter region has been shown to be important for expression in vitro. Two transcription factors, Sp1 and early growth response factor-1 (Egr-1), bind to the promoter in a series of tandem consensus sites located in a $G + C$-rich core promoter region between -179 and $-56\,bp$ relative to the transcriptional start site (91). The Sp1 binding sites are adjacent to the Egr-1 binding sites, and Egr-1 can displace Sp1 from this promoter region and increase transcription above basal levels by recruiting the transcriptional coactivator cyclic adenosine $3'$, $5'$-monophosphate response element (CREB)-binding protein. A family of *ALOX5* polymorphisms has been identified in this region that consists of a deletion of one or two Egr-1—GGGCGG—consensus binding sites or the addition of one of these sites (92). Approximately 78% of subjects have the wild-type allele at this microsatellite locus. Lack of the wild-type allele has been associated with decrements in FEV_1 upon receipt of leukotriene antagonists in two different studies (93,94). In a clinical drug trial of the zileuton-like 5-LO inhibitor, ABT-761, asthmatics with at least one wild-type allele had an average improvement in their FEV_1 of 19%, while patients with any two of the mutant alleles had an average decrement in their FEV_1 of 1% (Fig. 4) (94). Data demonstrating replication of these findings in a study of asthmatics on zafirlukast has been published in abstract form (93). A second leukotriene pathway pharmacogenetic locus has been described. A transversion SNP (A–C) at position –444 in the LTC_4 synthase gene (*LTC4S*) promoter results in the creation of an activator protein binding site that may be associated with enhanced production of cysteinyl-leukotrienes (95). In a small case control study, the presence of any C allele ($n = 13$) at this polymorphic site was associated with an increased FEV_1 response to zafirlukast therapy compared to those asthmatic individuals homozygous for the A allele ($n = 10$) (95). Of interest, Sanak et al. (96) have shown that this polymorphism may be associated with the diagnosis of aspirin-induced asthma; this may represent the first example of the idiosyncratic category of pharmacogenetic response to asthma therapy. Active investigation of other genes in the leukotriene pathway is underway.

Given the previous associations, Lima et al. (97) genotyped on 28 SNPs in five leukotriene pathway genes in subjects participating in a clinical trail comparing the efficacy of montelukast versus low dose theophylline versus placebo as add on therapy in mild-moderate asthma. DNA was obtained in 248 participants, and the primary analysis was performed on 61 Caucasians taking montelukast. Outcomes assessed included change in FEV_1 and presence of exacerbations over one, three, and six months time. At six months, two SNPs were associated with change in FEV_1, one in the MRP1 gene

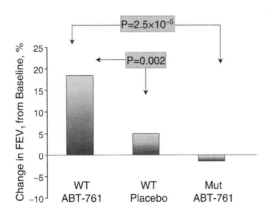

Figure 4 Response to leukotriene antagonist therapy in asthma, stratified by presence or absence of 5-lipoxygenase promoter wild-type tandem repeat. Those individuals with any copies of the wild type (five repeats) exhibit significant response to therapy with leukotriene antagonists, while those with two variant forms of the promoter do not respond to this class of therapy. *Source*: From Ref. 94.

(rs119774) and the second in ALOX5 (rs2115819). Of potentially greater interest, variants from three genes were associated with risk of exacerbations. Variation in one LTA4H SNP (rs2660845) was associated with a fourfold increase in the risk of at least one exacerbation over the six-month follow-up, whereas variation in the previously described ALOX5 promoter repeat and the LTC4S A-444C SNP was associated with a 73% and a 76% reduction in exacerbations, respectively. Although these findings require replication, they provide evidence of multiple leukotriene pathway pharmacogenetic loci in modulating the therapeutic response to these agents.

The Corticosteroid Pathway

Inhaled corticosteroids are the most effective and commonly used drugs for the chronic treatment of asthma but may be associated with serious adverse effects (53,61,98). The therapeutic response to inhaled corticosteroids in asthma generally increases with time. Many of the major benefits are achieved within the first two weeks of therapy; but some patients require more than a year of treatment before the therapeutic response plateaus (99). A number of family and twin studies have demonstrated that endogenous levels of glucocorticoids, usually measured as plasma cortisol levels, are heritable (100–103). In turn, decrements in endogenous plasma cortisol levels at night (104,105) and during periods of stress (106) have been associated with nocturnal and stress-related asthma, respectively. Furthermore, cortisol levels in nocturnal asthma may be partially resistant to the effects of corticotropin (104). In adults, subjects with low basal morning cortisol levels have longitudinal decrements in FEV_1 comparable to the effects of smoking, when compared to individuals with higher morning cortisol levels (107). Overall, these studies suggest a role for genetic factors regulating endogenous cortisol production in the pathogenesis and long-term treatment response of asthma.

Glucocorticoid resistance, defined in asthma as the failure to improve baseline morning prebronchodilator FEV_1 values by more than 15% after 7 to 14 days of 20 mg oral prednisone twice daily (108), is prevalent in approximately 25% of patients with difficult to control asthma (109). One study evaluating the role of interleukin-4 (*IL4*) in glucocorticoid resistant asthma performed genotyping of the *IL4* C589T SNP in case–control fashion comparing 24 patients with glucocorticoid resistant asthma to 682 glucocorticoid sensitive asthmatics (110). The *IL4* C589T SNP is associated with increased *IL4* gene transcription (111). Overexpression of the T allele was significantly associated with glucocorticoid resistant asthma ($p = 0.009$).

In a study of 14 candidate genes selected for their biologic relevance to the entire corticosteroid pathway, including synthesis, binding, and metabolism, we found a significant association between eight-week response to inhaled steroids and SNPs from the corticotropin releasing hormone receptor 1 (*CRHR1*) gene in adult asthmatics (112). *CRHR1* was also significantly associated with eight-week response to inhaled steroids in a clinical trial of children with asthma. Moreover, one particular SNP and one specific haplotype [utilizing haplotype-tag SNPs (113)] in the *CRHR1* gene that predicted good response to inhaled steroids in both populations were noted. The SNP, rs242941 (minor allele frequency approximately 30%) was associated with positive treatment response in both the Adult Study and the pediatric study, CAMP ($p = 0.025$ and 0.006, respectively). In the Adult Study, the mean percent change in FEV_1 for those homozygous for the minor allele was 13.28 ± 3.11, compared to 5.49 ± 1.40 for those homozygous for the wild-type allele. Similarly, in CAMP, the percent change was 17.80 ± 6.77 versus 7.57 ± 1.50 for the variant and wild-type homozygotes, respectively. In CAMP, evaluation of the placebo arm revealed no association of rs242941 or any of the other genotyped SNPs with change in lung function. Moreover, while inhaled corticosteroid usage was associated with improved FEV_1 at eight weeks ($p < 0.001$), variation in rs242941 significantly enhanced the improvement in lung function associated with this form of therapy (interaction $p = 0.02$).

The haplotype of interest had similar but larger improvements in FEV_1 on inhaled steroids. On average, those imputed to have the haplotype of interest had two to three times the short-term response to inhaled steroids compared to those without the haplotype (Fig. 5). The overall explained phenotypic variance was small ($<5\%$ in both populations), however, suggesting that multiple other factors (including additional genes) are responsible for the variability in the response to inhaled corticosteroids. As CRHR1 is the primary receptor for corticotropin releasing factor in the brain and modulates adrenocorticotropic hormone and endogenous cortisol levels, these results confirm the role of genetics in the asthma outcomes related to endogenous steroid levels. Further work along these lines, including the finding that the corticotropin releasing hormone knockout mouse demonstrates marked increases in airway inflammation in response to ovalbumin inhalational challenge (114), is progressing.

TBX21 encodes for the transcription factor T-bet, which is crucial in the development of naïve T-lymphocyte production. The T-bet knockout mouse spontaneously develops airways inflammation and hyperresponsiveness suggestive of asthma (115). Only one common nonsynonymous SNP has been identified in the *TBX21* gene, encoding for a replacement of histidine by glutamine at amino acid position 33 (H33Q). In a study of 701 CAMP children, 4.5% were noted to be heterozygous for this variant. After limiting the analysis to the Caucasian children, each of the H33Q individuals on inhaled corticosteroids was noted to demonstrate a marked improvement in airways hyperresponsiveness as measured by the PC_{20}, compared to either the steroid H33H homozygotes or any individual not taking inhaled steroids (interaction $p = 0.0002$) (116). The average improvement in the level of PC_{20}

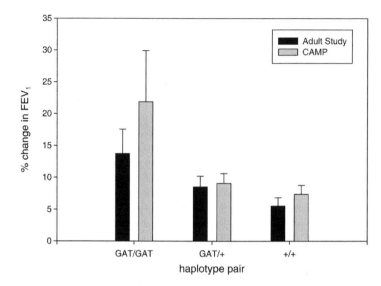

Figure 5 Eight-week response to inhaled corticosteroids, stratified by *CRHR1* GAT haplotype status in the adult study and Childhood Asthma Management Program (CAMP). Utilizing the htSNPs rs1876828, rs242939, and rs242941, the mean forced expiratory volume at one second improvement in an adult and a pediatric population was two to three times great for those imputed with the GAT/GAT homozygous haplotype than that for those homozygous for two non-GAT haplotypes. Improvement in those heterozygous for the GAT haplotype was intermediate between the two groups, suggesting an additive effect. Mean values ± SEM are shown. *Source:* From Ref. 112.

in those H33Q individuals taking inhaled corticosteroids was to the level associated with nonasthmatics.

As with the leukotrienes, pharmacogenetic investigations into the response to inhaled corticosteroid therapies remain in their formative stages. Several gene expression arrays evaluating response to the corticosteroid dexamethasone have now been performed, generating hundreds of novel potential candidate genes, with dozens of the assays now confirmed as being up- or down-regulated upon exposure to corticosteroids by quantitative reverse transcriptase polymerase chain reaction (rt-PCR) (117–119). One interesting potential candidate gene identified via gene expression work is histone deacetylase 2. Histone deacetylase is a corepressor of gene activity and is an important regulator of glucocorticoid transcriptional activity (111,120). Recruitment of histone deacetylase by glucocorticoid receptors to the activated transcriptional complex results in a decrease in inflammatory gene transcription (121). Histone deacetylase expression is decreased in cells from asthmatic airways (122,123), but, interestingly, increases upon the administration of oral (122) and inhaled corticosteroids (123). Active investigation of this and other genes in this complex pathway is underway.

D. The Pharmacogenetics of Asthma Disease Susceptibility

As noted previously, the final pharmacogenetic category is that of genetic factors influencing disease pathogenesis. In the case of asthma, it is easy to imagine that a gene influencing the inflammatory response within the airways could be an asthma susceptibility gene. However, by altering the inflammatory environment within the airways, variation in the same gene may also influence the relative effectiveness of anti-inflammatory asthma medications, such as leukotriene modifiers or inhaled corticosteroids. A similar story can be told for genes influencing airway tone and response to bronchodilator medications.

While no studies to date have specifically focused on the identification of asthma pharmacogenetic loci by focusing exclusively on asthma susceptibility loci, there are examples of genes, i.e., both asthma susceptibility genes and pharmacogenetic loci, from each of the three major classes of asthma therapy. The *ADRB2* gene has been associated with pediatric and nocturnal asthma in two recent meta-analyses of this gene (124,125). In the leukotriene pathway, the *LTC4S* promoter polymorphism has been associated with aspirin-intolerant asthma in a Polish population (126). Finally, in the corticosteroid pathway, *TBX21* has recently been described as a locus for both asthma susceptibility and methacholine responsiveness (127).

E. Asthma Pharmacogenetics—A Glimpse into the Future

Before beginning a discussion that optimistically describes the future of asthma pharmacogenetics, it is prudent to look back with a cautious eye upon the limitations of the studies performed to date. Active reading of the literature surrounding association studies related to this field should focus not only on the results of the association being evaluated within the study, but also the quality control of the study itself. In particular, many studies clearly suffer from problems related to inadequate sample size, improper matching of cases to controls, imprecise phenotypic definitions, potential population stratification, multiple comparisons, or the inability to replicate findings (128). As noted with regard to the *ADRB2* gene, these problems are beginning to gain the increasing attention that they deserve (83). One additional "limitation" to the asthma pharmacogenetics studies to date is the relatively small proportion of phenotypic variability that any one described genetic variant explains. No singular genetic marker, or for that matter, candidate gene, has been demonstrated to account for any more than a few percent of the variability for a given therapeutic outcome.

However, even given these limitations, the search for the genetic basis for asthma treatment response is becoming increasingly informative and closer to clinical applicability. In the near future, the field of asthma pharmacogenetics should continue to grow along four prominent lines. First, a better understanding of the molecular mechanisms of therapeutic agents will help to better elucidate exactly what constitutes a therapeutic "responder" from a "nonresponder." As noted previously, no singular or optimal phenotypic definition of response to any of the three well-established asthma medication classes has been established. Second, continued work into the known therapeutic pathways for novel candidate genes and functional variants influencing drug-treatment response will need to continue. Novel candidate genes may be identified through known pathways, by use of expression array profiling, or by the improved understanding of asthma disease pathogenesis. Along similar lines, pharmacogenetic investigations will also commence into the clarification of those at risk for asthma medication–related side effects. Third, for each of the drug classes, considerations must be given to predictive modeling incorporating both additive (two loci contributing equally to a given outcome) and epistatic (multiplicative) effects of multiple genes and loci. Finally, work toward the identification of pharmacogenetic loci predictive of response to new therapies, including omalizumaub (anti-IgE), will commence once reasonable test populations have been identified.

In conclusion, despite significant progress, with associations of genetic variation with therapeutic response to each the three major classes of asthma medications having now been reported, the field asthma pharmacogenetics remains in its infancy. However, the outlook to this field remains very promising. The increasing knowledge related to the human genome (129) and support of the research community (130) will only serve to promote efforts toward the discovery of the genetic basis of drug-treatment response in asthma. It is certainly possible that a prognostic test that is based upon an individual's genetic makeup, which will serve to optimize therapeutic response in asthma, while minimizing potential for side effects, may be developed in the foreseeable future.

III. The Pharmacogenetics of COPD

COPD is the fourth leading cause of morbidity and mortality in the United States (131). Worldwide projections note that COPD is likely to be fifth in burden of disease and third with respect to mortality by 2020 (132,133). COPD is a clinical disease consisting of cough, sputum production, and/ or dyspnea. The diagnosis is confirmed by an obstructive defect on spirometry that does not fully reverse upon administration of a short-acting bronchodilator (132). In the United States in 1993, COPD accounted for an estimated $23.9 billion in health care costs, of which $14.7 billion were direct costs (132). After hospitalizations, medication costs are the largest component of direct medical expenditures for COPD (134). Medication usage in COPD has traditionally been to control symptoms and complications related to the disease, because no medications have been demonstrated to modify the long-term decline in lung function that is the hallmark of the disease (132,135). Given the higher prevalence of the disease as well as proportion of nonresponders to medication therapy in COPD as compared to asthma, the ability to predict those individuals most likely to benefit from therapy would have far-reaching global implications.

Like asthma, COPD is a genetic disease (136), with α_1-antitrypsin deficiency providing the classic example of a Mendelian disorder resulting in emphysema. However, even in COPD that is not related to α_1-antitrypsin deficiency, there is a significant genetic component, with the heritability estimates of FEV_1, FEV_1/forced vital capacity (FVC), and FEF25–75/ FVC ratio between 0.31 and 0.45 in families of patients with COPD (137). There are currently three major classes of therapeutic agents available for the treatment of COPD, including β-agonists (both short and long acting), inhaled corticosteroids, and anticholinergic agents (also both short and long acting) (135). Theophylline is now an accepted second-line agent for the treatment of COPD. Like asthma, large interindividual variation exists in the treatment response to both corticosteroids (138) and to bronchodilator agents (Fig. 6) (139). This variability in response may have prognostic significance; patients on the long-acting anticholinergic agent, tiotropium, with a large short-term improvement in FEV_1 had improved lung function and fewer exacerbations at the end of the one-year therapy compared to those with a poor short-term response (140). Finally, there appears to be high repeatability of the response to therapy in COPD (141).

Given the genetic nature of COPD and the similarities to asthma in both medications and treatment response, much of the rationale behind pharmacogenetic studies in asthma also pertains to COPD. Nevertheless, few pharmacogenetic studies of COPD have been performed to date. This may be due to a relative scientific de-emphasis on medical therapies, given the failure, on average, to pharmacologically modify lung function in COPD (135). However, one could argue that, given the burden of disease and the lack of therapeutic response, it would be even more important to be able to readily identify those genetically most likely to benefit from medications. And while there is some evidence that there may be some common disease susceptibility genes for both COPD and asthma, including the β2-adrenergic receptor (142,143), there have been no studies that provide evidence that findings from asthma pharmacogenetic studies can be generalized to include COPD. In this section, after briefly reviewing potential COPD pharmacogenetic phenotypes, we discuss the pharmacogenetics of smoking cessation. While treatment to assist smoking cessation is clearly not equivalent to pharmacologic therapy directed at the disease, smoking cessation remains the single most effective way to stop the progression of COPD (132). Therefore, understanding the genetics of smoking cessation is paramount to COPD

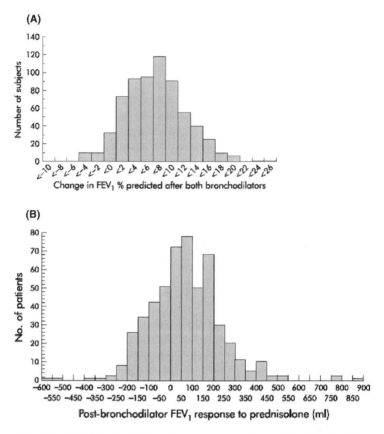

Figure 6 Interindividual variation in response to therapy for chronic obstructive pulmonary disease (COPD). Although the average response to treatment for COPD is often cited as no different than placebo, there is significant interindividual variability in the response to both bronchodilators (**A**) and corticosteroids (**B**). As with asthma, this suggests that factors other than the medications, including genetics, contribute to the therapeutic response. *Abbreviation*: FEV_1, forced expiratory volume at one second. *Source*: From Refs. 138,139.

management. We also review the data to date on the pharmacogenetics of COPD-related pulmonary hypertension. Other COPD pharmacogenetic studies focusing on bronchodilator and corticosteroid medications are clearly warranted.

A. COPD Pharmacogenetic Phenotypes

Despite the differences in pathophysiology, many of the phenotypes used in asthma pharmacogenetic studies would also be appropriate phenotypes for COPD. The pharmacogenetic determinants of the proposed variation in bioavailable levels of inhaled corticosteroids and β-agonists, as well as those demonstrated for theophylline, for COPD should parallel those of asthma (or normals), assuming that the prevalence of the pharmacokinetic SNPs of interest is constant. In the case of pharmacodynamic studies of COPD therapies, the intermediate phenotypes or measures of disease severity tend to parallel those of asthma, including measurements of lung function, airways responsiveness, and exacerbations (132,135). Therefore, the methodologic approach toward the pharmacogenetic investigation of these intermediate phenotypes would also parallel those of asthma. However, because the spectrum of COPD and its potential complications is wider, other phenotypes may also be useful. As an example, we briefly review the potential role for genetic variation to influence therapeutic response in the treatment of COPD-related pulmonary hypertension below. Perhaps more so than asthma, the therapy of COPD is also often specifically directed toward minimization of symptoms and avoiding exacerbations (132,135). As such, genetic studies predicting relative therapeutic success of a given medication using exacerbations or health care utilization as an outcome would be of interest.

COPD "Surgicogenetics"

In addition to the medication-related phenotypes noted above, one other potentially interesting COPD pharmacogenetic phenotype may, in reality, actually represent a "surgicogenetic" phenotype instead. The treatment of COPD now includes various methods aimed at removing severely emphysematous portions of the lung, allowing fuller expansion of the underlying lung tissue. Lung volume reduction surgery has been associated with increased exercise capacity, and with decreased mortality in patients with upper lobe predominance and low exercise capacity (144). In contrast, patients with homogeneous distribution of their underlying COPD and high baseline exercise capacity were at increased risk of surgical mortality with negligible functional improvement (144). Thus, the ability to predict who may respond to this surgical intervention may partially reside in the genetic determinants of upper versus homogenous emphysema. Recently, Ito et al. (145) described the association of a functional promoter polymorphism in the matrix metalloproteinase-9 gene with upper lobe predominance in emphysema in 84 Japanese subjects with emphysema. Presence of the variant allele was significantly associated with two radiographic parameters for upper lung field involvement by computed tomography. Investigation of the genetic factors influencing lobar predominance and exercise capacity in COPD in other populations is underway.

B. The Pharmacogenetics of Smoking Cessation

Cigarette smoking is the single most preventable cause of disease and death in the United States (146,147). Smoking cigarettes is also clearly the single greatest risk factor in the development of COPD (148). It is well established that smoking cessation has substantial immediate and long-term health benefits, regardless of the age or relative health of the individual (149). There is evolving evidence that smoking behavior and response to pharmacologic therapy designed to assist with smoking cessation may be influenced by genetics. Nicotine as a drug is known to exert its addictive effects through activation of the mesolimbic dopaminergic pathway (150). Genetic differences influencing both nicotine metabolism and nicotine's effect at its target site have been investigated, primarily to identify genetic risk factors for smoking behavior and nicotine addiction.

There are two principal classes of medications for the assistance of smoking cessation efforts. Currently, the most common pharmacologic interventions for smoking cessation are alternative forms of nicotine replacement, including gums, inhalational sprays, lozenges, and transdermal patches (151). Bupropion is an antidepressant that inhibits reuptake of dopamine, noradrenaline, and serotonin in the central nervous system and is a noncompetitive nicotine receptor antagonist (152). It is not clear which of these effects accounts for the antismoking activity of the drug, but inhibition of the reductions in levels of dopamine and noradrenaline levels in the central nervous system that accompany nicotine withdrawal is likely important. In double-blind, placebo-controlled trials of bupropion versus placebo, the one-year rates of smoking abstinence were significantly greater for individuals who took bupropion than for individuals who took placebo (153,154). In the paragraphs that follow, we shall briefly review the pharmacogenetic studies that have focused on both nicotine replacement therapy and bupropion.

Pharmacokinetic Paradigm

Nicotine is primarily metabolized by the CYP system. Specifically, *CYP2A6* and *CYP2D6* mediate the conversion of nicotine to cotinine (155,156). Recent heritability estimates derived from twin nicotine metabolism studies noted that 59.4% (95% CI = 44.7, 70.7) of the weight-adjusted rate of total clearance of nicotine may be attributable to additive genetic influences (157). Similar figures (60.8%, 95% CI = 46.9, 71.5) were noted for clearance of nicotine by the cotinine pathway. It was hypothesized over a decade ago that nicotine dependence might be modified by variation in *CYP2D6* (156). Additionally, *CYP2D6* also catalyzes the conversion of tyramine to dopamine (158); increased levels of dopamine available for the dopaminergic receptors would then be associated with decreased nicotine binding, forming another mechanism by which variation in *CYP2D6* might influence smoking behavior. As with many drug metabolizing enzymes, studies focusing on *CYP2D6* have combined genetic variations into groups, focusing on the variant ability to metabolize compared to the wild type. Homozygotes for the *CYP2D6*5*, *CYP2D6*4*, and *CYP2D6*3* alleles are associated with poor metabolism (159), whereas those for *CYP2D6*2* and *CYP2D6*1* are associated with ultrarapid metabolism (160). Overall, studies generally support the hypothesis that level of metabolism correlates with addiction to cigarettes, with rapid metabolizers more likely to become nicotine dependent than slow metabolizers (161,162). For instance, Saarikoski et al. examined 976 individuals (302 never smokers, 383 variable smokers, and 292 heavy smokers). The odds ratio (OR) for the presence of an ultra-rapid CYP2D6 metabolism phenotype in heavy smokers versus never smokers was 4.2 (95% CI: 1.8–9.8) (163).

The association of *CYP2A6* with smoking behavior has also been investigated. CYP2A6 may account for up to 90% of the nicotine → coti-nine conversion (155). Normal, as compared to slow, metabolism of nicotine by *CYP2A6* variants has been associated with increased daily amount of cigarettes smoked in French (164) and Canadian (165) adults. In contrast to the *CYP2D6* studies above, two studies demonstrated that it is actually slower not normal *CYP2A6* metabolizers that tend to become nicotine dependent (166,167). None of the studies measured nicotine or cotinine levels in association with smoking dependence and genotype.

Recently, the above studies of smoking behavior have extended into an interest in how drug metabolism genetics might affect pharmacologic efforts at smoking cessation. As one of the primary therapeutic approaches toward smoking cessation is via the use of nicotine replacement medications, it is reasonable to hypothesize that genetic variation in drug metabolism could have a direct influence on the ability to respond to nicotine replacement therapy. Unfortunately, this hypothesis has not yet been formally tested.

Bupropion is metabolized by *CYP2B6* (168). A *CYP2B6* polymor-phism (1459C > T) and its association with success of bupropion therapy for smoking cessation have been evaluated. This SNP has been associated with decreased CYP2B6 protein expression (169). Lerman et al. (170) exam-ined the 1459C > T variant in a trial of 197 subjects taking bupropion along with 229 placebo controls. Overall, the minor allele (lower activity variant) was associated with less abstinence at the end of therapy than the wild-type variant (OR 1.56, 95% CI: 1.01–2.41 for relapse). At the end of six months, the men, but not women, harboring the variant allele had a significantly higher relapse rate in those taking bupropion.

Pharmacodynamic Paradigm

Genetic variation at the site of the dopaminergic receptor in the central nervous system and its ability to influence therapeutic response to smoking cessation efforts have also recently been investigated (171). These studies have investigated pharmacogenetic effects in association with both nico-tine replacement therapy and bupropion. Not surprisingly, the studies have focused on the associations of genes within the dopamine pathway. The

D2 dopamine receptor gene (*DRD2*) is a G protein–coupled receptor located on postsynaptic dopaminergic neurons that is centrally involved in reward-mediating pathways and is felt to modulate the effects of nicotine. In addition to smoking, variants of the *DRD2* gene have also been associated with cocaine and opioid dependence, obesity, and gambling (172).

In a pharmacogenetic study of 755 smokers participating in a placebo-controlled trial of transdermal nicotine, nicotine replacement therapy was significantly more effective than placebo for carriers of the alternatively spliced A1 allele of *DRD2* but not for A2 homozygotes (173). The difference in the ORs for the treatment effect between the genotype groups was significant after the first week of treatment (patch/placebo OR 2.8, 95% CI = 1.7, 4.6 for any A1 allele vs. OR 1.4, 0.9–2.1 for A2 homozygotes; *p* for difference in ORs 0.04). This study also examined a polymorphism in the dopamine β-hydroxylase gene (*DBH*). Transdermal nicotine was more effective (OR of 3.6 for transdermal nicotine vs. placebo) in producing abstinence among smokers with both the *DRD2*∗*A1* allele and the *DBH*∗*A* allele when compared to smokers with other genotypes. This genetic association with treatment response was significant at both 1 and 12 weeks of treatment. This study was continued longitudinally and suggested that abstinence at 6 and 12 months posttreatment was associated with the *DRD2*∗*A1* variant. However, the effect was observed only among women (174). Two other functional variants of *DRD2* have been evaluated with respect to nicotine replacement therapy, an indel of the C allele at position –141 and a [C/T] SNP at position 957 (175). Both the deletion and the C957T variant alleles were associated with significantly higher quit rates on nicotine replacement therapy, compared to the wild-type alleles.

The μ opioid receptor is the primary site of action for the rewarding effects of the endogenous opioid peptide, β-endorphin, which is released after acute and short-term nicotine administration (176). A common (25–30% of Caucasians) Asn40Asp polymorphism of the μ opioid receptor gene (*OPRM1*) increases the binding affinity of β-endorphin for this receptor threefold, relative to the wild-type Asn40 *OPRM1* (177). Among 320 Caucasian smokers, persons carrying the Asp40 variant were significantly more likely than those homozygous for the Asn40 to be abstinent at the end of the nicotine replacement treatment (178). The treatment response differed by therapy type, and was significant among smokers who received transdermal nicotine (quit rates of 52% vs. 33% for the Asp40 and Asn40 groups, respectively; OR = 2.4) but not among smokers who received nicotine nasal spray. Further studies are warranted to investigate the reasons behind these differences.

Variants of the dopamine pathway have also been associated with differential response to smoking cessation with the use of bupropion. The *DRD2*-141C insertion (as compared to the deletion's association with nicotine replacement therapy) was significantly associated with higher quit rates in a placebo-controlled trial of 414 smokers taking bupropion (175). Additionally, the *DRD2* gene may interact with the dopamine transporter (*SLC6A3*) gene. In the same placebo-controlled study, smokers with both the *DRD2*∗*A2* and *SLC6A3*∗*9* variants had significantly higher abstinence rates at the end of treatment, as well as longer latency periods until relapse. Although confirmatory studies are needed, the development of genetic prediction models of response to smoking cessation therapies will likely be forthcoming in the near future.

C. Pharmacogenetic Studies of Pulmonary Hypertension in COPD

Pulmonary hypertension is a common sequelae in COPD, with 5% to 10% of patients developing severe pulmonary hypertension resulting in right heart failure (cor pulmonale) and a progressive worsening of their clinical course (179). Response to oxygen therapy has generally been poor, while vasodilators in COPD have the potential to worsen gas exchange due to alterations in hypoxic regulation of ventilation balance (132). In a series of studies evaluating alterations in pulmonary hemodynamics during exercise in COPD, Kanazawa and colleagues focused on the role of the *ACE* gene. The *ACE* gene contains an intronic indel of a 287 base pair nonsense DNA domain resulting in three genotypes (DD and II homozygotes and ID heterozygotes); the deletion (D) allele is associated with higher ACE activity and higher angiotensin II levels (6,21). The *ACE* DD genotype is associated with exaggerated pulmonary hypertension and disturbance of tissue oxygenation during exercise in patients with COPD (180). Kanazawa et al. then proceeded to investigate whether these genotypes influenced response to therapeutic agents.

As captopril is a vasodilator that inhibits the ACE's actions, the initial investigation focused on this medication (181). There were 13 patients with the II genotype, 11 with the ID genotype, and 12 with the DD genotype who underwent incremental exercise testing in a placebo-controlled double-blinded, crossover fashion. There were no significant differences between the groups in the mean pulmonary artery pressure (mPAP), peripheral vascular resistance (PVR), mixed venous oxygen (PvO_2), and lactate concentration at rest. After exercise, mPAP was significantly higher in patients with the DD genotype [placebo: 53.7 (3.7) mmHg, $p < 0.0001$; captopril: 52.7 (2.6) mmHg, $p < 0.0001$] than in those with the II [41.1 (3.8) mmHg; 37.8 (3.8) mmHg] or ID genotypes [46.2 (5.9) mmHg; 41.4 (5.8) mmHg; Fig. 1]. Additionally, mPAP after exercise was significantly lower with captopril than with placebo in patients with the II genotype (mean difference 3.308; 95% CI 2.405–4.210, $p < 0.0001$) or the ID genotype (mean difference 4.818; 95% CI 4.231–5.405, $p < 0.0001$) but not in those with the DD genotype (181). The II genotype also demonstrated significant improvements in PVR, PvO_2, and lactate levels while exercising after captopril compared to both ID and DD genotypes, as well as compared to placebo. The authors concluded that the II genotype may be a sensitive predictor of response to captopril in COPD-related pulmonary hypertension.

These investigators subsequently used a similar study design to investigate the role of oxygen therapy (182) and nifedipine administration (183) in relation to *ACE* genotype in the pulmonary hypertension of COPD. Oxygen did not influence mPAP or PVR but did result in improvements in PvO_2 and lactate. As with captopril, these improvements were limited to the *ACE* II genotype. While nifedipine improved mPAP in all three genotypic groups, no other differences were noted and the effect did not vary by genotype.

D. The Future of COPD Pharmacogenetics

The field of COPD pharmacogenetics is truly in its infancy. There are an increasing number of surgical therapeutic options, including LVRS and lung transplantation, in the treatment of COPD. However, the potential to predict those patients with COPD who are most likely to continue to maintain their functional status from medications alone would have a huge impact on the potential timing and benefit of such interventions. Moreover, pharmacogenetic prediction of therapeutic response would also help to alleviate the potentially devastating side effects of long-term therapy in these patients. Finally, pharmacogenetic predictors related to the ability to minimize symptoms and/or health care utilization would be of tremendous benefit. While we know of no large-scale COPD pharmacogenetic studies that are underway, implementation of these types of studies is clearly warranted.

IV. Conclusion

Asthma and COPD are on the rise and contribute to significant morbidity, mortality, and cost in the United States and worldwide. Much of this cost is drug related. Variation in response to drugs in these diseases has a significant heritable component. Although the time required to decipher the genetics of drug response adequately to result in "individualized medicine" is still likely to be years, investigations have begun into each of the major categories of pharmacogenetic response within these important obstructive airways diseases.

References

1. Ingelman-Sundberg M. Pharmacogenetics: an opportunity for a safer and more efficient pharmacotherapy. J Intern Med 2001; 250:186–200.
2. Maitland-van der Zee AH, de Boer A, Leufkens HG. The interface between pharmacoepidemiology and pharmacogenetics. Eur J Pharmacol 2000; 410:121–130.

3. Vesell ES. Therapeutic lessons from pharmacogenetics. Ann Intern Med 1997; 126:653–655.
4. Lazarou J, Pomeranz BH, Corey PN. Incidence of adverse drug reactions in hospitalized patients: a meta-analysis of prospective studies. JAMA 1998; 279:1200–1205.
5. Ernst FR, Grizzle AJ. Drug-related morbidity and mortality: updating the cost-of-illness model. J Am Pharm Assoc (Wash) 2001; 41:192–199.
6. Meisel C, Gerloff T, Kirchheiner J, et al. Implications of pharmacogenetics for individualizing drug treatment and for study design. J Mol Med 2003; 81: 154–167.
7. Drazen JM, Silverman EK, Lee TH. Heterogeneity of therapeutic responses in asthma. Br Med Bull 2000; 56:1054–1070.
8. Evans WE, McLeod HL. Pharmacogenomics–drug disposition, drug targets, and side effects. N Engl J Med 2003; 348:538–549.
9. Silverman ES, Hjoberg J, Palmer LJ, et al. Application of pharmacogenetics to the therapeutics of asthma. In: Eissa NT, Huston D, eds. Therapeutic Targets of Airway Inflammation. New York: Marcel Dekker, 2003:1000.
10. Steimer W, Potter JM. Pharmacogenetic screening and therapeutic drugs. Clin Chim Acta 2002; 315:137–155.
11. Brockmoller J, Kirchheiner J, Meisel C, et al. Pharmacogenetic diagnostics of cytochrome P450 polymorphisms in clinical drug development and in drug treatment. Pharmacogenomics 2000; 1:125–151.
12. Kirchheiner J, Brosen K, Dahl ML, et al. CYP2D6 and CYP2C19 genotype-based dose recommendations for antidepressants: a first step towards subpopulation-specific dosages. Acta Psychiatr Scand 2001; 104:173–192.
13. Cooke GE, Bray PF, Hamlington JD, et al. PlA2 polymorphism and efficacy of aspirin. Lancet 1998; 351:1253.
14. Johnson JA, Lima JJ. Drug receptor/effector polymorphisms and pharmaco-genetics: current status and challenges. Pharmacogenetics 2003; 13:525–534.
15. Meyer UA. Pharmacogenetics: the slow, the rapid, and the ultrarapid. Proc Natl Acad Sci USA 1994; 91:1983–1984.
16. Nebert DW. Pharmacogenetics and pharmacogenomics: why is this relevant to the clinical geneticist? Clin Genet 1999; 56:247–258.
17. Spielberg SP. *N*-acetyltransferases: pharmacogenetics and clinical conse-quences of polymorphic drug metabolism. J Pharmacokinet Biopharm 1996; 24:509–519.
18. Zielinska E, Niewiarowski W, Bodalski J. The arylamine *N*-acetyltransferase (NAT2) polymorphism and the risk of adverse reactions to co-trimoxazole in children. Eur J Clin Pharmacol 1998; 54:779–785.
19. O'Neil WM, MacArthur RD, Farrough MJ, et al. Acetylator phenotype and gen-otype in HIV-infected patients with and without sulfonamide hypersensitivity. J Clin Pharmacol 2002; 42:613–619.
20. Zielinska E, Bodalski J, Niewiarowski W, et al. Comparison of acetylation phe-notype with genotype coding for *N*-acetyltransferase (NAT2) in children. Pediatr Res 1999; 45:403–408.
21. McNamara DM, Holubkov R, Janosko K, et al. Pharmacogenetic interactions between beta-blocker therapy and the angiotensin-converting enzyme deletion

polymorphism in patients with congestive heart failure. Circulation 2001; 103:1644–1648.

22. Ueda S, Meredith PA, Morton JJ, et al. ACE (I/D) genotype as a predictor of the magnitude and duration of the response to an ACE inhibitor drug (enalaprilat) in humans. Circulation 1998; 98:2148–2153.

23. Masoli M, Fabian D, Holt S, et al. The global burden of asthma: executive summary of the GINA Dissemination Committee report. Allergy 2004; 59:469–478.

24. Chung F, Fabbri LM. Asthma. Sheffield: ERS Journals Ltd., 2003.

25. Centers for Disease Control. Surveillance for Asthma—United States, 1960–1995. Morbid Mortal Wkly Rep 1998; 47:1–27.

26. Beasley R, Crane J, Lai CK, et al. Prevalence and etiology of asthma. J Allergy Clin Immunol 2000; 105:S466–S472.

27. Weiss KB, Gergen PJ, Wagener DK. Breathing better or wheezing worse? The changing epidemiology of asthma morbidity and mortality. Annu Rev Public Health 1993; 14:491–513.

28. Akinbami LJ, Schoendorf KC. Trends in childhood asthma: prevalence, health care utilization, and mortality. Pediatrics 2002; 110:315–322.

29. Sullivan SD, Strassels SA. Health economics. In: Barnes PJ, Drazen JM, Rennard S, Thomson NC, eds. Asthma and COPD. Basic Mechanisms and Clinical Management. San Diego: Academic Press, 2002:657–671.

30. Lanes SF, Garcia Rodriguez LA, Huerta C. Respiratory medications and risk of asthma death. Thorax 2002; 57:683–686.

31. Dunlop KA, Carson DJ, Shields MD. Hypoglycemia due to adrenal suppression secondary to high-dose nebulized corticosteroid. Pediatr Pulmonol 2002; 34:85–86.

32. Blumenthal MN. Historical perspectives. In: Blumenthal MN, Bjorksten B, eds. Genetics of Allergy and Asthma: Methods for Investigative Studies. New York: Marcel Dekker, 1997:1–18.

33. Nieminen MM, Kaprio J, Koskenvuo M. A population-based study of bronchial asthma in adult twin pairs. Chest 1991; 100:70–75.

34. Duffy DL, Martin NG, Battistutta D, et al. Genetics of asthma and hay fever in Australian twins. Am Rev Respir Dis 1990; 142:1351–1358.

35. Malmstrom K, Rodriguez-Gomez G, Guerra J, et al. Oral montelukast, inhaled beclomethasone, and placebo for chronic asthma. A randomized, controlled trial. Montelukast/Beclomethasone Study Group. Ann Intern Med 1999; 130:487–495.

36. Lemanske RF Jr., Allen DB. Choosing a long-term controller medication in childhood asthma. The proverbial two-edged sword. Am J Respir Crit Care Med 1997; 156:685–687.

37. Wilk JB, Djousse L, Arnett DK, et al. Evidence for major genes influencing pulmonary function in the NHLBI family heart study. Genet Epidemiol 2000; 19:81–94.

38. Palmer LJ, Burton PR, James AL, et al. Familial aggregation and heritability of asthma-associated quantitative traits in a population-based sample of nuclear families. Eur J Hum Genet 2000; 8:853–860.

39. Szatmari P, Jones MB. Effects of misclassification on estimates of relative risk in family history studies. Genet Epidemiol 1999; 16:368–381.

40. Rothman N, Garcia-Closas M, Stewart WT, et al. The impact of misclassification in case-control studies of gene-environment interactions. IARC Sci Publ 1999; 148:89–96.
41. Gross NJ. What is this thing called love?—or, defining asthma. Am Rev Respir Dis 1980; 121:203–204.
42. Pacifici GM, Giulianetti B, Quilici MC, et al. (-)-Salbutamol sulphation in the human liver and duodenal mucosa: interindividual variability. Xenobiotica 1997; 27:279–286.
43. Abel SM, Maggs JL, Back DJ, et al. Cortisol metabolism by human liver in vitro—I. Metabolite identification and inter-individual variability. J Steroid Biochem Mol Biol 1992; 43:713–719.
44. Dube LM, Swanson LJ, Awni W. Zileuton, a leukotriene synthesis inhibitor in the management of chronic asthma. Clinical pharmacokinetics and safety. Clin Rev Allergy Immunol 1999; 17:213–221.
45. Winkler J, Hochhaus G, Derendorf H. How the lung handles drugs: pharmacokinetics and pharmacodynamics of inhaled corticosteroids. Proc Am Thorac Soc 2004; 1:356–363.
46. Handley D. The asthma-like pharmacology and toxicology of (S)-isomers of beta agonists. J Allergy Clin Immunol 1999; 104:S69–S76.
47. Szefler SJ, Martin RJ, King TS, et al. Significant variability in response to inhaled corticosteroids for persistent asthma. J Allergy Clin Immunol 2002; 109:410–418.
48. Enright PL, Lebowitz MD, Cockroft DW. Physiologic measures: pulmonary function tests. Asthma outcome. Am J Respir Crit Care Med 1994; 149: S9–S18; discussion S19–S20.
49. Rosias PP, Dompeling E, Dentener MA, et al. Childhood asthma: exhaled markers of airway inflammation, asthma control score, and lung function tests. Pediatr Pulmonol 2004; 38:107–114.
50. Brand PL, Duiverman EJ, Waalkens HJ, et al. Peak flow variation in childhood asthma: correlation with symptoms, airways obstruction, and hyperresponsiveness during long-term treatment with inhaled corticosteroids. Dutch CNSLD Study Group. Thorax 1999; 54:103–107.
51. Vargas MH, Ruiz-Gutierrez HH, Espinosa-Serafin C, et al. Underestimation of the peak flow variability in asthmatic children: evaluation of a new formula. Pediatr Pulmonol 2005; 39:325–331.
52. Frischer T, Meinert R, Urbanek R, et al. Variability of peak expiratory flow rate in children: short and long term reproducibility. Thorax 1995; 50:35–39.
53. NHLBI. Highlights of the Expert Panel Report 2: Guidelines for the Diagnosis and Management of Asthma. Bethesda: NIH Publications, 1997:50.
54. Smith AD, Taylor DR. Is exhaled nitric oxide measurement a useful clinical test in asthma? Curr Opin Allergy Clin Immunol 2005; 5:49–56.
55. Vercelli D. Arginase: marker, effector, or candidate gene for asthma? J Clin Invest 2003; 111:1815–1817.
56. Zimmermann N, King NE, Laporte J, et al. Dissection of experimental asthma with DNA microarray analysis identifies arginase in asthma pathogenesis. J Clin Invest 2003; 111:1863–1874.

57. Miller CA, Slusher LB, Vesell ES. Polymorphism of theophylline metabolism in man. J Clin Invest 1985; 75:1415–1425.
58. Obase Y, Shimoda T, Kawano T, et al. Polymorphisms in the CYP1A2 gene and theophylline metabolism in patients with asthma. Clin Pharmacol Ther 2003; 73:468–474.
59. Raby BA, Weiss ST. Beta2-adrenergic receptor genetics. Curr Opin Mol Ther 2001; 3:554–566.
60. Osler's Principles and Practice of Medicine. 14th ed. New York: D. Appleton-Century Company, 1942.
61. Chung KF, O'Byrne P. Pharmacological agents used to treat asthma. In: Chung KF, Fabbri LM, eds. Asthma. Sheffield: European Respiratory Society Journals Ltd., 2003:458.
62. Kobilka BK, Dixon RA, Frielle T, et al. cDNA for the human beta 2-adrenergic receptor: a protein with multiple membrane-spanning domains and encoded by a gene whose chromosomal location is shared with that of the receptor for platelet-derived growth factor. Proc Natl Acad Sci USA 1987; 84:46–50.
63. Reihsaus E, Innis M, MacIntyre N, et al. Mutations in the gene encoding for the beta 2-adrenergic receptor in normal and asthmatic subjects. Am J Respir Cell Mol Biol 1993; 8:334–339.
64. Ohe M, Munakata M, Hizawa N, et al. Beta 2 adrenergic receptor gene restriction fragment length polymorphism and bronchial asthma. Thorax 1995; 50:353–359.
65. Aziz I, McFarlane LC, Lipworth BJ. Comparative trough effects of formoterol and salmeterol on lymphocyte beta2-adrenoceptor—regulation and bronchodilatation. Eur J Clin Pharmacol 1999; 55:431–436.
66. Hancox RJ, Sears MR, Taylor DR. Polymorphism of the beta2-adrenoceptor and the response to long-term beta2-agonist therapy in asthma. Eur Respir J 1998; 11:589–593.
67. Martinez FD, Graves PE, Baldini M, et al. Association between genetic polymorphisms of the beta2-adrenoceptor and response to albuterol in children with and without a history of wheezing. J Clin Invest 1997; 100:3184–3188.
68. Lima JJ, Thomason DB, Mohamed MH, et al. Impact of genetic polymorphisms of the beta2-adrenergic receptor on albuterol bronchodilator pharmacodynamics. Clin Pharmacol Ther 1999; 65:519–525.
69. Choudhry S, Ung N, Avila PC, et al. Pharmacogenetic differences in response to albuterol between Puerto Rican and Mexican asthmatics. Am J Respir Crit Care Med 2004; 171:563–570.
70. Drazen JM, Israel E, Boushey HA, et al. Comparison of regularly scheduled with as-needed use of albuterol in mild asthma. Asthma Clinical Research Network. N Engl J Med 1996; 335:841–847.
71. Israel E, Drazen JM, Liggett SB, et al. The effect of polymorphisms of the beta(2)-adrenergic receptor on the response to regular use of albuterol in asthma. Am J Respir Crit Care Med 2000; 162:75–80.
72. Dishy V, Sofowora GG, Xie HG, et al. The effect of common polymorphisms of the beta2-adrenergic receptor on agonist-mediated vascular desensitization. N Engl J Med 2001; 345:1030–1035.

73. Israel E, Chinchilli VM, Ford JG, et al. Use of regularly scheduled albuterol treatment in asthma: genotype-stratified, randomised, placebo-controlled cross-over trial. Lancet 2004; 364:1505–1512.

74. Tattersfield AE, Hall IP. Are beta2-adrenoceptor polymorphisms important in asthma—an unravelling story. Lancet 2004; 364:1464–1466.

75. Taylor DR, Drazen JM, Herbison GP, et al. Asthma exacerbations during long term beta agonist use: influence of beta(2) adrenoceptor polymorphism. Thorax 2000; 55:762–767.

76. Lee DK, Currie GP, Hall IP, et al. The arginine-16 beta2-adrenoceptor polymorphism predisposes to bronchoprotective subsensitivity in patients treated with formoterol and salmeterol. Br J Clin Pharmacol 2004; 57:68–75.

77. Drysdale CM, McGraw DW, Stack CB, et al. Complex promoter and coding region beta 2-adrenergic receptor haplotypes alter receptor expression and predict in vivo responsiveness. Proc Natl Acad Sci USA 2000; 97: 10,483–10,488.

78. Taylor DR, Epton MJ, Kennedy MA, et al. Bronchodilator response in relation to beta2-adrenoceptor haplotype in patients with asthma. Am J Respir Crit Care Med 2005; 172:700–703.

79. Silverman EK, Kwiatkowski DJ, Sylvia JS, et al. Family-based association analysis of beta2-adrenergic receptor polymorphisms in the childhood asthma management program. J Allergy Clin Immunol 2003; 112:870–876.

80. Hawkins GA, Tantisira KG, Meyers DA, et al. Analysis of ADRB2 polymorphisms and haplotypes in caucasian and african american populations. Proceedings of the American Thoracic Society. 2005; 2:A30.

81. Small KM, Brown KM, Theiss CT, et al. An Ile to Met polymorphism in the catalytic domain of adenylyl cyclase type 9 confers reduced beta2-adrenergic receptor stimulation. Pharmacogenetics 2003; 13:535–541.

82. Tantisira KG, Small KM, Litonjua AA, et al. Molecular properties and pharmacogenetics of a polymorphism of adenylyl cyclase type 9 in asthma: interaction between beta-agonist and corticosteroid pathways. Hum Mol Genet 2005; 14: 1671–1677.

83. Contopoulos-Ioannidis DG, Alexiou G, Gouvias T, et al. An empirical evaluation of multifarious outcomes in pharmacogenetics: beta2 adrenoreceptor polymorphisms and asthma treatment. Pharmacogenet Genomics, 2006, In Press.

84. Samuelsson B, Dahlen SE, Lindgren JA, et al. Leukotrienes and lipoxins: structures, biosynthesis, and biological effects. Science 1987; 237:1171–1176.

85. Drazen JM. Cysteinyl leukotrienes. In: Barnes PJ, Rodger IW, Thomson NC, eds. Asthma: Basic Mechanisms and Clinical Management. San Diego: Academic Press, 1998:281–295.

86. Figueroa DJ, Breyer RM, Defoe SK, et al. Expression of the cysteinyl leukotriene 1 receptor in normal human lung and peripheral blood leukocytes. Am J Respir Crit Care Med 2001; 163:226–233.

87. Lewis RA, Austen KF, Soberman RJ. Leukotrienes and other products of the 5-lipoxygenase pathway. Biochemistry and relation to pathobiology in human diseases. N Engl J Med 1990; 323:645–655.

88. Holgate ST, Bradding P, Sampson AP. Leukotriene antagonists and synthesis inhibitors: new directions in asthma therapy. J Allergy Clin Immunol 1996; 98:1–13.
89. Drazen JM, Israel E, O'Byrne PM. Treatment of asthma with drugs modifying the leukotriene pathway. N Engl J Med 1999; 340:197–206.
90. Silverman ES, Drazen JM. The biology of 5-lipoxygenase: function, structure, and regulatory mechanisms. Proc Assoc Am Physicians 1999; 111:525–536.
91. Silverman ES, Du J, De Sanctis GT, et al. Egr-1 and Sp1 interact functionally with the 5-lipoxygenase promoter and its naturally occurring mutants. Am J Respir Cell Mol Biol 1998; 19:316–323.
92. In KH, Asano K, Beier D, et al. Naturally occurring mutations in the human 5-lipoxygenase gene promoter that modify transcription factor binding and reporter gene transcription. J Clin Invest 1997; 99:1130–1137.
93. Anderson W, Kalberg C, Edwards L, et al. Effects of polymorphisms in the promoter region of 5-lipoxygenase and LTC4 synthase on the clinical response to zafirlukast and fluticasone. Eur Respir J 2000; 16(suppl B):183s.
94. Drazen JM, Yandava CN, Dube L, et al. Pharmacogenetic association between ALOX5 promoter genotype and the response to anti-asthma treatment. Nat Genet 1999; 22:168–170.
95. Sampson AP, Siddiqui S, Buchanan D, et al. Variant LTC(4) synthase allele modifies cysteinyl leukotriene synthesis in eosinophils and predicts clinical response to zafirlukast. Thorax 2000; 55(suppl 2):S28–S31.
96. Sanak M, Pierzchalska M, Bazan-Socha S, et al. Enhanced expression of the leukotriene C(4) synthase due to overactive transcription of an allelic variant associated with aspirin-intolerant asthma. Am J Respir Cell Mol Biol 2000; 23:290–296.
97. Lima JJ, Zhang S, Grant A, et al. Influence of leukotriene pathway polymorphisms on response to montelukast in asthma. Am J Respir Crit Care Med 2006; 173:379–385.
98. Bousquet J. Global initiative for asthma (GINA) and its objectives. Clin Exp Allergy 2000; 30(suppl 1):2–5.
99. Barnes PJ, Grunstein MM, Leff AR, et al. Asthma. Philadelphia: Lippincott-Raven, 1997.
100. Levene RZ, Schwartz B, Workman PL. Heritability of plasma cortisol. Arch Ophthalmol 1972; 87:389–391.
101. Meikle AW, Stringham JD, Woodward MG, et al. Heritability of variation of plasma cortisol levels. Metabolism 1988; 37:514–517.
102. Inglis GC, Ingram MC, Holloway CD, et al. Familial pattern of corticosteroids and their metabolism in adult human subjects—the Scottish Adult Twin Study. J Clin Endocrinol Metab 1999; 84:4132–4137.
103. Bartels M, Van den Berg M, Sluyter F, et al. Heritability of cortisol levels: review and simultaneous analysis of twin studies. Psychoneuroendocrinology 2003; 28:121–137.
104. Sutherland ER, Ellison MC, Kraft M, et al. Altered pituitary-adrenal interaction in nocturnal asthma. J Allergy Clin Immunol 2003; 112:52–57.
105. Landstra AM, Postma DS, Boezen HM, et al. Role of serum cortisol levels in children with asthma. Am J Respir Crit Care Med 2002; 165:708–712.

106. Laube BL, Curbow BA, Costello RW, et al. A pilot study examining the relationship between stress and serum cortisol concentrations in women with asthma. Respir Med 2002; 96:823–828.

107. Sparrow D, O'Connor GT, Rosner B, et al. A longitudinal study of plasma cortisol concentration and pulmonary function decline in men. The Normative Aging Study. Am Rev Respir Dis 1993; 147:1345–1348.

108. Sher ER, Leung DY, Surs W, et al. Steroid-resistant asthma. Cellular mechanisms contributing to inadequate response to glucocorticoid therapy. J Clin Invest 1994; 93:33–39.

109. Chan MT, Leung DY, Szefler SJ, et al. Difficult-to-control asthma: clinical characteristics of steroid-insensitive asthma. J Allergy Clin Immunol 1998; 101:594–601.

110. Rosenwasser L, Klemm JD, Klemm DJ, et al. Association of asthmatic steroid insensitivity with an IL-4 gene promoter polymorphism [abstract 771]. J Allergy Clin Immunol 2001; 107:S235.

111. Leung DY, Bloom JW. Update on glucocorticoid action and resistance. J Allergy Clin Immunol 2003; 111:3–22; quiz 23.

112. Tantisira KG, Lake S, Silverman ES, et al. Corticosteroid Pharmacogenetics: association of sequence variants in CRHR1 with improved lung function in asthmatics treated with inhaled corticosteroids. Hum Mol Genet 2004; 13: 1353–1359.

113. Johnson GC, Esposito L, Barratt BJ, et al. Haplotype tagging for the identification of common disease genes. Nat Genet 2001; 29:233–237.

114. Silverman ES, Breault DT, Vallone J, et al. Corticotropin-releasing hormone deficiency increases allergen-induced airway inflammation in a mouse model of asthma. J Allergy Clin Immunol 2004; 114:747–754.

115. Finotto S, Neurath MF, Glickman JN, et al. Development of spontaneous airway changes consistent with human asthma in mice lacking T-bet. Science 2002; 295:336–338.

116. Tantisira KG, Hwang ES, Raby BA, et al. TBX21: a functional variant predicts improvement in asthma with the use of inhaled corticosteroids. Proc Natl Acad Sci USA 2004; 101:18099–18104.

117. Galon J, Franchimont D, Hiroi N, et al. Gene profiling reveals unknown enhancing and suppressive actions of glucocorticoids on immune cells. FASEB J 2002; 16:61–71.

118. Wang JC, Derynck MK, Nonaka DF, et al. Chromatin immunoprecipitation (ChIP) scanning identifies primary glucocorticoid receptor target genes. Proc Natl Acad Sci USA 2004; 101:15,603–15,608.

119. Yoshida NL, Miyashita T, Mami U, et al. Analysis of gene expression patterns during glucocorticoid-induced apoptosis using oligonucleotide arrays. Biochem Biophys Res Commun 2002; 293:1254–1261.

120. Barnes PJ, Adcock IM, Ito K. Histone acetylation and deacetylation: importance in inflammatory lung diseases. Eur Respir J 2005; 25:552–563.

121. Ito K, Barnes PJ, Adcock IM. Glucocorticoid receptor recruitment of histone deacetylase 2 inhibits interleukin-1beta-induced histone H4 acetylation on lysines 8 and 12. Mol Cell Biol 2000; 20:6891–6903.

122. Cosio BG, Mann B, Ito K, et al. Histone acetylase and deacetylase activity in alveolar macrophages and blood monocytes in asthma. Am J Respir Crit Care Med 2004; 170:141–147.

123. Ito K, Caramori G, Lim S, et al. Expression and activity of histone deacetylases in human asthmatic airways. Am J Respir Crit Care Med 2002; 166:392–396.

124. Thakkinstian A, McEvoy M, Minelli C, et al. Systematic review and meta-analysis of the association between beta2-adrenoceptor polymorphisms and asthma: a HuGE review. Am J Epidemiol 2005; 162:201–211.

125. Contopoulos-Ioannidis DG, Manoli EN, Ioannidis JP. Meta-analysis of the association of beta2-adrenergic receptor polymorphisms with asthma pheno-types. J Allergy Clin Immunol 2005; 115:963–972.

126. Penrose JF, Baldasaro MH. Leukotriene C4 synthase: a candidate gene for the aspirin-intolerant asthmatic phenotype. Allergy Asthma Proc 1999; 20:353–360.

127. Raby BA, Hwang ES, Van Steen K, et al. T-Bet polymorphisms are associated with asthma and airway hyperresponsiveness. Am J Respir Crit Care Med 2006; 173:64–70.

128. Weiss ST, Silverman EK, Palmer LJ. Case-control association studies in phar-macogenetics. Pharmacogenomics J 2001; 1:157–158.

129. Drazen JM. Asthma and the human genome project: summary of the 45th Annual Thomas L. Petty Aspen Lung Conference. Chest 2003; 123:447S–449S.

130. Busse W, Banks-Schlegel S, Noel P, et al. Future research directions in asthma: an NHLBI Working Group report. Am J Respir Crit Care Med 2004; 170: 683–690.

131. Mannino DM, Homa DM, Akinbami LJ, et al. Chronic obstructive pulmonary disease surveillance—United States, 1971–2000. MMWR Surveill Summ 2002; 51:1–16.

132. Pauwels RA, Buist AS, Calverley PM, et al. Global strategy for the diagnosis, management, and prevention of chronic obstructive pulmonary disease. NHLBI/WHO Global Initiative for Chronic Obstructive Lung Disease (GOLD) Workshop summary. Am J Respir Crit Care Med 2001; 163:1256–1276.

133. Murray CJ, Lopez AD. Alternative projections of mortality and disability by cause 1990–2020: Global Burden of Disease Study. Lancet 1997; 349:1498–1504.

134. Wilson L, Devine EB, So K. Direct medical costs of chronic obstructive pulmonary disease: chronic bronchitis and emphysema. Respir Med 2000; 94: 204–213.

135. Rodriguez-Roisin R. The airway pathophysiology of COPD: implications for treatment. J COPD 2005; 2:253–262.

136. DeMeo DL, Silverman EK. Genetics of chronic obstructive pulmonary disease. Semin Respir Crit Care Med 2003; 24:151–160.

137. DeMeo DL, Carey VJ, Chapman HA, et al. Familial aggregation of FEF(25–75) and FEF(25–75)/FVC in families with severe, early onset COPD. Thorax 2004; 59:396–400.

138. Burge PS, Calverley PM, Jones PW, et al. Prednisolone response in patients with chronic obstructive pulmonary disease: results from the ISOLDE study. Thorax 2003; 58:654–658.

139. Calverley PM, Burge PS, Spencer S, et al. Bronchodilator reversibility testing in chronic obstructive pulmonary disease. Thorax 2003; 58:659–664.

140. Tashkin D, Kesten S. Long-term treatment benefits with tiotropium in COPD patients with and without short-term bronchodilator responses. Chest 2003; 123:1441–1449.

141. Ihre E, Larsson K. Airways responses to ipratropium bromide do not vary with time in asthmatic subjects. Studies of interindividual and intraindividual variation of bronchodilatation and protection against histamine-induced bronchoconstriction. Chest 1990; 97:46–51.

142. Meyers DA, Larj MJ, Lange L. Genetics of asthma and COPD. Similar results for different phenotypes. Chest 2004; 126:105S–110S; discussion 159S–161S.

143. Hegab AE, Sakamoto T, Saitoh W, et al. Polymorphisms of IL4, IL13, and ADRB2 genes in COPD. Chest 2004; 126:1832–1839.

144. Fishman A, Martinez F, Naunheim K, et al. A randomized trial comparing lung-volume-reduction surgery with medical therapy for severe emphysema. N Engl J Med 2003; 348:2059–2073.

145. Ito I, Nagai S, Handa T, et al. Matrix metalloproteinase-9 promoter polymorphism associated with upper lung dominant emphysema. Am J Respir Crit Care Med 2005; 172:1378–1382.

146. U.S. Department of Health and Human Services. Healthy People 2010: Understanding and Improving Health. 2nd ed. Washington, DC: U.S. Government Printing Office, November 2000.

147. Mokdad AH, Marks JS, Stroup DF, et al. Actual causes of death in the United States, 2000. JAMA 2004; 291:1238–1245.

148. Mannino DM. Epidemiology and global impact of chronic obstructive pulmonary disease. Semin Respir Crit Care Med 2005; 26:204–210.

149. Edwards R. The problem of tobacco smoking. BMJ 2004; 328:217–219.

150. Dani JA, Heinemann S. Molecular and cellular aspects of nicotine abuse. Neuron 1996; 16:905–908.

151. Molyneux A. Nicotine replacement therapy. BMJ 2004; 328:454–456.

152. Roddy E. Bupropion and other non-nicotine pharmacotherapies. BMJ 2004; 328:509–511.

153. Hurt RD, Sachs DP, Glover ED, et al. A comparison of sustained-release bupropion and placebo for smoking cessation. N Engl J Med 1997; 337: 1195–1202.

154. Jorenby DE, Leischow SJ, Nides MA, et al. A controlled trial of sustained-release bupropion, a nicotine patch, or both for smoking cessation. N Engl J Med 1999; 340:685–691.

155. Malaiyandi V, Sellers EM, Tyndale RF. Implications of CYP2A6 genetic variation for smoking behaviors and nicotine dependence. Clin Pharmacol Ther 2005; 77:145–158.

156. Cholerton S, Arpanahi A, McCracken N, et al. Poor metabolisers of nicotine and CYP2D6 polymorphism. Lancet 1994; 343:62–63.

157. Swan GE, Benowitz NL, Lessov CN, et al. Nicotine metabolism: the impact of CYP2A6 on estimates of additive genetic influence. Pharmacogenet Genomics 2005; 15:115–125.

158. Hiroi T, Imaoka S, Funae Y. Dopamine formation from tyramine by CYP2D6. Biochem Biophys Res Commun 1998; 249:838–843.

159. Daly AK, Brockmoller J, Broly F, et al. Nomenclature for human CYP2D6 alleles. Pharmacogenetics 1996; 6:193–201.

160. Johansson I, Lundqvist E, Bertilsson L, et al. Inherited amplification of an active gene in the cytochrome P450 CYP2D locus as a cause of ultrarapid metabolism of debrisoquine. Proc Natl Acad Sci USA 1993; 90:11825–11829.

161. Cholerton S, Boustead C, Taber H, et al. CYP2D6 genotypes in cigarette smokers and non-tobacco users. Pharmacogenetics 1996; 6:261–263.

162. Boustead C, Taber H, Idle JR, et al. CYP2D6 genotype and smoking behaviour in cigarette smokers. Pharmacogenetics 1997; 7:411–414.

163. Saarikoski ST, Sata F, Husgafvel-Pursiainen K, et al. CYP2D6 ultrarapid metabolizer genotype as a potential modifier of smoking behaviour. Pharmacogenetics 2000; 10:5–10.

164. Gambier N, Batt AM, Marie B, et al. Association of CYP2A6*1B genetic variant with the amount of smoking in French adults from the Stanislas cohort. Pharmacogenomics J 2005; 5:271–275.

165. Schoedel KA, Hoffmann EB, Rao Y, et al. Ethnic variation in CYP2A6 and association of genetically slow nicotine metabolism and smoking in adult Caucasians. Pharmacogenetics 2004; 14:615–626.

166. O'Loughlin J, Paradis G, Kim W, et al. Genetically decreased CYP2A6 and the risk of tobacco dependence: a prospective study of novice smokers. Tob Control 2004; 13:422–428.

167. Vasconcelos GM, Struchiner CJ, Suarez-Kurtz G. CYP2A6 genetic polymorphisms and correlation with smoking status in Brazilians. Pharmacogenomics J 2005; 5:42–48.

168. Faucette SR, Hawke RL, Lecluyse EL, et al. Validation of bupropion hydroxylation as a selective marker of human cytochrome P450 2B6 catalytic activity. Drug Metab Dispos 2000; 28:1222–1230.

169. Lang T, Klein K, Fischer J, et al. Extensive genetic polymorphism in the human CYP2B6 gene with impact on expression and function in human liver. Pharmacogenetics 2001; 11:399–415.

170. Lerman C, Shields PG, Wileyto EP, et al. Pharmacogenetic investigation of smoking cessation treatment. Pharmacogenetics 2002; 12:627–634.

171. Berrettini WH, Lerman CE. Pharmacotherapy and pharmacogenetics of nicotine dependence. Am J Psychiatr 2005; 162:1441–1451.

172. Noble EP. The DRD2 gene in psychiatric and neurological disorders and its phenotypes. Pharmacogenomics 2000; 1:309–333.

173. Johnstone EC, Yudkin PL, Hey K, et al. Genetic variation in dopaminergic pathways and short-term effectiveness of the nicotine patch. Pharmacogenetics 2004; 14:83–90.

174. Yudkin P, Munafo M, Hey K, et al. Effectiveness of nicotine patches in relation to genotype in women versus men: randomised controlled trial. BMJ 2004; 328:989–990.

175. Lerman C, Jepson C, Wileyto EP, et al. Role of functional genetic variation in the dopamine D2 receptor (DRD2) in response to bupropion and nicotine replacement therapy for tobacco dependence: results of two randomized clinical trials. Neuropsychopharmacology 2006; 31:231–242.

176. Davenport KE, Houdi AA, Van Loon GR. Nicotine protects against mu-opioid receptor antagonism by beta-funaltrexamine: evidence for nicotine-induced release of endogenous opioids in brain. Neurosci Lett 1990; 113:40–46.

177. Bond C, LaForge KS, Tian M, et al. Single-nucleotide polymorphism in the human mu opioid receptor gene alters beta-endorphin binding and activity: possible implications for opiate addiction. Proc Natl Acad Sci USA 1998; 95:9608–9613.

178. Lerman C, Wileyto EP, Patterson F, et al. The functional mu opioid receptor (OPRM1) Asn40Asp variant predicts short-term response to nicotine replacement therapy in a clinical trial. Pharmacogenomics J 2004; 4:184–192.

179. Wright JL, Levy RD, Churg A. Pulmonary hypertension in chronic obstructive pulmonary disease: current theories of pathogenesis and their implications for treatment. Thorax 2005; 60:605–609.

180. Kanazawa H, Otsuka T, Hirata K, et al. Association between the angiotensin-converting enzyme gene polymorphisms and tissue oxygenation during exercise in patients with COPD. Chest 2002; 121:697–701.

181. Kanazawa H, Hirata K, Yoshikawa J. Effects of captopril administration on pulmonary haemodynamics and tissue oxygenation during exercise in ACE gene subtypes in patients with COPD: a preliminary study. Thorax 2003; 58:629–631.

182. Kanazawa H, Hirata K, Yoshikawa J. Influence of oxygen administration on pulmonary haemodynamics and tissue oxygenation during exercise in COPD patients with different ACE genotypes. Clin Physiol Funct Imaging 2003; 23:332–336.

183. Kanazawa H, Tateishi Y, Yoshikawa J. Acute effects of nifedipine administration in pulmonary haemodynamics and oxygen delivery during exercise in patients with chronic obstructive pulmonary disease: implication of the angiotensin-converting enzyme gene polymorphisms. Clin Physiol Funct Imaging 2004; 24:224–228.

Index